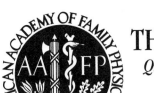

THE ACADEMY COLLECTION
Quick Reference Guides for Family Physicians

Skin Disorders

EUGENE J. BARONE, MD
Adjunct Associate Professor
Department of Family Practice
Creighton University;
Active Staff
Department of Family Practice
St. Joseph Hospital at the Creighton University Medical Center
Omaha, Nebraska

JUDSON C. JONES, MD
Assistant Professor
Department of Family Practice
Creighton University;
Full Active Staff
St. Joseph Hospital/Bergan Mercy Hospital
Omaha, Nebraska

JOANN E. SCHAEFER, MD
Assistant Professor
Department of Family Practice
Creighton University Medical School;
Full Active Staff
Family Practice
St. Joseph Hospital/Bergan Mercy Hospital
Omaha, Nebraska

Series Medical Editor
Richard Sadovsky, M.D.
Associate Professor of Family Medicine
State University of New York Health Science Center
Brooklyn, New York

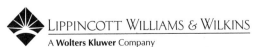

LIPPINCOTT WILLIAMS & WILKINS
A **Wolters Kluwer** Company
Philadelphia · Baltimore · New York · London
Buenos Aires · Hong Kong · Sydney · Tokyo

Project Manager: Leigh McKinney
Acquisitions Editor: Richard Winters
Developmental Editor: Paula Brown
Production Editor: Emily Harkavy
Manufacturing Manager: Kevin Watt
Cover Designer: Mark Lerner
Compositor: Lippincott Williams & Wilkins Desktop Division
Printer: Edwards Brothers

© **2000 by LIPPINCOTT WILLIAMS & WILKINS**
227 East Washington Square
Philadelphia, PA 19106-3780 USA
LWW.com

Printed in the USA

Library of Congress Cataloging-in-Publication Data
Barone, Eugene J.
  Skin disorders / Eugene J. Barone, Judson C. Jones, Joann E. Schaefer.
    p.   cm. — (The Academy collection—quick reference guides for family physicians)
  Includes bibliographical references and index.
  ISBN 0-683-30420-8 (alk. paper)
  1. Skin—Diseases Handbooks, manuals, etc.   I. Jones, Judson C.
II. Schaefer, Joann E.   III. Title.   IV. Series.
  [DNLM: 1. Skin Diseases Handbooks.   WR 39 B265s 1999]
RL74.B36 1999
616.5—dc21
DNLM/DLC
For Library of Congress   99-26966
                                                                        CIP

10   9   8   7   6   5   4   3   2   1

Coventry University

To our families for their love and support.

CONTENTS

....

ACKNOWLEDGMENTS

Writing a book is a massive, time-consuming undertaking which requires the support of many individuals. The authors acknowledge the following people.

We thank the series editor, Richard Sadovsky, M.D., M.S.; Leigh McKinney, special projects department manager at the American Academy of Family Practice; the staff at the American Academy of Family Practice; and Paula Brown, Associate Developmental Editor, and Jane Velker, Manager of Clinical Development, both at Lippincott Williams & Wilkins.

The support staff at Creighton University and from the Omaha community was also a tremendous help and greatly appreciated. In the Department of Family Practice, we thank Tyrone Jones, secretary; Gail Burns, secretary; and Deborah Badura, curriculum coordinator for their ability to organize this large task into a manageable endeavor. Technical support at any time of the day or night was willingly given by Gary N. Elsasser, Pharm.D., B.C.P.S., our clinical pharmacist in the Department of Family Practice at Creighton University, as well as by Thomas A. Ourada, B.S., R.P., our local pharmacist, who kept us in touch with reality.

Finally, we cannot say enough about the support we received from our spouses and families, who endured a lot from us in our efforts to complete this dermatology textbook.

Again, to all, thank you very much.

SERIES INTRODUCTION

Family practice is a unique clinical specialty encompassing a philosophy of care rather than a modality of care provided to a specific segment of the population. This philosophy of providing longitudinal care for persons of all ages in the complete context of their physical, emotional, and social environments was modeled by general practitioners, the parents of our modern specialty. To provide this kind of care, the family physician needs a broad knowledge base, appropriate evaluation tools, effective interventions, and patient education.

The knowledge base needed by a family physician is extraordinarily large. The American Academy of Family Physicians and other organizations provide clinical education to practitioners through conferences and journals. Individual family physicians have written journal articles about specific clinical topics or have tried to cover the broad knowledge base of family medicine in a single volume. The former are helpful, but may cover only a narrow segment of medicine, while the latter may not provide the depth needed to be useful in actual patient care.

The Academy Collection: Quick Reference Guides for Family Physicians is a series of books designed to assist family physicians with the broad knowledge base unique to our specialty. The books in this series have all been written by practicing family physicians who have special interest in the topics, and the chapters have been formatted to provide easy access to information needed at varying stages in the physician-patient encounter. Each volume is unique because each author has personalized the volume and provided a unique family physician perspective.

This series is not meant to be a final reference for the family physician who seeks a comprehensive text. The series also does not cover every topic that may be encountered by the family physician. The series does offer, in a depth deemed appropriate by the authors, the information needed by the physician to handle most patient encounters. The series also provides information to make patient care a combined doctor-patient effort. Specific patient education materials have been included where appropriate. Readers can contact the American Academy of Family Physicians Foundation for other resources.

The topics selected for *The Academy Collection* were chosen based on what family physicians said they needed. The first group of books covers office procedures, conditions of aging, and some of the most challenging diagnoses seen in family practice. Future books in the series will address musculoskeletal problems, environmental medicine, children's health, gastrointestinal problems, and women's health issues.

I welcome your comments. Please contact me at the American Academy of Family Physicians with your suggestions (Rick Sadovsky, MD, Series Editor, *The Academy Collection*, c/o AAFP, 8880 Ward Parkway, Kansas City, MO 64116; e-mail: academycollection@aafp.org). This collection is meant to be useful to you and your patients.

Richard Sadovsky, M.D., M.S.
Series Editor

DIAGNOSTIC CHART

Symptom: Rash, flat (macule or patches)

Related Findings	Differential Diagnosis
Skin-colored, scaling	Actinic keratosis (p. 105) (solar keratosis)
Tan-brown-black, nonscaling	Cafe-au-lait spots (neurofibromatosis), freckles (ephelides), junctional melanocytic nevi (p. 75), lentigo maligna, lentigo simplex, melanoma (p. 116), melasma (p. 152), nevi (p. 75), solar lentigo, tinea versicolor
White, nonscaling	Candidiasis (p. 300), tinea versicolor (p. 309), tuberous sclerosis, vitiligo (p. 149)
Blue-gray, nonscaling	Fixed drug eruption (p. 230), mongolian spot (p. 79)
Pink-red, scaling	Candidiasis (Intertrigo & Balanitis) (p. 300), erythrasma (p. 264), Pityriasis rosea (p. 137), seborrheic dermatitis (p. 42).
Pink-red, nonscaling	Aphthous ulcers (p. 61), erythema multiforme (p. 169), erythema chronica migrans (Lyme disease) (p. 271), exanthematous drug eruption (p. 225), fixed drug eruption (p. 230), infectious exanthems, Kawasaki's disease (p. 329), Rocky Mountain Spotted Fever

Symptom: Rash, raised (papule/nodule/plaque)

Related Findings	Differential Diagnosis
Nonpigmented, scaling	Actinic keratosis, ichthyosis vulgaris, (p. 55)
Nonpigmented, nonscaling	Acne vulgaris (p. 1), basal cell carcinoma (p. 113), condylomata accuminata, dermato-fibroma (p. 85), granuloma annulare (p. 141), keratoacanthoma (p. 83), keratosis pilaris (p. 58), melanocytic nevi (p. 75), molluscum contagiosum (p. 326), neurofibromatosis, nevi, skin tag (p. 87) (acrochordon) (p. 87), squamous cell carcinoma (p. 110), tuberous sclerosis (angiofibroma), verruca vulgaris, plantaris & plana (warts) (p. 318)
Pigmented, brown-black	Acanthosis nigricans, black head (comedone) (p. 1), dermatofibroma (p. 85), lichen simplex chronicus, malignant melanoma (p. 116), melanocytic nevi (p. 75), neurofibromatosis, nevi, pigmented basal cell carcinoma (p. 113), seborrheic keratosis (p. 81), skin tag (p. 87)
Pigmented, white	Aphthous ulcers (p. 61), leukoplakia (p. 108), milia (p. 99), molluscum contagiosum (p. 326), lichen planus (mouth) (p. 143), white head (comedone) (p. 1)
Pigmented, blue-gray	Blue nevus (p. 77), hemangiomas (cavernous) (p. 91) Kaposi's sarcoma (p. 380), pyogenic granuloma (p. 96)

Pigmented, yellow, scaling	Actinic keratosis (p. 105)
Pigmented, yellow, nonscaling	Xanthelasma
Pigmented, red/pink, scaling	
Pruritic	Atopic dermatitis (eczema), contact dermatitis, dyshidrotic eczema, impetigo, Paget's disease of the breast, Perioral dermatitis, pityriasis rosea, psoriasis, seborrheic dermatotis, tinea (capitis, corporis, pedis, cruris), erhythema chronica migrans, nummular eczema
Nonpruritic	Bowen disease (scaly)
Pigmented, red/pink, nonscaling	
Pruritic	Atopic dermatitis (eczema) (p. 27), bullous pemphigoid (p. 183), cercarial dermatitis (p. 344), dermatitis herpetiformis (p. 166), erysipeloid (p. 261), erythema multiforme (p. 169), exanthematous drug eruption (p. 225), fixed drug eruption (p. 230), insect bites & stings (p. 335), lichen planus (p. 143), lichen simplex chronicus (p. 35), pediculosis pubis (p. 335), perioral dermatitis (p. 18), polymorphous light eruption (p. 132), scabies (p. 340), seabathers eruption (p. 347)
Nonpruritic	Acne vulgaris (p. 1), cystic acne (p. 1), apthous ulcer (p. 61), basal cell carcinoma (p. 113), cherry angioma (p. 93), condyloma, diaper rash (p. 304), epidermoid (p. 100), epidermal inclusion & trichilemmal cysts (p. 102), erysipelas & cellulitis (p. 253), erythema multiforme (p. 169), erythema nodosum (p. 174), furuncle (p. 239), granuloma annulare (p. 141), hemangioma of infancy (p. 91), hidradenitis suppurativa (p. 21), infectious exanthems, infectious folliculitis (p. 244), Kaposi's sarcoma, Lyme disease, neurofibromatosis, pyogenic granuloma (p. 96), rosacea (acne rosacea) (p. 11), spider angioma (p. 94), sporotrichosis (p. 261), squamous cell carcinoma (p. 110), stasis dermatitis, Tuberous sclerosis (angiofibroma), verruca (warts)

Symptom: Rash, crustules

Related Findings	**Differential Diagnosis**
	Contact dermatitis (p. 32), herpes simplex (p. 316), herpes zoster (p. 316), infectious folliculitis (p. 244), impetigo and ecthyma (p. 233)

Symptom: Rash, vesicular/bullous

Related Findings	**Differential Diagnosis**
Clear fluid, pruritic	Bullous pemphigoid (p. 183), cercarial dermatitis (p. 344), contact dermatitis (p. 32),

	dermatitis herpetiformis, dyshidrotic eczema (pompholyx) (p. 46), eczema (atopic dermatitis) (p. 27), erythema multiforme (p. 169), fixed drug eruption (p. 230), herpes zoster, impetigo, phototoxicity (p. 127), Rhus dermatitis, seabather's eruption, vasculitis (p. 177), varicella
Clear fluid, nonpruritic	Hand-foot-mouth disease (p. 323), herpes simplex, pemphigus vulgaris (p. 186)

Symptom: Rash, pustules

Related Findings	**Differential Diagnosis**
Pigmented fluid, pruritic	Candidiasis (intertrigo, interdigital, Balanitis & follicular) (p. 300), dermatophytosis(p. 283), herpes zoster, impetigo, infectious folliculitis (p. 244)
Pigmented fluid, nonpruritic	Acne vulgaris (p. 1), erythema toxicum neonatorum (p. 375), furruncle (p. 239), carbuncle (p. 239), hidradenitis suppurativa (p. 21), infectious folliculitis, rosacea (acne rosacea) (p. 11)

Symptom: Rash, wheal

Related Findings	**Differential Diagnosis**
Red/pink	Angiodema, urticaria (p. 157), contact dermatitis (p. 32), insect bites

Symptom: Rash, ulcerations & erosions

Related Findings	**Differential Diagnosis**
Painful	Aphthous ulcer (p. 61), chancroid, fixed drug eruption (p. 230), impetigo (ecthyma), leg ulcer (arterial & venous), pressure ulcer
Nonpainful	Chancre (primary syphilis), granuloma inguinale, melanoma (p. 116)

Symptom: Rash, purpura

Related Findings and Differential Diagnosis	
Palpable	Henoch-Schonlein purpura, vasculitis (hypersensitivity)

Symptom: Nail disorders

Related Findings	**Differential Diagnosis**
Nail plate abnormalities	Junctional nevus (p. 75), nicotine habituation, tinea unguium (p. 287), yellow nail syndrome (p. 196)
Nail bed abnormalities	Malignant melanoma (p. 116), psoriasis (p. 51), splinter hemorrhage, subungual hematoma (p. 194)
Pitting disorders	Alopecia areata (p. 206), eczema, psoriasis
Ridges, transverse	Beau's lines (p. 192), chronic paronchyia (p. 192), eczema (p. 27)
Ridges, longitudinal	Habit tic deformity, lichen planus

Symptom: Hair disorder

Related Findings	**Differential Diagnosis**
Growth disturbance	Alopecia areata (p. 206), anagen effluvium (p. 216), male pattern baldness (p. 210), telogen effluvium (p. 214)
Infectious	Folliculitis, fungal infections (kerion) (p. 283), pseudofolliculitis barbae (p. 221)

Symptom: Pruritis

Related Findings	**Differential Diagnosis**
Systemic/generalized, renal	Uremia/chronic renal failure
Systemic/generalized, biliary	Biliary cirrhosis, intrahepatic cholestasis of pregnancy, extrahepatic biliary obstruction
Systemic/generalized, vascular	Hypersensitivity vasculitis
Systemic/generalized, endocrine	Hyperthyroidism, hypothyroidism, diabetes, mastocytosis
Systemic/generalized, malignancy	Hodgkins lymphoma, non-Hodgkins lymphoma, cutaneous T-cell lymphoma (mycosis fungoides), gastric carcinoma, pancreatic carcinoma, breast carcinoma, lung carcinoma, vulvar carcinoma, CNS tumors, multiple myeloma, leukemia, extramammary Paget's disease
Systemic/generalized, hematologic	Polycythemia vera, iron deficiency anemia
Systemic/generalized, neurologic	Multiple sclerosis
Systemic/generalized, infectious	HIV virus (AIDS), viral exanthems: varicella, herpes zoster, herpes simplex (genitalis) (p. 315)
Systemic/generalized, psychiatric	Depression, neurotic excoriations, stress (intense)
Systemic/generalized, medications	Quinidine, aspirin, morphine, codeine, scopolamine, dextran, phenothiazines, hormones, erythromycin estolate
Cutaneous, inflammatory	Atopic dermatitis (p. 27), lichen simplex chronicus (p. 85), seborrheic dermatitis (p. 42), psoriasis, irritant dermatitis (p. 32), contact dermatitis (p. 32), lichen planus, exanthematous drug reaction (p. 225), fixed drug reaction (p. 230), nummular eczema (p. 39), dyshidrotic eczema (p. 46), perioral dermatitis (p. 18), pityriasis rosea, sunburn (p. 123)
Cutaneous, infectious	Candidiasis (p. 300), dermatophytosis (p. 283), erythrasma (p. 264), impetigo (p. 233), erysipeloid (p. 261), condyloma acuminata, vulvitis/vaginitis, folliculitis, erythema chronica migrans (Lyme disease)
Cutaneous, infestations	Seabather's eruption (p. 347), scabies (p. 340), trichinosis, pediculosis (p. 335), pinworms, insect bites and stings, cercarial dermatitis (p. 344)
Cutaneous, mechanical	Hemorrhoids
Cutaneous, immunologically mediated	Dermatitis herpetiformis (p. 166), pemphigus, bullous pemphigoid (p. 183), herpes gestationis (p. 374)

Cutaneous, environmental	Xerosis, polymorphous light eruption (p. 132), eczema craquelé (p. 27)
Cutaneous, vascular reactions	Urticaria
Cutaneous, miscellaneous	Pruritis ani, pruritic urticarial papules and plaques of pregnancy (PUPPP) (p. 374)

Symptom: Fever

Related Findings	Differential Diagnosis
Rash (macules, papules, or nodules)	Streptococcal cellulitis, meningococcemia, erythema in chronica migrans, HIV, drug hypersensitivity, viral exanthems (erythema infectiosum, roseola, rubeola, rubella) (p. 315), secondary syphyllis, Rocky Mountain Spotted Fever, erythema multiforme (p. 169), erythema nodosum (p. 174), serum sickness, urticaria secondary to viral hepatitis, typhoid fever, enterovirus, adenovirus, systemic lupus erythematosus
Rash (vesicles, pustules, or bullae)	Contact dermatitis (p. 32), gonococcemia, viral exanthems (varicella) (p. 315), herpes zoster, herpes simplex, eczema herpeticum, hand-foot-mouth disease (p. 323), herpangina (p. 70), staphylococcal scalded-skin syndrome (SSS) (p. 233), erythema multiforme (p. 169), Kawasaki's disease (p. 329), drug hypersensitivity
Rash (desquamation)	Drug hypersensitivity, scarlet fever, staphylococcal scalded-skin syndrome (SSS), toxic shock syndrome, Kawasaki's disease (p. 329), toxic epidermal necrolysis (p. 169)
Rash (purpura)	Bacteremia, meningococcemia, gonococcemia, subacute bacterial endocarditis enterovirus, Rocky Mountain spotted fever, vasculitis, disseminated intravascular coagulation, drug hypersensitivity, Henoch-Schönlein purpura

Symptom: Joint pain/Arthritis

Related Findings	Differential Diagnosis
Rash, raised (papules, plaques, and nodules)	Psoriasis, Lyme disease, Reiter's syndrome
Rash, nodules	Erythema nosodum (p. 174)
Rash, ulcers	
Mouth and genitalia	Behçet's syndrome
Lower extremities	Rheumatoid arthritis

Symptom/Sign: Telangiectasia

Related Findings	Differential Diagnosis
Rash, red macules	
Fingers, lips, and mucosa	Osler-Weber-Rendu syndrome, CRST syndrome (calcinosis, Reynaud's phenomenon, scleroderma, and telangiectasia)

Symptom/Sign: Gastrointestinal disease (polyps)

Related Findings	**Differential Diagnosis**
Rash, brown/black	
Freckles around the lips and on the fingertips	Peutz-Jeghers Syndrome

Symptom/Sign: Gastrointestinal disease (inflammatory)

Related Findings	**Differential Diagnosis**
Rash, ulcerations	
Lower extremities	Pyoderma gangrenosum (inflammatory bowel disease)

Symptom/Signs: Eczematous lesions (red papules and plaques with scales)

Related Findings	**Differential Diagnosis**
Hand	Dyshidrotic eczema (p. 46), atopic dermatitis (p. 27), contact dermatitis (p. 32), scabies (p. 340)
Foot	Dyshidrotic eczema (p. 46), atopic dermatitis (p. 27), tinea pedis, contact dermatitis (p. 32), stasis dermatitis
Groin, Adult	Atopic dermatitis (p. 27), tinea cruris, candidiasis (p. 300)
Groin, Infants	Contact dermatitis (diaper dermatitis) (p. 32), seborrheic dermatitis (p. 42), candidiasis (p. 300), atopic dermatitis (p.27)
Extremities	Atopic dermatitis (p. 27), stasis dermatitis, contact dermatitis (p. 32), xerosis

Symptom/Sign: Alopecia

Related Findings	**Differential Diagnosis**
Restricted to the top of the scalp	Male pattern baldness, female pattern baldness
Entire scalp	Alopecia areata (p. 206), medications (coumadin, antithyroid), hypothyroidism, anemia, secondary syphilis, systemic lupus erythematosis
Discreet areas of the scalp	
No scarring	Alopecia areata (p. 206), traction alopecia (p. 207), tinea capitis (p. 287), lichen simplex (p. 35), psoriasis
Scarring	Burn, kerion, herpes zoster, squamous cell cancer (p. 110), solar keratosis, folliculitis, lichen planus, discoid lupus

Symptom/Sign: Hyperpigmentation

Related Findings	**Differential Diagnosis**
Face	Porphyria cutanea tarda
Upper extremities	Porphyria cutanea tarda
Generalized	Addison's disease, scleroderma, Hemochromatosis, carcinoma of the lung, acanthosis nigricans, neurofibromatosis
Intertriginous	Acanthosis nigricans

Symptom/Sign: Flushing, skin

Related Findings	Differential Diagnosis
Face	Carcinoid tumor
Trunk	Pheochromocytoma
Generalized	Mastocytosis

Symptom/Sign: Hirsutism

Related Findings	Differential Diagnosis
Face/generalized	Porphyria cutanea tarda, Cushing's disease, virilizing tumors, polycystic ovarian syndrome, anorexia nervosa, medications (dilantin, minoxidil, cyclosporine, phenothiazines), familial

Symptom/Sign: Pupura (petechiae and eccymosis)

Related Findings	Differential Diagnosis
Intravascular	Thrombocytopenia purpura, hemophilia, anticoagulant administration, diffuse intravascular coagulation
Extravascular	"Senile" pupura, steroid-induced, scurvy, primary amyloidosis
Vascular wall	Vasculitis, Henoch-Schonlein purpura

Symptom/Sign: Jaundice

Related Findings	Differential Diagnosis
Adults (generalized)	Sickle cell anemia, hemolytic anemia, resorption of hematoma, pulmonary infarction, hepatitis—viral (alcoholic), drugs, septicemia, congestive heart failure, cholelithiasis, choledocholithiasis, toxic shock syndrome, lymphoma, pancreatic cancer, prostate cancer, amyloidosis, cholangitis, pregnancy, cholangitis, cancer of the bile duct, biliary cirrhosis, sarcoidosis, Rocky Mountain Spotted Fever
Infants (generalized)	Physiologic, medication, septicemia, breast milk, biliary atresia, Crigler-Najjar syndrome, ABO incompatability, Rh incompatability, metabolic disorders, Infectious-viral (toxoplasmosis, listeriosis, and syphillis), Down syndrome, trisomy E, G-6-PD deficiency, sickle cell anemia, thalassemia, polycythemia, Lucey-Driscoll syndrome, hypothyroidism, hypoxia, acidosis, hematoma

Symptom/Sign: Carotenemia

Related Findings	Differential Diagnosis
Adults (yellow/orange skin sparing sclera and oral cavity)	Hypothyroidism, hypopituitarism, diabetes mellitus, hepatic disease, anorexia nervosa, β–carotene supplements
Children (yellow/orange skin sparing sclera and oral cavity)	Inborn errors of metabolism, carotene-rich food ingestion

Symptom/Sign: Spider nevus (angioma)

Related Findings	**Differential Diagnosis**
Adults	Pregnancy, estrogen-containing medication, viral hepatitis, alcoholic cirrhosis
Children	Idiopathic

Diagnostic Test	
Low iron	
Related Findings	**Differential Diagnosis**
Spoon-shaped nails (koilonychia)	Iron-deficiency anemia
Hair loss	Alopecia (p. 205)

Diagnostic Test	
Increased Lipids	
Related Findings	**Differential Diagnosis**
Yellow/brown macules, papules, or nodules	Hyperlipidemia (xanthelasma)

Diagnostic Test	
Decreased T4	
Related Findings	**Differential Diagnosis**
Loss of hair	Alopecia (p. 205)
Hypopigmentation	Vitiligo (p. 149)
Dry, coarse, pale skin	Hypothyroidism

Diagnostic Test	
Increased T4	
Related Findings	**Differential Diagnosis**
Loss of hair	Alopecia (p. 205)
Pink/skin-colored papules and nodules in pretibial regions	Hyperthyroidism (Graves)

Diagnostic Test	
Decreased Platelets	
Related Findings	**Differential Diagnosis**
Asymptomatic petechiae or ecchymosis	Thrombocytopenic purpura

Diagnostic Test	
Increased Glucose	
Related Findings	**Differential Diagnosis**
Painful plaques/ulcers on the lower extremities	Necrobiosis lipoidica

Diagnostic Test	
Increased Cortisol	
Related Findings	**Differential Diagnosis**
Purple striae, erythema, and telangiectases of the face and neck	Cushing's syndrome

Diagnostic Test	
Serum uric acid	
Related Findings	**Differential Diagnosis**
White/skin-colored papules and nodules of the ear helix, digits, or bony prominences	Tophaceous gout

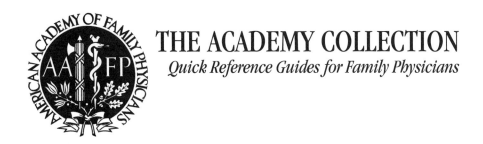

THE ACADEMY COLLECTION
Quick Reference Guides for Family Physicians

Skin Disorders

CHAPTER 1
....

Acne and Related Disorders

ACNE

Acne is a common chronic skin disease of adolescents and young adults. Its etiology is multifactorial and involves overproduction of sebum, proliferation of skin bacteria, and abnormal follicular keratinization. Psychosocial factors are inherent in the condition, and the patient may feel socially isolated and emotionally distressed as a result of appearance.

Chief Complaint
- A 17-year-old boy arrives at your office with red and inflamed, and sometimes painful, lesions on his face and shoulders. He relates to you that he is embarrassed by his zits.
- A 25-year-old woman has an appointment the same day. She has red blotches on her cheeks and chin and around her mouth, which worsen just before her period.

Clinical Manifestations
- *Lesions of acne vulgaris* can be single, discrete (nodules) or multiple, scattered lesions (papules, cysts, and nodules).
- *Comedones* can be closed (**whiteheads** are keratin plugs that form at the opening of the sebaceous gland; Figure 1.1, see color insert following page 170) or open, with a darker color (**blackheads**; Figure 1.2, see color insert following page 170). Usually erythema and pustules surround the comedones.
- *Papules* and *papulopustules* can be red and inflamed and, at times, painful.
- *Nodules/cysts* can be 1 to 4 cm in diameter. At times, the nodules tend to be painful.
- *Nodular cystic acne* occurs when comedones rupture into the dermis, giving rise to an intense inflammatory response, often with erythema (Figure 1.3, see color insert following page 170).
- *Scarring* can occur when sebaceous cysts become atrophic and cause pitting. Sometimes the scar becomes hypertrophic, causing keloids.

    It is not unusual to see a patient with acne vulgaris who exhibits simultaneously inflammatory papules, pustules, and crustules in areas with a high number of sebaceous glands [e.g., on the face (cheeks, chin, forehead, and nose)] and, to a lesser extent, on the neck, upper arms, and trunk.

Epidemiology
Family History
Severe acne tends to run in families, but the exact mode of inheritance is unknown.

Age
- Acne usually first occurs in early adolescence, at ages 10 to 17 years in girls and 14 to 19 years in boys. After the age of 25, the incidence of acne decreases in both sexes; however, acne can occur initially at age 25 and persist to age 35 to 40.

- Mild acne can be present in up to 20% of newborns, spontaneously resolving in 1 to 3 months. Infantile acne can occur around 3 to 6 months of age; boys are affected more often than girls. It can persist up to age 5 years. Children with infantile acne may have an increased risk of developing severe acne in adolescence.

Race
There is a lower incidence of acne in Asians and African Americans.

Sex
Acne is more severe in males.

Risk Factors
- *Emotional stress* can exacerbate acne.
- *Diet* has little effect on acne. Contrary to popular belief, diets rich in fat (chocolate, greasy food) usually do not exacerbate the condition.
- *Endocrine factors.* Women can have flare-ups of acne premenstrually.
- Pregnancy can either exacerbate acne or cause a regression.
- *Hygiene.* Acne is not caused by dirt or poor hygiene.
- *Environmental factors.* Sweating can cause flare-ups in 15% of acne patients, probably because sweat causes partial follicular obstruction, leading to inflammation.
- Humid environments (humid climates, kitchens, steam rooms) can cause acne flare-ups.
- There is no scientific documentation that the effects of ultraviolet radiation (i.e., sun exposure) are beneficial in controlling acne, although patient perceptions suggest a beneficial effect.
- *Occupational factors.* Some people using mineral oils, petroleum products, or coal tar can develop acne when in contact with these chemicals on a regular basis.
- *Chloracne* is a type of acne induced by external contact to or inhalation of certain chlorinated hydrocarbons (e.g., Agent Orange, naphthalenes, benzenes), which causes comedones that can persist for years.
- *Drugs.* Lithium, hydantoins, corticosteroids (including topical agents), and certain oral contraceptives (those with higher androgenic activity such as those which contain norethindrone, levonorgestrel, norgestrel, or desogestrel) have a tendency to contribute to acne.
- *Occlusion.* Repeated pressure from headbands, bra straps, and chin straps and repeated occlusion of the skin with the hand or helmets can worsen acne.
- *Cosmetics* containing lanolin, petrolatum, vegetable oils, lauryl alcohol, butyl stearate, and oleic acid can induce comedone formation on the face. These products include oily or greasy sunblocks and hair oils or pomades (used to defrizz curly hair), which may cause comedone formation along the hairline.

PATHOLOGY

Acne is thought to be caused by a variety of factors, including hormones (androgens) and bacteria *(Propionibacterium acnes)*. Androgens stimulate the sebaceous gland to produce large amounts of sebum, which the bacteria convert into fatty acids. The fatty acids cause an inflammatory response in the sebaceous gland, resulting in hyperkeratinization of the lining of the follicle, which in turn causes plugging. The excessive keratin causes whitehead and blackhead formation. The follicular wall may break down, and its contents (the sebum and fatty acids) enter the dermis, provoking a foreign body inflammatory response, which causes formation of papules, pustules, and nodules. This intense inflammation and rupture of the sebaceous cyst can lead to scar formation.

T ABLE 1.1.   Categorization of Acne

Category	Comedones	Papules/pustules	Nodules
Noninflammatory			
Minimal	Few	Rare, small papules	None
Inflammatory			
Mild	Few to many	Few to several	None
Moderate	Few to many	Several to many	Few to several
Severe	Few to many	Numerous, extensive	Many

From Lookingbill D, Egan N, Santen R, et al. Correlation of serum 3α-androstanediol glucuronide with acne and chest hair density in men. *J Clin Endocrinol Metab* 1988;67:986–991; Pochi PE, Shalita AR, Strauss JS, et al. Report of the consensus conference on acne classification. *J Am Acad Dermatol* 1991;24(3):495–500.

Diagnosis

Clinical presentation is distinctive and sufficient for diagnosis (Table 1.1).

Diagnostic Tests
- *Acne vulgaris.* No specific tests are needed to make a diagnosis of acne vulgaris.
- *Acne caused by polycystic ovarian disease.* An evaluation of the adrenal ovarian androgens *dehydroepiandrosterone sulfate (DHEA)*, free testosterone, and *follicle-stimulating hormone/leutinizing hormone (FSH/LH)* are needed to make this diagnosis.

Differential Diagnosis
See Table 1.2.

T ABLE 1.2.   Acne Vulgaris: Differential Diagnosis

Staphylococcus aureus folliculitis	*S. aureus* folliculitis is usually characterized by a single acute, erythematous, slightly tender cyst.
	No comedones are present.
	It is associated with diabetes and the use of topical corticosteroids.
Perioral dermatitis	Perioral dermatitis is characterized by papulopustules on an erythematous background surrounding the mouth but with a clear zone around the vermillion border of the lips.
	There are no comedones.
	Acne does not have a chronic erythematous background.
Rosacea	Rosacea has confluent red papulopustules and can be distinguished from acne, which has more discrete lesions.
	There are no comedones.
Pseudofolliculitis barbae	The main distinguishing characteristic is the presence of ingrown hair shafts, which are absent in acne.

T ABLE 1.3.   Topical Acne Medication

Benzoyl peroxide 2.5%, 5%, 10%

Availability:	Over the counter (OTC) or prescription.
Form:	Gel, cream, lotion, soap, or wash.
Activity:	Potent antibacterial and mildly comedolytic.
Dosage:	Applied once or twice daily.
Side effects:	Mild redness, pruritus, and scaling of skin. Sometimes increased erythema secondary to contact (irritant) dermatitis; stop treatment if this occurs.
Duration:	Results in 1 to 2 months.
Comments:	Liquid and cream formulations are more irritating but more useful in oily-skinned individuals. First-line therapy for noninflammatory and mild inflammatory acne. Start with 5% or 10% strength.

Benzoyl peroxide 5%/erythromycin 3% (Benzamycin)

Availability:	Prescription only.
Form:	Gel.
Activity:	Potent antibacterial and mildly comedolytic.
Dosage:	Applied twice daily.
Side effects:	Mild redness, pruritus, and scaling of skin. Sometimes increased erythema secondary to contact (irritant) dermatitis; stop treatment if this occurs. Allergic reaction to erythromycin.
Duration:	Results in 1 to 2 months.
Comments:	Combination useful when using both agents separately. Cannot tell which agent patient may be sensitive to if erythema develops.

Sodium sulfacetamide 10%/sulfur 5% (Sulfacet-R)

Availability:	Prescription only.
Form:	Lotion.
Activity:	Antibacterial (sulfacetamide) and keratolytic (sulfur).
Dosage:	Applied 1 to 3 times daily.
Side effects:	Allergic reaction to sodium sulfacetamide.
Duration:	Results in 1 to 2 months.
Comments:	Does not blend in with skin; comes with a blending kit to match the lotion to skin tone.

Topical antibiotics
Agents

Tetracycline	
Clindamycin	
Eythromycin	
Availability:	Prescription only.

Forms

Tetracylcine	Solution.
Clindamycin	Solution and gel.
Erythromycin	Solution, gel, swabs.
Activity:	Reduces bacterial colonization.

continued

TABLE 1.3. *continued.*   **Topical Acne Medication**

Dosage: Applied once daily.
Side effects: May irritate skin (gel probably more than solution).
Duration: Results in 1 to 2 months.

Tretinoin (Retin-A)

Availability: Prescription only.
Forms: Cream 0.025%, 0.05%, 0.1%; gel 0.01%, 0.025%.
                 Liquid 0.5%.
                 Microsphere gel 0.1% (Retin-A Micro).
Activity: Induces desquamation of the follicles and reduces comedones.
Dosage: Applied once daily at bedtime.
Side effects: Retin-A can sting the skin; it also causes dryness and erythema. Use lower
                 concentrations to start; initially use 2 to 3 times per week to allow the patient to
                 adjust to the irritating and drying sensation, then increase to daily use as tolerated.
                 Can make skin more susceptible to sunburn; should protect with sunblock.
Duration: Slow improvement over 1 to 2 months.
Comments: Retin-A Micro gel was developed to decrease the dryness, stinging, and erythema. Not
                 enough personal experience to confirm this claim.

Adapalene 0.1% (Differin)

Availability: Prescription only.
Form: Gel.
Activity: Retinoid-like compound that decreases comedone formation.
Dosage: Applied once nightly to affected areas.
Side effects: Pruritus, scaling of skin, burning, erythema, and dryness of skin reported in 10% to
                 40% of patients.
Duration: Results in 1 to 2 months.
Comments: Not enough personal experience to confirm efficacy.

Salicylic acid 2%

Availability: OTC.
Activity: Removes excess sebum.
Dosage: Face washed 2 to 3 times daily.
Side effects: Skin dryness or irritation.
Duration: Results in 1 to 2 months.

Azelaic acid 20% (Azelex)

Availability: Prescription only.
Form: Cream.
Activity: Both antibacterial and anticomedonal effect.
Dosage: Applied topically twice daily.
Side effects: In 1% to 5% of patients, pruritus, burning, stinging, or tingling. Erythema and rash in
                 less than 1% of patients. Isolated reports of hypopigmentation.
Duration: Results in 1 to 2 months.
Comments: Naturally occurring product found in cereal grains. Not enough personal experience
                 to confirm efficacy.

Referral

The treatment of acne is an art as much as a science. If the family physician takes the time and energy to educate the patient and family about the various treatment modalities, it is not necessary to refer the patient to a dermatologist. A patient with an intense inflammatory response to therapy or an inadequate response to what the family physician believes to be aggressive therapy may require referral to a dermatologist.

Management

- The treatment of acne involves reduction of colonizing bacteria in the follicles, unblocking plugged follicles, and induction of desquamation to open the comedones. There is no single best treatment modality for acne. Therapy should be individualized based on the classification of acne described in Table 1.1 and in close communication with the patient regarding side effects.
- *Noninflammatory and mild inflammatory acne* is amenable to topical treatment (Table 1.3) with medications such as benzoyl peroxide (some of the over-the-counter products include Clearasil and Oxy-5), keratolytic agents, and topical antibiotics.
- *Moderate inflammatory acne* is usually managed by using topical antibiotics and keratolytic agents together. Moderate acne resistant to topical therapy can also be managed by starting the patient on a regimen of systemic antibiotics (Table 1.4) along with the keratolytic agents (the antibiotics can potentiate the effects of the keratolytic agents).
- *Severe inflammatory acne* should be treated with systemic antibiotics, and different antibiotics can be tried in resistant cases. Severe acne can be treated with more potent strengths of topical tretinoin (Retin-A) along with the systemic antibiotics. Oral isotretinoin (Accutane) is also useful (Table 1.4).

Other Treatment Modalities

- *Alternative treatments* for acne are widely available to the lay person via the Internet and the lay press. Vitamin and mineral supplements (such as beta-carotene, vitamin E, zinc chromium picolinate, vitamin B complex, and selenium) have been suggested to improve skin health. Patients should be cautioned about using these alternative treatments in high doses because they can be toxic.
- Even *herbs* have been suggested to clear the skin. Dandelion root, milk thistle, and burdock root have been used to clear the skin. Since these herbs have not been tested for their efficacy in the treatment of acne, their use is not recommended.
- Table 1.5 presents additional treatment modalities.

Follow-up
Monitoring Disease Course

- *Reduction of pustules and nodules.* In recalcitrant cases of mild to moderate inflammatory acne, different topical or systemic antibiotics can be used. Sometimes antibiotic resistance develops to *P. acnes.* Also, using an increased strength of topical tretinoin is helpful in difficult cases.
- *Endocrine-associated complications.* Women resistant to treatment who have signs of hirsutism or irregular menstruation should be investigated for a possible endocrine cause. Screening with DHEA and free/total testosterone is helpful in determining whether a patient has an adrenal or ovarian tumor. In these women, alternative treatments such as oral contraceptives, low-dose glucocorticoids, or spironolactone may be helpful.

T ABLE 1.4.   Systemic Acne Treatment

Oral antibiotics

Availability:	Prescription only.
Activity:	Predominately antibacterial; also intrinsic antiinflammatory effects.
Dosage:	
Tetracycline	250 to 1,500 mg/day, two divided doses.
Doxycycline	50 to 200 mg/day, once daily.
Erythromycin	250 to 1,500 mg/day, two divided doses.
Minocycline	50 to 200 mg/day, 1 to 2 divided doses.
Trimethoprim-suflamethoxazole	One double-strength pill daily.
Side effects:	
Tetracycline	Must be taken on empty stomach, otherwise, absorption is impaired. Can cause gastrointestinal tract upset, candidal overgrowth, bone/tooth discoloration, and photosensitivity. Should not be used in pregnant women and children under 12 years of age. Possible interference with oral birth control efficacy.
Doxycycline	Can be taken with food with fewer gastrointestinal tract side effects; otherwise, similar side effects as tetracycline. Should not be used in pregnant women and children under 12 years of age.
Erythromycin	Predominant gastrointestinal tract side effects.
Minocycline	Can be taken with food. Can cause pseudotumor cerebri, skin hyperpigmentation, gastrointestinal tract upset, tooth/bone discoloration, and vertigo. Possible interference with oral birth control efficacy. Should not be used in pregnant women and children under 12 years of age.
Trimethoprim-sulfamethoxazole	Can cause agranulocytosis and severe allergic reactions. Do not use in pregnant patients, especially at term, or in nursing mothers.
Duration:	Can range from 1 month to years.
Comments:	The initial oral antibiotic of choice is tetracycline, with its low cost and minimal side effects. Avoid in pregnant women and in children under 12 years. Women on oral birth control should be warned about potential for reduced efficacy. Taper oral antibiotics to the lowest dose tolerated once the acne improves, and maintain at that level. If acne is no longer controlled by the current oral antibiotic used, suspect bacterial resistance; switching to another antibiotic is indicated. Minocycline is costly but useful in resistant acne.

Isotretinoin (Accutane)

Availability:	Prescription only.
Activity:	Oral retinoid that inhibits sebaceous gland function and keratinization.
Dosage:	1 to 1.5 mg/kg orally per day taken with food. In more severe cases of acne, 2.0 mg/kg may be required.
Side effects:	Isotretinoin is *teratogenic;* pregnancy should be avoided. Contraception is necessary for women of child-bearing age 1 month before starting treatment and continued for 2 months beyond cessation of therapy. A serum pregnancy test should be obtained before the start of treatment, and then monthly.

continued

T ABLE 1.4. *continued.* **Systemic Acne Treatment**

Isotretinoin (Accutane) *continued*

Tetracyline and isotretinoin should not be taken together; the combination can cause pseudotumor cerebri.

The blood lipids (cholesterol and triglycerides) should be monitored at the start of treatment (baseline), 1 to 2 weeks after starting the course, and at monthly intervals thereafter. The drug can increase plasma triglycerides, increase total cholesterol, and decrease high-density lipoproteins.

Isotretinoin can also cause an elevated platelet count, neutropenia, and elevated levels of hepatic enzymes, which will return to normal after cessation of drug administration. Liver function tests (AST, GGTP, ALT, LDH) should be determined at the start of treatment and 1 to 2 weeks after starting course, and checked at monthly intervals thereafter. If elevation of liver enzyme values or hepatitis occurs, the medication should undergo a dosage reduction, or in the case of hepatitis, be discontinued. A CBC should be obtained initially and 1 to 2 weeks after starting course, and then at monthly intervals thereafter.

Other side effects include cheilitis, dry skin, pruritus, headaches, epistaxis, and photosensitivity. These are relatively frequent and are dose related.

Duration:	4- to 5-month course.
Comments:	Isotretinoin can induce a long-lasting remission in about 90% of patients.

Hormone therapy
   Birth control pills

Availability:	Prescription only.
Form:	Recommend oral estrogen-progesterone birth control pills.
Activity:	Suppression of ovarian androgen production.
Dosage:	Norgestimate 0.025 mg and ethinyl estradiol 0.035 mg or other low-androgenic combinations (avoid norgestrel, levonorgestrel, and norethindrone).
Duration:	Improvement will take 3 to 4 months.
Comments:	Hormone therapy should be limited to female patients who have severe acne and are unresponsive to all medications used previously.

Other less commonly used hormones
   Prednisone

Activity:	Suppresses adrenal overproduction of androgens.
Dosage:	5 mg daily.
Side effects:	Long-term use can cause serious systemic side effects.

   Spironolactone

Activity:	Reduces sebum production by follicles.
Dosage:	150 to 200 mg/day in 3 to 4 divided doses.
Side effects:	Can cause hyperkalemia.

continued

T ABLE 1.4. *continued.* **Systemic Acne Treatment**

Acetazolamide (Diamox)
Premenstrual flaring of acne may be prevented with the use of acetazolamide 125 to 250 mg every morning for 10 days before menstruation.

Oral prednisone
Oral prednisone, 20 to 40 mg daily, is also effective in reducing premenstrual flares when used in conjunction with other acne treatments. Its use should be limited to 2 weeks just before menstruation.

Nonsteroidal antiinflammatory agents
Nonsteroidal antiinflammatory agents, such as ibuprofen (Motrin) and piroxicam (Feldene), either alone or in conjunction with oral tetracycline, have also been useful to reduce the inflammatory response in acne.

AST, aspartate transaminase; GGTP, gamma-glutamyl transpeptidase; ALT, alanine aminotransferase; LDH, lactate dehydrogenase; CBC, complete blood cell count.

T ABLE 1.5.   **Other Treatment Modalities for Acne**

Physical and environmental measures
Sometimes the physician can extract the comedones using a comedone extractor. This will remove the keratin plugs and allow the sebum to flow freely.

Exfoliants
Salicylic acid 2%, elemental sulfur, resorcinol, alpha-hydroxy acids (fruit acids), glycolic acid, and lactic acid are exfoliants that cause desquamation of the stratum corneum, which is thought to improve the look of the skin. These agents are available over the counter as acne soaps, scrubs, creams, lotions, and gels.

Intralesional corticosteroids
Intralesional injections of 0.05 to 0.2 mL triamcinolone acetonide (1 to 2.5 mg/mL concentration) using a 27- or 30-gauge needle can help reduce cystic acne lesions in several days. Side effects include skin atrophy and hypopigmentation.

Dermabrasion
Hypertrophic scars can be reduced by dermabrasion, a technique best left to those with experience in this exfoliative technique. It is usually offered to the patient after the acne is no longer active. Some scars resembling pits can be treated by the experienced dermatologist with collagen injections as well.

Bleaching
Acne can leave the face with hyperpigmentation following the inflammatory response. Hydroquinone and topical tretinoin have been useful to reduce the pigmentation. Bleaching techniques should be undertaken by the experienced practitioner.

continued

T ABLE 1.5. *continued.* **Other Treatment Modalities for Acne**

Ultraviolet therapy

Patients perceive an improvement of their acne when they are exposed to ultraviolet radiation (UVR). Acne is
perceived to improve in summertime and worsen in winter. Although exposure to UVR may improve
inflammatory lesions, it can worsen comedonal lesions, according to some experts. UVR can also interact
with the medication often used to treat acne. Because of the negative effects of UVR, we do not
recommend exposing acne patients to UVR as a routine treatment.

Cosmetics

Recommend cosmetics that are noncomedogenic, realizing that a small portion of patients will react to these types
of cosmetics with an acne flare. A noncomedogenic cosmetic usually contains silicone derivatives (cyclome-
thicone, dimethicone) or a small amount of mineral oil. Cosmetics should be labeled "oil-free" and "water-
based." Avoid fatty, comedogenic emollients such as octyl stearate and isocetyl stearate, detergents such as
sodium lauryl sulfate, and moisturizers such as mineral oil, petrolatum, sesame oil, and cocoa butter.

Cleanliness

Excessive scrubbing and facial washing with abrasive lotions or soaps, facial sponges, or harsh washcloths may
actually worsen acne and should be avoided. The face should be cleansed with mild, unscented soap and water.

Moisturizers

The topical treatment of acne can cause skin dryness and erythema, often a major reason patients discontinue
acne treatment. Facial dryness can be corrected with a noncomedogenic moisturizer (used once daily). Moisturizers are also useful for patients with facial dryness from isotretinoin. Lip balm is helpful for lip dryness.

Psychosocial support

Diminished self-esteem, social withdrawal, and a negative self-image have been reported by acne patients.
These factors can lead to anxiety and depression. Ambulatory screening techniques for anxiety and for
depression (e.g., Zung, Beck, Hamilton) would be useful to detect the impact of acne on the patient's mental
state. Supportive counseling by the interested family physician or psychologist would be indicated. Successful
treatment of the acne has been shown to significantly diminish the symptoms of anxiety and depression.

- In *severe acne,* higher doses of isotretinoin can be used. However, increased dosage
  may cause more skin drying, erythema, and xerostomia. Isotretinoin therapy can be
  stopped when approximately 70% to 80% of the acne lesions are reduced. Its
  action continues for 1 to 2 months after cessation of the medication.

Potential Problems and Complications

- Advise the patient and family to look for painful boils that suggest the need for systemic antibiotics. Patients with *pustules, abscesses,* and *furuncles on the face,*
  especially those arising in the facial triangle surrounding the nose in which the
  venous drainage flows directly into the cavernous sinus, are predisposed to cavernous sinus thrombosis or meningitis, or both, and should be treated with systemic antibiotics. Patients and their families should be warned not to pick at or
  squeeze lesions anywhere on the face.
- *Noncompliance* is usually evident when the patient fails to improve. Ask concrete
  questions about when and how much of the acne therapy prescribed is being followed. Keep the regimen simple. Patient education is a key factor in compliance.

- *Overuse of acne medication* is as bad as noncompliance. Overuse of topical agents like benzoyl peroxide and tretinoin can lead to skin dryness and erythema. Photosensitivity can also be caused by medication overuse and sun exposure.

Patient Education
Compliance
It is wise to tell patients and their family members that the treatment of acne is only as good as daily patient compliance with the prescribed regimen of medication and cleansing. Without the necessary investment of time in treatment, the acne will not show any improvement. The patient and family should be told that the treatment of acne will take 6 to 8 weeks before an improvement is noticed. Acne can be expected to *regress after adolescence.* The exact mechanism is unknown but is related to a decrease in sebum excretion.

Lifestyle Changes
- The patient should be advised to *keep the face clean* and free from sebum by washing twice daily with a mild soap. The patient should *avoid scrubbing* and rubbing the skin with abrasive cleansers and pads.
- *Oily materials should be kept off the face.* This includes cover-up cosmetics as well as oil-based cosmetics. Water-based cosmetics should be recommended.
- *Greasy lotions* applied to the hair can spread to the face with perspiration and aggravate the acne. Hair should brushed away from the face.
- *Stressful situations should be avoided.*
- The patient must *avoid popping the pustules* and picking at the crustules. Serious infections can result from this behavior.
- *Certain foods,* such as fried, greasy foods, chocolate, and caffeinated drinks have been implicated as a cause of acne; however, there is no proof that these foods are linked to acne flare-ups. Patients should be encouraged to eat a diet low in fat and refined sugars, which supports healthy living in general.
- *Photosensitivity* can be a side effect of some of the acne medications. Tetracycline and tretinoin use can cause photosensitivity when the patient is exposed to the sun. Patients using tretinoin should use a noncomedogenic sun-blocking agent with a skin protection factor (SPF) of 15 or higher to eliminate this possibility.
- *Ultraviolet radiation (UVR)* has not been scientifically proved to help reduce the inflammatory aspects of acne. However, if patients relate or perceive an improvement in their acne following sun exposure, the author finds it acceptable. Caution should be given to the patient to use adequate sun block (SPF of 15 or higher) to reduce UVR effects on the skin and prevent photosensitivity.

Family and Community Support
- A family physician involved in the treatment of an adolescent with acne should caution the family not to put undue pressure on the patient regarding the acne and its treatment. This can cause psychological damage.
- Nearly all adolescents develop acne to some degree, and it is difficult to reduce the risk of developing acne in this group of patients.

ROSACEA

Rosacea is an acneiform disorder of the skin, *usually* involving the middle third of the face; it is an increased susceptibility to a variety of stimuli such as heat, alcohol ingestion, certain foods, and stress. The etiology is unknown, and the condition may appear with or without a preceding history of acne or seborrhea.

Chief Complaint

A 47-year-old man, embarrassed by a red maculopapular rash on both cheeks and nose, has come to you for treatment (Figure 1.4, see color insert following page 170).

Clinical Manifestations

- Presenting signs include frequent episodes of facial flushing and blushing.
- Eventually, these signs lead to persistent erythema, which involves the cheeks, nose, forehead, chin, and, occasionally, the upper trunk.
- There is a feeling of heat in the face.
- The erythema is usually symmetric with paranasal telangiectasia formation. (Paranasal telangiectasia is not always indicative of rosacea; it is seen with chronic liver disease.)
- Occasionally, facial lesions progress to papules, tiny pustules, and even solid nodules, which appear similar to the lesions of acne vulgaris. Lesions can persist for days to months.
- Some patients, mostly men, develop rhinophyma, which is hyperplasia (bulbous enlargement) of the soft tissue of the nose.
- Eye involvement may occur, causing a red eye secondary to blepharitis, conjunctivitis, scleritis, or keratitis.
- There are no open or closed comedones, which distinguishes rosacea from acne vulgaris.

Epidemiology

Age

Rosacea usually begins at approximately age 40, and it can develop as early as 30 years of age.

Race

Celtic people, northern Europeans, and southern Italians are predisposed to rosacea.

Sex

Women are predominately affected, although rhinophyma is more common in men.

Risk Factors

- *Diet. Hot beverages* (such as coffee and tea), *spicy foods,* and *alcoholic beverages* can trigger transient flushing (erythema) of the face.
- *Emotional stress* can trigger rosacea.
- *Drugs.* Persistent use of potent topical fluorinated steroids on the face can cause rosacea. The condition is rarely seen with the use of oral (systemic) steroids.
- *Associated conditions.* Rosacea can develop with cases of carcinoid syndrome or mastocytosis.
- *Environment.* Heat sources such as the sun and hot kitchens can trigger symptoms.

PATHOLOGY

Histologic changes vary according to the stage of the disease. Commonly, a lymphohistiocytic infiltrate occurs around the upper dermal blood vessels, causing a disruption of the dermal structure. There is no involvement of the hair follicles or sebaceous glands; therefore there are no comedones.

Diagnosis

- A bilateral, symmetric erythematous rash on the face with some papules and pustules without comedones should direct the investigator to a diagnosis of rosacea instead of common acne. A history of facial flushing in response to hot liquids, spicy foods, or alcohol is noted. Skin changes include persistent facial erythema, papules, pustules, and/or nodules. Some patients develop telangiectasias of the paranasal region or rhinophyma.
- No specific testing needs to be performed.
- If there are pustules, rule out *Staphylococcus aureus* infection with a bacterial culture.

Differential Diagnosis

See Table 1.6.

Referral

Rosacea can be adequately treated by the family physician. In patients who are unresponsive to treatment, which means the inflammatory response is not controlled with mainstream medication, a referral to a dermatologist is warranted. Patients with moderate to severe ocular symptoms should be referred to an ophthalmologist. Rhinophyma and telangiectasias are almost always treated by a specialist.

Management

Several topical medications can be used to treat rosacea. Topical treatment is ideal for papular and pustular lesions. Systemic treatments are used if topical treatments fail or when the disease is very severe. Medication is usually used long term to control the disease, since curing rosacea is not possible. Flare-ups may require higher dosages of the antibiotics, which should then be tapered to the lowest dose to control the disease (Tables 1.7–1.9).

T ABLE 1.6.   Rosacea: Differential Diagnosis

Perioral dermatitis	There are tiny papules, erythema, scaling, and pustules around the mouth and chin. Perioral dermatitis is seen in younger individuals than is rosacea.
Staphylococcus aureus folliculitis	Pustules are culture positive. Lesions are discrete, not symmetric.
Systemic lupus erythematosus	The rash is bilateral, symmetric, and erythematous, with redness, papules, or pustules. Systemic complaints are present.
Acne vulgaris	Acne is seen in younger patients. Comedones are present. There is no flushing or diffuse facial erythema as is seen in rosacea.
Carcinoid syndrome	The patient has transient flushing, whereas persistent flushing is noted in rosacea. Urinary 5-HIAA levels are increased in carcinoid syndrome.
Seborrheic dermatitis	There are no comedones, and there are red scales around the nose, eye brow, ears, and scalp in seborrheic dermatitis. No flushing is noted.

5-HIAA, 5-hydroxyindoleacetic acid.

T ABLE 1.7.   Topical Rosacea Medication

Metronidazole (MetroGel) 0.75%

Availability:	Prescription only.
Form:	Gel or cream.
Dosage:	Applied twice daily.
Side effects:	Can cause a flare-up of the rash, with additional redness, sometimes with itching and skin irritation.
Duration:	1 to 2 months or until lesions are gone.
Comments:	First choice for topical treatment.

Erythromycin 2%

Availability:	Prescription only.
Form:	Gel or solution.
Dosage:	Applied twice daily.
Side effects:	May irritate skin (gel probably more than solution).
Duration:	1 to 2 months or until lesions are gone.
Comments:	Not as effective as metronidazole.

Sodium sulfacetamide 10%/sulfur 5% (Sulfacet-R)

Availability:	Prescription only.
Form:	Lotion.
Dosage:	Applied twice daily.
Side effects:	Allergic reaction to sodium sulfacetamide.
Duration:	1 to 2 months or until lesions are gone.
Comments:	Not as effective as metronidazole. Does not blend in with skin; comes with a blending kit to match the lotion to skin tone.

Clindamycin 2%

Availability:	Prescription only.
Form:	Gel or solution.
Dosage:	Applied twice daily.
Side effects:	May irritate the skin.
Duration:	1 to 2 months or until lesions are gone.
Comments:	Not as effective as metronidazole.

Benzoyl peroxide 2.5%, 5%, 10%

Availability:	Over the counter and prescription.
Form:	Gel, cream, or lotion.
Dosage:	Applied once or twice daily.
Side effects:	Mild redness, pruritus, dry skin, or scaling of skin. Sometimes increased erythema secondary to contact (irritant) dermatitis; stop treatment if this occurs.
Duration:	1 to 2 months or until lesions are gone.
Comments:	Usually start at 5%, may increase to 10% after several weeks if there is no improvement and there are no symptoms of skin dryness or erythema. Start at 2.5% strength in patients with history of sensitive skin.

continued

T ABLE 1.7. *continued.* **Topical Rosacea Medication**

Tretinoin (Retin-A)

Availability:	Prescription only.
Forms:	Cream 0.025%, 0.05%, 0.1%; gel 0.01%, 0.025%.
	Liquid 0.05%.
Dosage:	Applied 2 to 3 times weekly initially, increasing over several weeks to nightly use.
Side effects:	Can sting the skin; can also cause skin dryness and erythema. Start with lowest concentrations 2 to 3 times weekly and increase in response to the lesions. Retin-A can make skin more susceptible to sunburn; should protect with sunblock.
Duration:	1 to 2 months or until lesions are gone.
Comments:	Can be used in conjunction with topical antibiotics.

T ABLE 1.8.   **Systemic Rosacea Treatment**

Tetracycline

Availability:	Prescription only.
Dosage:	1 to 1.5 g daily in two divided doses.
Side effects:	Can cause gastrointestinal tract upset, candidal overgrowth, bone/tooth discoloration, and photosensitivity. Possible interference with oral birth control efficacy.
Duration:	Used for 1 to 2 months, then dosage tapered to 250 to 500 mg/day over 1 to 2 months as rosacea improves.
Comments:	First choice in severe nodular rosacea. To be taken on an empty stomach; otherwise, absorption can be impaired. Should not be used in pregnant women and children under 12 years of age.

Doxycycline

Availability:	Prescription only.
Dosage:	50 to 100 mg twice daily.
Side effects:	Fewer gastrointestinal tract side effects; otherwise, has side effects similar to tetracycline.
Duration:	Once the rash is controlled in 1 to 2 months, doxycycline is decreased to 50 mg/day, if possible.
Comments:	Alternative antibiotic choice. Can be taken with food. Should not be used in pregnant women and children under 12 years of age.

Minocycline

Availability:	Prescription only.
Dosage:	50 to 100 mg in 1 to 2 divided doses.
Side effects:	Can be taken with food. Can cause pseudotumor cerebri, skin hyperpigmentation, tooth/bone discoloration, possible interference with oral birth control efficacy, and vertigo.
Duration:	1 to 2 months, then decreased to 50 mg/day once the rash is controlled.
Comments:	Costly. Should not be used in pregnant women and children under 12 years of age.

Erythromycin

Availability:	Prescription only.
Dosage:	500 mg twice daily.

continued

T ABLE 1.8. *continued.*   **Systemic Rosacea Treatment**

Erythromycin *continued*
Side effects: Gastrointestinal tract side effects are predominant.
Duration: 1 to 2 months.

Isotretinoin (Accutane)
Availability: Prescription only.
Dosage: 0.5 to 1.0 mg/kg daily, taken with food.
Side effects: Isotretinoin is *teratogenic;* pregnancy should be avoided. Contraception is necessary for women of child-bearing age 1 month before starting treatment and continued for 2 months beyond cessation of therapy.
Tetracycline and isotretinoin should not be taken together; the combination can cause pseudotumor cerebri.
The blood lipids (cholesterol and triglycerides) should be monitored at the start of treatment (baseline), 1 to 2 weeks after starting the course, and at monthly intervals thereafter.
Isotretinoin can increase levels of plasma triglycerides, increase total cholesterol, and decrease high-density lipoproteins.
Isotretinoin can also cause an elevated platelet count, neutropenia, and elevated levels of hepatic enzymes, which will return to normal after cessation of drug administration.
Other side effects include cheilitis, dry skin, pruritus, headaches, epistaxis, and photosensitivity. These are relatively frequent and dose related.
Duration: 4- to 5-month course.
Comments: Not first-line therapy for rosacea.

Follow-up
Monitoring Disease Course
- Monitor the rash for 2 to 3 weeks during the initial treatment phase. Three percent of patients using topical metronidazole (MetroGel) develop a flare of rosacea with this medication. If this occurs, the medication should be withdrawn and another medication used.
- Expect to see therapeutic results with the use of topical medication within 6 to 8 weeks.
- Schedule a return visit within the first 6- to 8-week period.

Potential Problems and Complications
- Periodic exacerbations of rosacea can be expected with the use of topical antibiotics, and the patient should be instructed to return during these periods. These flare-ups can be managed by starting a regimen of oral antibiotics for 6 to 8 weeks or by increasing the dose of the current oral antibiotic for 2 weeks and then tapering it to the lowest dose for the remaining 4 to 6 weeks.
- If the patient has no response to either topical or oral medication within 3 to 4 months of treatment, isotretinoin should be considered.

T ABLE 1.9.   Other Treatment Modalities for Rosacea

Physical and environmental measures

Patients should be reminded to reduce or eliminate alcohol, spicy foods, and hot beverages from the diet, as this will help to reduce the erythema.

Areas with a great deal of heat (e.g., kitchens) should be avoided.

Patients should stay out of the sun and use sunscreens.

Emotional stress should be reduced.

Water-based, noncomedogenic cosmetics only should be used.

Astringents or other skin lotions containing alcohol, abrasives, menthol, peppermint, eucalyptus oil, clove oil, or witch hazel should be avoided.

Abrasive clothing and excessive facial rubbing are to be avoided as well.

Treatment of rhinophyma

Patients with unresponsive rhinophyma that is increasing in size should be referred for surgical intervention. The progression of rhinophyma can be controlled by aggressively treating the rosacea and avoiding any provocative triggers. The experienced dermatologist or plastic surgeon can offer the patient electrosurgery, excision (scalpel), dermabrasion, or carbon dioxide laser treatment to reduce the rhinophyma.

Treatment of telantiectasias

Likewise, patients with resistant telangiectasias should be referred to skin specialists for pulsed-dye or continuous-wave laser therapy. Patients can cover the telangiectasias with yellow-or green-tinted coverup cosmetics (prefoundation base). The tint neutralizes the erythema (redness) of the rash.

Psychosocial support

Rosacea rash causes a great deal of redness and brings attention to the face and eyes. Patients often ask for immediate relief of this cosmetically unpleasant disease. Counsel patients to accept themselves as they are, and accept and be compliant with medical treatment. Since stress, anxiety, and anger can trigger rosacea, teach your patients simple relaxation techniques or encourage them to engage in moderate exercise. The National Rosacea Society is a good patient support group (www.rosacea.org).

Patient Education

Compliance

As with acne treatment, the treatment of rosacea is lengthy and patients must comply with daily treatments if this rash is to be controlled. Anticipatory guidance should be given to alert patients to flare-ups occasionally caused by the environment, emotional distress, certain foods, and sometimes the medication used for treatment.

Family and Community Support

Advise patients with rosacea that the physical effects of the disease can lead to embarrassing or rude comments from people. Patients may feel self-conscious, increasing stress, which in turn may lead to a flare-up of the condition.

PERIORAL DERMATITIS

Perioral dermatitis is an erythematous papular disease of the perioral area that can occasionally cause itching or burning. Etiology is unknown.

Chief Complaint

Patients often present with perioral papules and report a feeling of tightness around the mouth.

Clinical Manifestations

- The rash occurs over a few weeks to months and is usually self-limited (Figure 1.5, see color insert following page 170).
- Sometimes the rash causes itching or burning and a feeling of tightness in the perioral area. Uncommonly, it can involve the periorbital or paranasal area.
- The rash can also be nonpruritic.
- The rash usually spares the vermilion border of the lips.
- Discrete erythematous papules can become confluent, forming inflammatory plaques on the perioral skin area.
- Occasionally, the rash can cause scaling.
- Sometimes pustules may arise.
- The rash may appear in a nongranulomatous and granulomatous (rare) form.

Epidemiology

Perioral dermatitis involves children and adults (most frequently women) 20 to 30 years of age.

Risk Factors

- The rash can be caused by long-standing topical corticosteroid use on the face and often is indistinguishable from steroid acne.
- The rash can be caused by fluoridated and tartar-control toothpaste.

PATHOLOGY

Perifollicular inflammation and perivascular infiltrate are seen; often, only the degree of inflammation differentiates perioral dermatitis from rosacea.

Diagnosis

- Diagnosis of the rash is usually clinical, based on the history and physical examination.
- Culture of the pustules can be obtained to rule out an *S. aureus* infection when there is no response using common treatment.
- Biopsy can be helpful to distinguish the granulomatous form of perioral dermatitis.

Differential Diagnosis

See Table 1.10.

Referral

Referral is appropriate if there is no substantial improvement after several months of adequate treatment.

TABLE 1.10.   **Perioral Dermatitis: Differential Diagnosis**

Allergic contact dermatitis	Usually a history of an offending irritating agent; no history associated with perioral dermatitis.
Atopic dermatitis	Usually there are symptoms of atopy, whereas none are associated with perioral dermatitis.
Seborrhea dermatitis	Usually includes scaly involvement of the scalp and periorbital region. Seborrhea rarely involves the perioral area.
Rosacea	Usually is seen in adults over 40 years of age. Lacks a clear zone around the vermillion border of the lips and is located paranasally.
Acne vulgaris	Rash is not confined to the perioral region. No comedones noted in perioral dermatitis.
Steroid acne	History of long-standing topical steroid use on the face. Can be indistinguishable from perioral dermatitis.

Management

- Discontinuing use of topical corticosteroids on the face should be the first step in the treatment process. However, a rebound flare-up of the rash may occur. Low-potency corticosteroid creams, such as 1% hydrocortisone cream, desonide (Des-Owen), or alclometasone (Aclovate), applied topically twice daily may ease the transition from the poststeroidal flare-up to controlling the rash with nonsteroidal topical or systemic medication.
- *Topical medication* is useful in mild to moderate cases of perioral dermatitis (Table 1.11).

TABLE 1.11.   **Topical Perioral Dermatitis Treatment**

Metronidazole (MetroGel) 0.75%

Availability:	Prescription only.
Form:	Gel or cream.
Dosage:	Applied topically to rash twice a day.
Side effects:	Some skin irritation and pruritus.
Duration:	1 to 3 months of treatment.
Comments:	First choice in mild to moderate cases in adults and preferred treatment in children under 12 years of age.

Erythromycin 2%

Availability:	Prescription only.
Form:	Gel.
Dosage:	Applied topically twice a day.
Side effects:	Skin dryness, erythema, burning, and pruritus.
Duration:	1 to 3 months of treatment.
Comments:	Alternate choice for mild to moderate cases when patients may be sensitive or unresponsive to metronidazole topically.

- *Systemic medication* is useful in severe cases of perioral dermatitis or when topical therapy is not effective (Table 1.12). Systemic therapy may be used alone or in resistant cases in conjunction with topical agents.

Follow-up

- Monitoring the course of the disease involves follow-up 1 month after initiation of therapy and monthly thereafter until the rash clears.
- The patient should be advised to return if there are mild recurrences and to be compliant with the daily use of the medication. Mild recurrences can be treated successfully with topical metronidazole or low-dose oral tetracycline or minocycline.

T ABLE 1.12. Systemic Perioral Dermatitis Treatment

Minocycline

Availability:	Prescription only.
Dosage:	50 to 100 mg orally twice daily.
Side effects:	Can be taken with food. Can cause pseudotumor cerebri, skin hyperpigmentation, tooth/bone discoloration. Possible interference with oral birth control efficacy. Vertigo.
Duration:	1 to 3 months.
Comments:	Costly. First choice in severe or resistant cases in adults. Should not be used in pregnant women or children under 12 years of age.

Tetracycline

Availability:	Prescription only.
Dosage:	250 to 500 mg orally 2 to 3 times daily.
Side effects:	Can cause gastrointestinal tract upset, candidal overgrowth, bone/tooth discoloration, and photosensitivity. Possible interference with oral birth control efficacy.
Duration:	1 to 3 months.
Comments:	Inexpensive. Must be taken on empty stomach; otherwise, absorption is impaired. Should not be used in pregnant women and children under 12 years of age.

Doxycycline

Availability:	Prescription only.
Dosage:	100 mg orally twice daily.
Side effects:	Fewer gastrointestinal tract side effects; otherwise, has side effects similar to those of tetracycline.
Duration:	1 to 3 months.
Comments:	Should not be used in pregnant women and children under 12 years of age.

Erythromycin

Availability:	Prescription only.
Dosage:	250 to 333 mg orally twice daily.
Duration:	1 to 3 months.
Side effects:	Gastrointestinal tract upset.
Comments:	Erythromycin is recommended if oral therapy is necessary in pregnant women and children under 12 years of age. Avoid the estolate salt in children and pregnancy.

Patient Education
Compliance
Perioral dermatitis is a chronic rash and can fluctuate in its severity over months and years; therefore, recurrences are possible. The patient should be educated in the treatment of the rash with topical or systemic medications.

Health Promotion
- Healthy skin can be achieved by cleansing the skin with mild soap and water, moisturizing the skin to protect it from excessive dryness, and preventing sun damage to the skin by using a sunscreen with an SPF of 15 or higher.
- Avoidance of potent topical corticosteroids on the face is an important preventive factor of this rash.

Psychosocial Support
The rash can cause cosmetic disfigurement. The patient should be advised of this and that the rash should be controlled by the treatment discussed.

HIDRADENITIS SUPPURATIVA

Hidradenitis suppurativa is a chronic disease of skin in the axilla and the anogenital regions involving the sweat glands. It causes intermittent pain and sometimes point tenderness because of recurrent abscesses in these locations. The etiology is unknown (Figure 1.6, see color insert following page 170).

Chief Complaint
A 27-year-old woman comes to you with recurrent, tender abscesses in the axillae.

Clinical Manifestations
- Intermittent pain and point tenderness are related to abscess formation in the axilla or anogenital region.
- Sometimes the pain is preceded by pruritus.
- Inflammatory nodules and/or abscesses may resolve or drain purulent material.
- Nodules are usually red and exquisitely tender to palpation.
- Hair follicles are usually spared.
- Sinus tracts can form.
- Hypertrophic or keloid scars can occur.
- Comedones are often seen.

Epidemiology
History
A high incidence of cases are associated with a positive family history.

Age
Hidradenitis suppurativa may occur at any time from puberty to the climacteric but usually dissipates after the age of 35 years.

Race
Although the disease occurs in all races, it is most severe in African Americans.

Sex
- The disease is more common in women.
- Men usually have more anogenital lesions.
- Women have more axillary involvement.

Risk Factors

- Obesity, smoking, and a genetic predisposition to acne.
- A positive family history.

PATHOLOGY

Keratinaceous plugging of the apocrine gland ducts leads to dilation of these structures and severe inflammatory changes. Secondary bacterial growth then occurs, resulting in rupture of the ductal/gland system and extending the inflammation and infection to surrounding tissue. Connecting sinus tracts can also form.

Diagnosis

- This diagnosis is mainly clinical, arising from history and physical examination.
- Bacterial cultures can reveal *S. aureus,* Streptococci, *Escherichia coli, Proteus mirabilis,* and *Pseudomonas aeruginosa.*
- A skin biopsy should be conducted on any chronic ulcerated lesion in the axilla or anogenital region to rule out squamous cell carcinoma.

Differential Diagnosis

See Table 1.13.

Referral

In its mild form, this disease can be treated by the family physician. In the progressive stages and severe disease involving extreme amounts of pain and scarring, a referral to a dermatologist or general surgeon may be necessary.

Management

Hidradenitis suppurativa may require several treatment combinations: antibiotics, intralesional corticosteroids, incision and drainage, excision of the fibrotic nodules or sinus tracts, and extensive excision of the axilla or anogenital area. Hidradenitis that does not respond initially to empiric antibiotics and recurs should be cultured to guide future antibiotic treatment.

T ABLE 1.13.   Hidradenitis Suppurativa: Differential Diagnosis

Simple furuncles and carbuncles	No comedones.
	Abscesses are usually distinguishable by location (they can occur anywhere on the body, not just in axilla or anogenital region).
Lymphadenitis	Usually the infection follows lymphatic channels and is not an abscess.
	Usually not recurrent.
Ruptured inclusion cysts	No comedones.
	Not limited to axilla or anogenital region.
	Usually not recurrent.

- *Painful nodules and lesions* can be treated with oral prednisone, initially at 60 mg daily and tapered over 14 days, administered concurrently with antibiotics. Many serious systemic side effects occur if prednisone is used on a regular basis, including the inhibition of the pituitary adrenal axis.
- *Early abscess* can be injected with a sufficient quantity (3 to 10 mg/mL) of intralesional triamcinolone acetonide to cause the abscess to blanch.
- *Painful nodules* can be injected with a sufficient quantity (3 to 10 mg/mL) of intralesional triamcinolone acetonide to cause the abscess to blanch.
- *Fluctuant abscess* walls can be injected with 2 to 3 cc (3 to 10 mg/mL) of intralesional triamcinolone acetonide after the abscess is incised and drained.
- *Recurrent disease* usually requires surgical management.

Medications
Table 1.14 discusses *medical management* of the disease.

Other Treatment Modalities
Surgical management for recurrent disease with fibrosis, scarring, or sinus tract formation includes the following:
- Incision and drainage of abscesses.
- Excision of fibrotic nodules or sinus tracts.
- Wide excision down to the fascia, which may be required with subsequent skin grafting in extensive disease.
- Tight-fitting clothing and undergarments should be avoided to prevent friction to the affected area, which could exacerbate the lesion.
- Lesions should be cleansed daily with a germicidal soap (e.g., chlorhexidine gluconate).
- Preventive measures include the topical application of 2% clindamycin or 2% erythromycin daily to the axilla or anogenital region.
- An effective antiperspirant and deodorant agent is 6.25% aluminum chloride hexahydrate ethanol (Xerac AC).
- Roll-on or stick deodorants and antiperspirants should be avoided because they can cause friction during application.

Follow-up
Monitoring Disease Course
In mild to moderate disease, patients should be followed up every several months to make sure no new nodules or abscesses are forming.

Potential Problems and Complications
With more severe disease involving pain and scarring, consultation with a general surgeon is advised.

Patient Education
Compliance
Patients usually do not have a problem with treatment compliance, since these lesions often are very painful, recurrent, and/or drain purulent material.

Lifestyle Changes
Patients should be counseled about weight reduction. They should be instructed to avoid frictional trauma to the affected areas and to cleanse the areas with antibacterial soaps.

T ABLE 1.14.   Medical Treatment of Hidradenitis Suppurativa

Tetracycline

Availability:	Prescription only.
Dosage:	1 to 1.5 g daily in 2 divided doses.
Side effects:	Can cause gastrointestinal tract upset, candidal overgrowth, bone/tooth discoloration, and photosensitivity. Possible interference with oral birth control efficacy.
Duration:	10 to 14 days.
Comments:	Inexpensive. Should be taken on an empty stomach; otherwise, absorption is impaired. Should not be used in pregnant women and children under 12 years of age.

Erythromycin

Availability:	Prescription only.
Dosage:	250 to 333 mg orally twice daily.
Duration:	10 to 14 days.
Side effects:	Gastrointestinal tract upset.
Comments:	Erythromycin is recommended if oral therapy is necessary in pregnant women and children under 12 years of age. Avoid the estolate salt in children and pregnancy.

Minoclycline

Availability:	Prescription only.
Dosage:	50 to 100 mg daily, 1 to 2 divided doses.
Side effects:	Can be taken with food. Can cause pseudotumor cerebri, skin hyperpigmentation, tooth/bone discoloration. Possible interference with oral birth control efficacy. Vertigo.
Duration:	10 to 14 days.
Comments:	Costly. First choice in severe or resistant cases in adults. Should not be used in pregnant women or children under 12 years of age.

Doxycycline

Availability:	Prescription only.
Dosage:	100 to 200 mg/day.
Side effects:	Fewer gastrointestinal tract side effects; otherwise, has side effects similar to those of tetracycline.
Duration:	10 to 14 days.
Comments:	Should not be used in pregnant women and children under 12 years of age.

Isotretinoin (Accutane)

Availability:	Prescription only.
Dosage:	1.0 mg/kg daily, taken with food.
Side effects:	Isotretinoin is *teratogenic;* pregnancy should be avoided. Contraception is necessary for women of child-bearing age 1 month before starting treatment and continued for 2 months beyond cessation of therapy.
	Tetracycline and isotretinoin should not be taken together; the combination can cause pseudotumor cerebri.

continued

TABLE 1.14. *continued.*   **Medical Treatment of Hidradenitis Suppurativa**

	The blood lipids (cholesterol and triglycerides) should be monitored at the start of treatment (baseline), 1 to 2 weeks after starting the course, and at monthly intervals thereafter.
	Isotretinoin can increase levels of plasma triglycerides, increase total cholesterol, and decrease high-density lipoproteins.
	Isotretinoin can also cause an elevated platelet count, neutropenia, and elevated levels of hepatic enzymes, which will return to normal after cessation of drug administration.
	Other side effects include cheilitis, dry skin, pruritus, headaches, epistaxis, and photosensitivity. These are relatively frequent and dose related.
Duration:	4- to 5-month course.
Comments:	Variable degree of success in early disease. Can be used in recurrent disease after surgical excision of lesions.

BIBLIOGRAPHY

Bergfeld WF. The evaluation and management of acne: Economic considerations. *J Am Acad Dermatol* 1995;32(5, Pt 3)S52–S56.

Berson DS, Shalita AR. The treatment of acne: the role of combination therapies. *J Am Acad Dermatol* 1995;32(5,Pt 3)S31–S41.

Draelos ZK. Patient compliance: enhancing clinician abilities and strategies. *J Am Acad Dermatol* 1995;32(5, Pt 3)S42–S48.

Drake LA. Guidelines of care for acne vulgaris. *J Am Acad Dermatol* 1989;22(4) 676–680.

Kaminer MS, Gilchrest BA. The many faces of acne. *J Am Acad Dermatol* 1995;32(5, Pt 3)S6–S14.

Leyden JJ. New understandings of the pathogenesis of acne. *J Am Acad Dermatol* 1995;32(5, Pt 3)S15–S25.

Lookingbill D, Egan N, Santen R, et al. Correlation of serum 3α-androstanediol glucuronide with acne and chest hair density in men. *J Clin Endocrinol Metab* 1988; 67:986–991.

Nguyen QH, Kim YA, Schwartz RD. Management of acne vulgaris. *Am Fam Physician* 1994;50(1)89–96.

Pochi PE, Shalita AR, Strauss JS, et al. Report of the Consensus Conference on Acne Classification. *J Am Acad Dermatol* 1991;24(3)495–500.

Thiboutot DM. Acne rosacea. *Am Fam Physician* 1994;50(8)1691–1697.

Thiboutot DM, Lookingbill DP. Acne: acute or chronic disease? *J Am Acad Dermatol* 1995;32(5, Pt 3)S2–S5.

Wu SF, Kinder BN, Trunnell TN, et al. Role of anxiety and anger in acne patients: a relationship with the severity of the disorder. *J Am Acad Dermatol* 1988;18(2, Pt 1) 325–333.

CHAPTER 2

. . . .

Eczematous Disorders

Eczematous disorders is a term used to describe a wide variety of cutaneous inflammatory conditions that may be characterized by erythema, papules, vesicles, pustules, crusts, or scales, depending on the type and stage of a particular disorder.

ATOPIC DERMATITIS

Atopic dermatitis is a common disorder characterized by lesions often accompanied by profound pruritus.

Chief Complaint

Patients complain of highly pruritic rash, rhinorrhea, sneezing, nasal congestion, lacrimation, and pharyngeal and conjunctival itching.

Clinical Manifestations

- Scaly skin eruption with inflammation is usually located on flexor or extensor surfaces or the face (Figures 2.1 and 2.2, see color insert following page 170).
- Symptoms may fluctuate seasonally in temperate climates, worsening in winter and improving in summer.
- Small vesicles on edematous and erythematous skin are often accompanied by plaques and patches that may be crusted and weeping.
- Lesions may be acute, with poorly defined erythematous plaques with scaling and excoriations, or demonstrate a more chronic appearance of lichenification, fissures, and erosions.
- In cases of *infantile atopic dermatitis* (in children up to 2 years of age) lesions are located in the extremities, popliteal and antecubital fossa, groin, wrists, and face (generally sparing the area around the mouth).
- In cases of *childhood atopic dermatitis* (in children 4 to 10 years of age) lesions are particularly prevalent in the antecubital and popliteal regions, but may also occur on the neck, wrists, and face. Perioral pallor and the Dennie-Morgan sign (a characteristic infraorbital fold in the eyelid) are often noted. Lichenification of the affected skin, as well as fissuring, may occur. Periorbital hyperpigmentation may result from chronic rubbing of the eyelids.
- In cases of *adult atopic dermatitis*, lesions are often located on the flexor aspects of the extremities as well as the sides and front of the neck, eyelids, face, forehead, wrists, hands, and feet. Adult-onset atopic dermatitis is characterized by remissions and exacerbations.

Epidemiology

Age

- Onset of atopic dermatitis begins before 1 year of age in roughly 60% of cases.
- Only 10% of cases of atopic dermatitis develop between 6 and 20 years of age.
- Adult onset is rare. In severe cases, childhood or infantile atopic dermatitis may persist into adulthood.

Sex

Atopic dermatitis is seen slightly more often in boys than in girls.

Risk Factors
Approximately two-thirds of patients with atopic dermatitis have a positive family or personal history of asthma, hay fever, allergic rhinitis, or allergic sinusitis.

PATHOLOGY
Type I [immunoglobulin E (IgE)–mediated] hypersensitivity reaction in the skin occurs from the release of vasoactive substances from mast cells and basophils that have been sensitized by the interaction of an antigen with IgE.

Diagnosis
- Diagnosis relies mainly on history and clinical findings.
- The diagnostic criteria of atopic dermatitis are listed in Table 2.1.

Diagnostic Tests
- Diagnostic testing is usually not needed. The diagnosis is made on clinical evidence.
- *Serum levels of IgE.* Increased levels are supportive evidence.
- Biopsies are usually not helpful because of the lack of specificity of the microscopic findings.

Differential Diagnosis
See Table 2.2.

Referral
If the physician is uncertain of the diagnosis, if the treatment plan has not been helpful, or if diffuse, severe pruritus is present, referral may be warranted.

Management
The treatments outlined in Table 2.3 are for atopic dermatitis, not for the variants mentioned in the Differential Diagnosis section. Additional treatment modalities and treatments for diseases or disorders that may accompany atopic dermatitis are discussed below.

Medications
See Table 2.3.

Other Treatment Modalities
Physical
- *Ultraviolet A-range* and *B-range (UVA and UVB) phototherapy* and *psoralen ultraviolet A-range (PUVA) photochemotherapy* have been shown to be effective in some cases.
- Patients with atopic dermatitis are at a higher risk for secondary skin infections in the affected areas. If any signs of infection are observed, treat promptly with oral antibiotics effective against Staphylococcus and Streptococcus for 10 days as follows:
  - *Cephalexin,* 250 mg 4 times daily;
  - *Dicloxacillin,* 250 mg 4 times daily;
  or
  - *Erythromycin,* 250 mg 4 times daily.

T ABLE 2.1.   Diagnostic Criteria of Atopic Dermatitis

Major features (must have 3 or more)	Minor features (must have 3 or more)
Pruritus	Cataracts (anterior subcapsular)
Characteristic morphology and distribution	Cheilitis
Adults: lichenification to flexor areas	Conjunctivitis (chronic or relapsing)
Children/infants: involvement of face	Cutaneous infection (chronic or recurrent)
and extensor areas	Dennie-Morgan lines (infraorbital fold)
Chronic or relapsing dermatitis	Eczema
Family or personal history of asthma, atopic	Elevated serum immunoglobulin E
dermatitis, allergic rhinitis	Facial pallor or erythema
	Food intolerance
	Hand dermatitis (following exposure to irritant)
	Ichthyosis
	Keratoconus
	Keratosis pilaris
	Nipple dermatitis
	Orbital darkening
	Pityriasis alba
	Pruritus with sweating
	Type 1 (immediate) skin test reactivity
	White dermatographism
	Wool intolerance
	Xerosis

From Hanifin JM, Rajka G. Diagnostic features of atopic dermatitis. *Acta Dermatol Suppl* 1980;92:44–47, with permission.

T ABLE 2.2.   Atopic Dermatitis: Differential Diagnosis

Seborrheic dermatitis	Seborrheic dermatitis is typically more greasy and scaly in appearance, with most lesions located on the scalp.
Contact dermatitis	There is a history of exposure to an inciting substance, causing a spontaneous eruption. Patch testing may be helpful.
Psoriasis	Psoriasis has a characteristic thicker scale and distribution on the extensor surfaces.
Nummular eczema	IgE level is normal, and history is characteristic.
	Lesions are typically singular, annular, and located on lower legs, trunk, and hands. It occurs mostly in winter months.
Dermatophytosis	KOH testing rules out this diagnosis.
Dry skin	IgE level is normal; history and environmental factors are diagnostic.

IgE, immunoglobulin E; KOH, potassium hydroxide.

T ABLE 2.3.   Medical Treatment of Atopic Dermatitis

Topical corticosteroids

Administration: Apply to lesions 2 to 3 times daily when using lower-potency agents; 1 to 2 times daily when using higher-potency agents.

Side effects: Long-term use may cause skin atrophy.

Comments: When rash is controlled, switch to lower potency for maintenance. Generally, choose the lowest potency according to the severity of disease. Avoid high- and super-high–potency corticosteroid use on face and groin because of increased risk of side effects.

Prednisone

Administration: *Adults:* 70 to 80 mg daily, tapering by 5 to 10 mg daily every 2 to 3 days.

 Children: 1 mg/kg daily tapering by 5 to 10 mg daily every 2 to 3 days.

Duration of use: 7 to 10 days maximum.

Side effects: Prednisone can cause many side effects; see *Physicians' Desk Reference.*

Comments: Prednisone is indicated for severe, refractory cases. Cessation often causes recurrence of symptoms.

Diphenhydramine (Benadryl)

Administration: *Adults:* 25 to 50 mg every 6 hours as needed.

 Children: 5 mg/kg daily divided into 4 doses.

Duration of use: As needed.

Side effects: Drowsiness and sedation are possible.

Comments: Patients should not drive or operate hazardous machinery. Alcohol should be avoided while using medication.

Hydroxyzine (Atarax)

Administration: *Adults:* 10 to 50 mg every 6 hours.

 Children: 2 mg/kg daily divided into 4 doses.

Duration of use: As needed.

Side effects: Drowsiness and sedation are possible.

Comments: Patients should not drive or operate hazardous machinery. Alcohol should be avoided while using medication.

Loratadine (Claritin), cetirizine (Zyrtec)

Administration: *Adults:* 10 mg daily.

 Children: 10 mg loratadine or 5 to 10 mg cetirizine daily.

Duration of use: As needed.

Comments: These agents are less sedating than diphenhydramine and hydroxyzine and are helpful for daytime pruritus.

Doxepin (Sinequan)

Administration: 10 to 50 mg at bedtime.

Duration of use: As needed for pruritus.

Comments: Sedation and anticholinergic effects are possible. Agents are useful for severe nighttime pruritus.

continued

TABLE 2.3. *continued.*   Medical Treatment of Atopic Dermatitis
_____

Tar ointments and preparations (T-Derm, Fototar cream, Zetar emulsion)
Administration: Apply a thin layer to affected areas once or twice daily.
Duration of use: As needed; best used as maintenance therapy.
Comments: Sunlight should be avoided; preparations increase tendency to sunburn. Tar preparations
                    may cause temporary staining of light-colored hair.

Emollients (Lubriderm, Nutraderm, Eucerin, or Moisturel)
Administration: Apply daily to damp skin immediately after bathing.
Duration of use: As needed for maintenance therapy.
Comments: Use lanolin-free, fragrance-free emollients only.
_____

- Treat any frank pyoderma promptly for ten days with *any* of the above three antibiotics; only use a long-term cyclic antibiotic regimen, perhaps 5-6 days with medication, followed by 2 to 3 weeks without medication, and so forth, to **prevent** Staphylococcal colonization or recurrent secondary bacterial infection.
- Patients with atopic dermatitis are at a higher risk for herpes simplex virus (HSV). If the patient has signs of HSV, an antiviral agent such as acyclovir [Zovirax (20 mg/kg daily in four divided doses in children)] or valacyclovir [Valtrex (500 mg two times daily for 5 to 7 days in adults)] should be added.

Environmental
- *Cold compresses* may be applied to rash; lukewarm baths with oatmeal (Aveeno) also relieve itching.
- *Mild skin cleansers* should be used (e.g., Dove, Aveeno soap, Cetaphil).
- *Mild, unscented laundry detergents* are recommended (several companies make laundry detergents free of dyes or perfumes, including Cheer-Free, Arm & Hammer, Purex, and Ivory Snow).
- *Sensitizing objects* such as wool, lanolin, cosmetics with fragrances, and bubble bath *should be avoided.*
- Patients should wear *100% cotton clothing* as much as possible.
- Make sure indoor environment has appropriate humidity.
- Although allergy testing is of limited benefit in the workup of atopic dermatitis, identification and efforts to limit exposure to a specific exacerbating allergen can be helpful.

Psychological
- Stress management education may prove beneficial for patients who have stress-related exacerbations.

Follow-up
- Patients undergoing topical treatment of atopic dermatitis should be followed closely for signs of skin atrophy.
- Once lesions are stable, the patient should be given a low-potency topical corticosteroid to control lesions.
- Patients should be followed monthly and offered emotional support as well as therapeutic advice. As the rash diminishes, follow-up visits for monitoring may be decreased to every 3 months in a 1-year period.

Patient Education

Compliance

- Rubbing, picking, or scratching of the affected areas should be strongly discouraged.
- Patients should be counseled to use warm, not hot, water for bathing and washing.
- Soap use should be kept to a minimum, except in the skin folds, when bathing.
- Physical contact with friends or relatives with obvious HSV infections (such as cold sores) should be avoided.

Family and Community Support

Patients should receive psychological support; in particular, children should be encouraged by their parents to discuss their feelings about having this disease.

CONTACT DERMATITIS

Contact dermatitis is an acute inflammatory reaction caused by a substance brought into contact with the skin. Contact dermatitis falls into two basic categories: *irritant contact dermatitis* and *allergic contact dermatitis*. Irritant contact dermatitis occurs when a substance (such as kerosene or strong detergent) causes direct damage and irritation to the epidermis. Allergic contact dermatitis occurs when a substance that serves as an allergen (such as poison ivy or nickel) elicits a type IV (cell-mediated, or delayed) hypersensitivity reaction.

Chief Complaint

A young man comes to your clinic and complains of burning and itching under his watchband.

Clinical Manifestations

- The *lesions are sharply defined areas of inflammation* confined to areas of contact exposure. Burning and itching may be associated. In severe cases of allergic contact dermatitis, some patients may complain of constitutional symptoms such as fever, chills, and headaches.
- *Onset of the localized itching and skin eruption* may be gradual or almost immediate. The cutaneous manifestations may be acute, lasting from days to weeks, or chronic, lasting from months to years.
- Physical findings are similar in both irritant and allergic contact dermatitis (Figures 2.3 and 2.4, see color insert following page 170). Erythema develops into papules and vesicles, eventually giving way to erosions with crusting and scaling.
- There is a notable difference between the two forms: The lesion of allergic contact dermatitis, although originally sharply defined, may eventually demonstrate peripheral spreading. This marginal spreading usually consists of tiny papules that cause the borders of the lesions to become ill-defined or even generalized.

Epidemiology

Irritant or allergic contact dermatitis may occur in any population and in any age group.

Risk Factors

- Exposure to any substances likely to cause a toxic or irritant dermatitis (often, organic solvents or soap) puts a person at risk. Table 2.4 lists common irritants and allergens.
- Degree of exposure needed to elicit a dermatologic response varies widely, depending on the individual's sensitivity to the irritant involved.
- Family history may also play a role.

PATHOLOGY

Allergic contact dermatitis is caused by contact with a substance that causes a type IV hypersensitivity reaction. The substance responsible is often a low molecular-weight hapten; very low concentrations may cause a reaction.

TABLE 2.4.   Common Substances Causing Contact Dermatitis

Irritants (irritant contact dermatitis)	Allergens (allergic contact dermatitis)
Lubricants	Latex
Cement (dichromate)	Rubber
Paint remover	Fragrance
Shampoos	Nickel sulfate
Detergents	Plastics
Alcohols	Disinfectants
Grease	Parabens (sunscreens)
Alkali (lye)	Poison ivy, oak, or sumac (rhus dermatitis)
Nitric acid	Benzocaine (in products such as Lanacaine, Solarcaine)
Turpentine	Formaldehyde
Laundry bleach	Neomycin (Neosporin)
Gasoline	Textile or hair dyes (paraphenylenediamine)
	Solvents
	Printer's ink

Diagnosis

Contact dermatitis typically shows inflammation and spongiosis. A noneczematous disease does not show this type of inflammation.

Differential Diagnosis

See Table 2.5.

Diagnostic Tests

Patch testing is indicated to determine the substance or allergen responsible for *allergic contact dermatitis* in order to avoid or eliminate future exposures to allergens. The standard patch test uses an assembly of 20 substances or chemicals. Because the standard patch test kit is not inclusive of every possible allergen, other substances may be used in the test. The basic technique is to place a possible allergen in a holding device, which is taped to the patient's skin (usually the back). The patches are removed after 48 hours. The areas tested are examined 20 minutes after removal of the patches and again in 3 to 7 days. The reactions may be rated negative (nonreactive), weakly positive (erythema with possible papules but no vesicles), strongly positive (erythema with edema and vesicles), and extremely positive

T ABLE 2.5.   Contact Dermatitis: Differential Diagnosis

Nummular eczema	Lesions are usually round (coin-shaped) rather than the conforming rash of contact dermatitis. There is no history of allergen exposure.
Atopic eczema	There is a chronic rash with a flexural distribution along with other atopic symptoms.
Dermatitis herpetiformis	Rash is localized to elbows, knees, scalp, and buttocks, with severe pruritus.
Scabies	Rash is localized to finger webs, wrists, and waist initially, then spreads to other areas. Also seen in other family members.

(spreading bullae and ulcerations). Patch testing is *not useful* in cases of *irritant contact dermatitis.*

Referral

Referral may be warranted for patch testing, if the physician has concerns about the diagnosis, if the treatment plan is ineffective, or if symptoms such as bronchospasm or angioedema are present.

Management
Medications
See Table 2.6.

Other Treatment Modalities
Physical
- Large vesicles and bullae may be drained, but tops should not be removed, to aid healing and prevent secondary infection.
- Cold compresses may help to control itching.

Environmental
- The most important aspect in managing contact dermatitis is identifying and removing the responsible agent.

Follow-up

Patients do not need close follow-up, since eliminating the offending agent and treating the rash usually eliminates the problem. Patients should, however, be advised to return if the rash does not resolve within 2 weeks.

Patient Education
- All patients should be counseled that contact dermatitis is not contagious and that the best protection is avoidance of the allergen or irritant.
- Patients should wear protective clothing such as gloves or long sleeves whenever repeated exposure to an allergen or irritant is necessary.
- Topical agents for associated pruritus, such as benzocaine and diphenhydramine, should be avoided, since these medications can also cause contact dermatitis.
- Patients with an allergic reaction to poison ivy should be advised to use Ivy B Block (a barrier cream) to prevent contact with poison ivy. Patients should reapply the cream often when sweating.

T ABLE 2.6. **Medical Treatment of Contact Dermatitis**

High-potency topical corticosteroids

Administration:	Apply 2 to 3 times daily.
Duration of use:	Use no longer than 3 weeks.
Side effects:	Long-term use may cause skin atrophy.
Comments:	Avoid use or use lower potency on face and groin because of increased risk of side effects.

Burow solution (dressings of aluminum acetate)

Administration:	Apply daily.
Duration of use:	Stop use when the lesion is dry and not weeping.
Side effects:	Burow solution can cause skin drying or fissuring.
Comments:	Mix solution per manufacturer's guidelines. Apply saturated gauze pad until dry, then remove.

Prednisone

Administration:	*Adults:* 60 mg daily initially, taper by 5 to 10 mg every 2 days over a 2-week period
	Children: 1 mg/kg daily; taper similarly as for adults.
Duration of use:	1 to 2 weeks.
Side effects:	Prednisone can cause many systemic side effects; see *Physicians' Desk Reference.*
Comments:	Avoid dose packs because steroid dose is insufficient (dosage lasts for only 6 days), thereby treating the rash inadequately.

Doxepin

Administration:	10 to 50 mg at bedtime.
Duration of use:	As needed for pruritus.
Side effects:	Sedation and anticholinergic effects.

Hydroxyzine (Atarax)

Administration:	*Adults:* 10 to 50 mg every 6 hours.
	Children: 2 mg/kg daily divided into 4 doses.
Duration of use:	As needed.
Side effects:	Sedation, drowsiness.
Comments:	Patients should not drive or operate hazardous machinery. Alcohol should be avoided whileusing this medication.

Loratadine (Claritin), cetirizine (Zyrtec)

Administration:	*Adults:* 10 mg daily.
	Children over 6: 10 mg loratadine or 5 to 10 mg cetirizine daily, 2.5 mg cetirizine daily from 2–5 years.
Duration of use:	As needed.
Comments:	These agents are less sedating than diphenhydramine and hydroxyzine and are helpful for daytime pruritus.

LICHEN SIMPLEX CHRONICUS

Lichen simplex chronicus, or circumscribed neurodermatitis, is a localized eruption of cutaneous inflammation characterized by a pruritic, lichenified plaque brought about by persistent and habitual scratching or rubbing of a well-circumscribed area.

Chief Complaint

Your patient presents with a well-demarcated area on her neck of thickened, raised, and intensely pruritic skin.

Clinical Manifestations

- A *thick, lichenified plaque with accentuated skin lines is common.* The plaques are generally sharply defined, although small papules may occur in the margins (Figure 2.5, see color insert following page 170).
- Lesions are usually *round or oval, but may be linear,* following the path of scratching, and generally solitary. Occasionally, there may be multiple, scattered lesions.
- The *localized plaque has little tendency to expand over time,* except in the case of lichen simplex nuchae. In this variant form of lichen simplex chronicus, the lesions may extend beyond the neck and into the scalp.
- Lesions are usually erythematous or a dull red, but may become *hyperpigmented* in more chronic conditions.
- Lesions appear on areas of the body that are easily reached for scratching and may be present for weeks to years (Table 2.7).
- Lesions are accompanied by *severe, often paroxysmal pruritus,* possibly resulting from minor stimuli such as rubbing from clothing or warming of the skin.
- A strong reflexive desire to scratch the inflamed skin occurs after it is lightly stroked with a cotton swab. This urge to scratch does not occur following the same test to normal skin.
- The patient often describes a profound pleasure from frantically scratching the area of inflammation. Many times, the scratching and rubbing of the affected area becomes subconscious and habitual.

Epidemiology

History

Recurrence, a salient feature of this disorder, is likely to be related to periods of remission in which scratching and rubbing are at a minimum because of lack of associated pleasure. In the absence of constant scratching, the eruption begins to resolve on its own.

Age

Lichen simplex chronicus is commonly seen in patients over 20 years of age.

Sex

Lichen simplex nuchae occurs almost exclusively in women and is characterized by lesions to the back of the neck brought about by persistent scratching of that area, especially in times of stress.

T ABLE 2.7. **Areas Most Commonly Affected by Lichen Simplex Chronicus**

• Lateral lower portion of leg	• Scalp
• Wrists and ankles	• Scrotum, anal area, vulva, pubis
• Back of neck (lichen simplex nuchae)	• Upper eyelids
• Side of neck	• Orifice of ear
• Extensor surface of forearms near elbow	• Fold behind ear

Risk Factors

Stress is a risk factor in some cases.

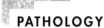
PATHOLOGY

Epidermal hyperplasia with scale, crust, and neutrophils is seen in the excoriated lesions.

Diagnosis

Extensive tests are generally not needed for diagnosis, which is usually based on *history* and *physical findings.*

Differential Diagnosis
See Table 2.8.

Diagnostic Tests
- The physician may wish to do a *potassium hydroxide (KOH) preparation* to confirm the absence of a dermatophytic etiology.
- Although usually not necessary for diagnosis, a *biopsy of the lesion* demonstrates generalized hyperplasia of all components of the epidermis, as well as chronic inflammatory infiltration of the dermis.

Referral

Referral to a dermatologist is warranted if the initial treatment is unsuccessful or if extensive disease or infection is associated. In the case of psychiatric issues, psychological dependence, or self-mutilation suggest referral to a psychiatrist.

Management
Medications
See Table 2.9.

Other Treatment Modalities
Physical

Patients with this disorder are at greater risk for bacterial infection, especially by *Staphylococcus aureus.* Any one of the oral antibiotics, as follows, are indicated at the first sign of secondary infection:
- *Cephalexin,* 250 to 500 mg 4 times daily for 10 days;
- *Dicloxacillin,* 250 mg 4 times daily for 10 days; *or*
- *Erythromycin,* 250 mg 4 times daily for 10 days.

T ABLE 2.8.   Lichen Simplex Chronicus: Differential Diagnosis

Psoriasis vulgaris	The characteristic silvery scales of psoriasis vulgaris are not apparent in lichen simplex.
Dermatophytosis	Dermatophytosis can be confirmed with KOH preparation.
Contact dermatitis	A causative substance can be identified.

KOH, potassium hydroxide.

T ABLE 2.9. Medical Treatment of Lichen Simplex Chronicus

Topical corticosteroids

Administration:	Apply twice daily.
Duration of use:	Use until lesion is resolved.
Side effects:	Long-term use may cause skin atrophy.
Comments:	Use a less potent form for intertriginous areas. Ointments work better than creams. Occlusion may be used overnight to improve skin penetration.

Intralesional triamcinolone acetonide

Administration:	2 to 3 mL injected intralesionally (2.5 to 5 mg/mL)
Duration of use:	Injection may need to be repeated every 6 to 8 weeks.
Side effects:	Intralesional use of steroids at higher concentrations may cause skin atrophy or adrenal suppression.

5% Crude oil tar in zinc oxide paste

Administration:	Apply once or twice daily and cover with dry occlusive dressing.
Duration of use:	As needed.
Comments:	Use in combination with corticosteroid, if possible. Tar may stain clothing.

Capsaicin 0.025% (Zostrix)

Administration:	Apply 2 to 3 times daily.
Duration of use:	Use until lesion resolves.
Comments:	Avoid use near eyes; it may cause stinging or burning.

Prednisone

Administration:	60 to 80 mg orally daily, tapered by 5 to 10 mg every 2 days.
Duration of use:	1 to 2 weeks.
Side effects:	Long-term use will suppress pituitary-adrenal axis; see *Physician's Desk Reference.*
Comments:	Prednisone may be indicated, especially in lichen simplex nuchae with extensive scalp inflammation.

Unna paste boot and topical corticosteroid [flurandrenolide (Cordran)] tape

Duration of use:	Tape and dressing may be left in place for up to 1 week and may be reapplied every 5 to 7 days as needed, until rash resolves.
Side effects:	Long-term use of corticosteroids may cause skin atrophy.

Doxepin 5% cream (for pruritus) (Zonalon)

Administration:	Apply topically up to 4 times daily.
Duration of use:	May be used for up to 8 days.
Side effects:	May cause localized burning sensation, dry mouth, drowsiness, or headache.

Loratidine (Claritin), cetirizine (Zyrtec) (for pruritus)

Administration:	To be taken orally. *Adults:* 10 mg daily. *Children over 6:* 10 mg loratadine or 5 to 10 mg cetirizine daily; use 2.5 mg cetirizine from 2–5 years..
Duration of use:	As needed.
Comments:	These agents are less sedating than other antihistamines and are helpful for daytime pruritus.

Psychological
- Therapy such as behavioral modification or biofeedback to reduce anxiety and stress may prove helpful in severe cases.

Follow-up
- Initial follow-up should occur in 1 to 2 weeks to check for secondary bacterial infection, unresponsiveness, or complications related to the topical corticosteroids.
- With the cyclic nature of this condition, *close management is not required* unless the patient is not improving after initial success.

Patient Education
The paramount issue in assisting patients with this disorder is to help them stop scratching and rubbing the lesions. It must be stressed that no resolution of symptoms can be hoped for until even minor scratching and rubbing are discontinued.

NUMMULAR ECZEMA

Nummular eczema is a pruritic, often chronic, cutaneous inflammatory disorder of uncertain etiology. Also known as discoid eczema, it is characterized by erythematous coin-shaped lesions (hence the adjective nummular, derived from the Latin word *nummularis,* which means "like a coin").

Chief Complaint
Patients report intense pruritus associated with an erythematous, raised, coin-shaped rash, which most often occurs in localized clusters. Some patients may develop a more generalized distribution of lesions.

Clinical Manifestations
- Pink to dull red, round skin eruptions are composed of small, closely grouped papules and vesicles coalescing to form a well-defined plaque with sharp, distinct borders (Figure 2.6, see color insert follwing page 170).
- Plaques may develop a crust from exudate and are often excoriated from repeated scratching. The plaques are usually 1 to 5 cm in diameter.
- Patients may have a solitary lesion or numerous lesions, which are usually symmetrically distributed; the lesions may have been present for weeks or months.
- The plaques generally stay in one location and demonstrate no tendency to enlarge, although, often, a single lesion demonstrates smaller satellite lesions nearby.

Epidemiology
Age
Nummular eczema is more likely to affect young adults and individuals over the age of 50 years.

Sex
- Older men usually develop the lesions on the lower legs.
- Young adult women usually develop these lesions on the trunk, hands, and fingers.

Seasonal Factors
Nummular eczema is more prevalent in the fall and winter months.

Risk Factors

Nummular eczema is idiopathic.

PATHOLOGY

The lesions are associated with small areas of intraepidermal, intercellular edema and nonspecific dermal inflammation.

Diagnosis

Nummular eczema is usually a clinical diagnosis based on the history and physical examination.

Differential Diagnosis

See Table 2.10.

Diagnostic Tests

- Tests are unnecessary for diagnosis, but may be performed to eliminate other diagnoses.
- *IgE levels* are normal in this condition, and *KOH preparation* eliminates a diagnosis of dermatophytosis.
- Although not necessary for diagnosis, a *biopsy of the lesion* shows subacute inflammation with acanthosis and spongiosis.

Referral

The physician may wish to refer patients to the dermatologist if the treatment plan is unsuccessful.

Management

Nummular eczema is a chronic condition with common recurrences and is often resistant to the treatment options currently available.

Medications

See Table 2.11.

T ABLE 2.10. Nummular Eczema: Differential Diagnosis

Dermatophytosis	Dermatophytosis can be confirmed with KOH preparation.
Contact dermatitis	A causative substance can be identified.
Psoriasis vulgaris	The characteristic silvery scales of psoriasis vulgaris are not apparent in nummular eczema.
Impetigo	A positive bacterial culture is associated with impetigo.
Erythema multiforme	Erythema multiforme has lesions of mucous membranes, palms, or soles of feet. These lesions are distributed differently than those of nummular eczema.
Lyme disease	Lyme disease has a characteristic prodrome, history of a tick bite, and joint involvement. Erythema migrans is typically not pruritic.

KOH, potassium hydroxide.

TABLE 2.11.   **Medical Treatment of Nummular Eczema**

Potent topical corticosteroids
Administration: Apply twice daily.
Duration of use: Use until rash resolves, usually 3 to 4 weeks.
Side effects: Avoid use of potent agents on face or groin because of increased risk of side effects.
                    Long-term use may cause skin atrophy.
Comments: Ointments are preferred; use lowest potency according to the severity of disease.

Intralesional triamcinolone acetonide
Administration: 1 to 3 mL of a 3 to 10 mg/mL solution, depending on size of lesions. Administer once.
Duration of use: Repeat injection may be necessary if the lesions have not resolved in a 4- to 6-week
                    period.
Side effects: Long-term use may cause adrenal suppression and skin atrophy.

Intramuscular triamcinolone acetonide
Administration: 40 to 60 mg. Administer once.
Side effects: Long-term use may cause adrenal suppression and skin atrophy.

2% Tar ointment combined with a potent topical steroid
Administration: Apply twice daily.
Duration of use: As needed.
Comments: Tar may stain clothing.

Prednisone
Administration: 40 mg daily initially, tapered by 5 to 10 mg every 2 to 3 days.
Duration of use: 3 weeks.
Side effects: See *Physicians' Desk Reference*.
Comments: Cessation often causes recurrence. Add a midpotency topical steroid for last 2 weeks to
                    decrease risk of rash flareup.

Diphenhydramine (Benadryl), hydroxyzine (Atarax)
Administration: 25 to 50 mg every 6 hours.
Duration of use: As needed for pruritis.
Side effects: Drowsiness, sedation.
Comments: Patients should not drive or operate hazardous machinery. Alcohol should be avoided
                    while using medication.

Loratidine (Claritin), cetrizine (Zyrtec)
Administration: 10 mg daily.
Duration of use: As needed for pruritis.
Comments: These agents are less sedating than diphenhydramine and hydroxyzine.

Other Treatment Modalities
  Physical
  • Mild cleansing agents, such as Dove soap, may be helpful.
  • Hydrating the skin with a moisturizing cream (such as Eucerin or Lubriderm)
    immediately after showering or bathing may also be of benefit.

- Patients should avoid skin irritants.
- There has been some success with PUVA treatment, but lesions still recur.
- Patients with nummular eczema are at greater risk of secondary infection; any one of the following oral antibiotics are indicated if culture for *S. aureus* is positive.
  - *Cephalexin,* 250 mg 4 times daily for 7 to 10 days;
  - *Dicloxacillin,* 250 mg 4 times daily for 7 to 10 days; *or*
  - *Erythromycin,* 250 mg 4 times daily for 7 to 10 days.

Environmental

- Maintaining proper humidity in the home may be of benefit.

Follow-up

Patients should be followed up in 3 to 4 weeks.

Patient Education

- Patients should be made aware of the risk of secondary infection and advised to notify the physician if any such signs should develop.
- Patients should be instructed to use lukewarm water and mild soap for bathing, to hydrate skin immediately after bathing, and to avoid skin irritants. For treatment to be successful, the underlying dry skin associated with nummular eczema must be controlled.

SEBORRHEIC DERMATITIS

Seborrheic dermatitis is a chronic eczematous disorder characterized by redness and scaling in areas of the body where the sebaceous glands are most active.

Chief Complaint

Patients report inflamed, erythematous areas with a greasy scale, often accompanied by burning or itching.

Clinical Manifestations

- Seborrheic lesions are relatively sharply defined macules, papules, or plaques, which are erythematous and usually covered by a yellow, red, or even white and often greasy crust. They are often fissured (Figure 2.7, see color insert following page 170).
- Onset is usually gradual.
- Seborrheic dermatitis occurs most often in infants, usually affecting the scalp (cradle cap, which is diffuse inflammation of the scalp with classic physical findings of scaling and even fissuring), face, groin, trunk, and/or axillary folds (diaper rash).
- In adults, areas most affected are the scalp, nasolabial folds, eyebrows, eyelashes, ears, groin, axilla, gluteal cleft, and submammary folds. Other common presentations include lesions affecting the follicular orifices of the beard, blepharitis affecting the eyelashes, and corona seborrheicia, affecting the forehead specifically. Seborrheic dermatitis of the scalp in adults causes flaking (pityriasis sicca, or dandruff).
- Many patients present with a history of an "oily" complexion, the so-called seborrheic diathesis.
- Pruritus is variable among individuals, but is often exacerbated by perspiration.
- If inflammation and fissuring are severe, a secondary infection may also be present.

Epidemiology

Seborrheic dermatitis is a common dermatosis, affecting 2% to 5% of the population.

Age

The condition occurs most frequently in infancy and generally is not seen in children past infancy; however, it may recur in adults.

Sex

The condition is most common in male patients.

Seasonal Factors

The disease course will often follow a pattern of recurrences and remissions, often improving in the summer, with flare-ups in the winter.

Risk Factors

- *Genetic factors.* Some role is played by genetic factors, such as Parkinson disease, which may precipitate a seborrheic dermatitis–like rash.
- *Diet.* Seborrheic dermatitis–like rashes may also be associated with riboflavin, biotin, pyridoxine, zinc, and niacin deficiencies.

PATHOLOGY

The dermatophyte *Pityrosporum ovale* is often involved in the pathologic features of seborrheic dermatitis; however, exact pathogenesis and pathophysiology are unclear. Microscopic findings of intercellular edema, parakeratosis, and acanthosis with dermal inflammation are nonspecific.

Diagnosis

Diagnosis is usually based on *history* and *physical examination.*

Differential Diagnosis

- See Table 2.12.
- A refractory rash with scaling lesions on the trunk, groin, or extremities may be a sign of human immunodeficiency virus (HIV).

T ABLE 2.12. Seborrheic Dermatitis: Differential Diagnosis

Psoriasis vulgaris	The characteristic silvery scales of psoriasis vulgaris are not apparent in seborrheic dermatitis.
Impetigo	Impetigo has a honey-colored crust; bacterial culture is positive.
Dermatophytosis	KOH preparation is positive.
Pityriasis versicolor	KOH preparation is positive.
Subacute lupus erythematous	DNA antibodies and ANA are positive in subacute lupus, and the rash lacks greasy scale.
Atopic dermatitis	Although the rash sites of atopic dermatitis are the same as those of seborrheic dermatitis, the former often are associated with an allergic history or elevated immunoglobulin E levels.
Rosacea	The rash of rosacea is similar to that of seborrheic dermatitis, but it does not involve the scalp or forehead.

KOH, potassium hydroxide; ANA, antinuclear antibodies.

Referral
The physician may wish to refer the patient to the dermatologist if rash is unresponsive to treatment.

Management
The treatment for seborrheic dermatitis is usually a twofold process of initial treatment followed by some type of continuing maintenance therapy.

Medications
See Table 2.13.

Other Treatment Modalities
Physical
- Castellani paint is beneficial, particularly for weeping lesions in intertriginous areas.
- Treatment of cradle cap should be focused on removal of scale, reducing the inflammation, and treating secondary infection. Once scales are removed (Table 2.13), inflammation can be controlled with the use of low-potency topical corticosteroids (see Appendix A). If there is evidence of a secondary infection, administer oral antistaphylococcal antibiotics such as cephalexin, dicloxacillin, or erythromycin. Maintenance therapy consists of routine use of salicylic acid or tar shampoos and attention to routine scale removal.

Environmental
- Ultraviolet radiation may be beneficial for controlling symptoms.

Follow-up
After the initial visit, close follow-up is unnecessary unless treatment is unsuccessful or the rash becomes resistant to treatment.

Patient Education
Compliance
Patients should be advised that seborrheic dermatitis can only be controlled, not cured. Maintenance entails continuing the use of medicated shampoos, which should be left on the scalp for 5 minutes before rinsing, in addition to the use of low-potency topical steroids.

Lifestyle Changes
Patients, particularly those who are alcoholics, should be informed that eating heavy meals may exacerbate the condition.

Family and Community Support
Family and patients should be advised that emotional or psychological factors may cause flare-ups of seborrheic dermatitis.

TABLE 2.13.   **Medical Treatment of Seborrheic Dermatitis**

Initial therapy
For scalp
Prepared OTC antiseborrheic shampoos containing selenium sulfide, zinc pyrithione, or tar; also, ketoconazole 2% shampoo (prescription) or 1% OTC.

Administration:	Shampoo 2 to 3 times weekly, using regular shampoo in between.
Duration of use:	As needed to control dandruff.
Comments:	In moderate to severe cases, a low-potency steroid lotion may be massaged into scalp following medicated shampoo.

For face
Ketoconazole 2% shampoo or cream; hydrocortisone cream 1% or 2.5%.

Administration:	Twice daily.
Duration of use:	As needed.
Comments:	Monitor carefully for skin atrophy when using corticosteroids.

For trunk
Midpotency topical corticosteroids.

Administration:	2 to 3 times daily.
Duration of use:	As needed.
Comments:	Monitor carefully for skin atrophy when using corticosteroids.

For refractory seborrheic blepharitis
Solution of 10% sodium sulfacetamide, 0.2% prednisone, and 0.12% phenylephrine (Blephamide).

Administration:	Apply once daily after cleaning eyelid with cotton swab saturated with diluted baby shampoo.
Duration of use:	As needed.
Comments:	Mild blepharitis responds to daily cleansing with diluted baby shampoo without need of Blephamide.

For cradle cap
Sulfur and salicylic acid shampoo (Sebulex).

Administration:	Shampoo daily.
Duration of use:	As needed.
Comments:	Thicker or refractory scales may also be removed with mineral oil, olive oil, or diluted dishwashing liquid.

Maintenance therapy
Ketoconazole 2% cream or shampoo.

Administration:	Once or twice weekly.
Duration of use:	Continuing, for maintenance.

Or

Topical corticosteroid.

Administration:	Apply daily.
Duration of use:	Continuing, for maintenance.
Comments:	Use lowest-potency steroids to achieve results and lessen risk of side effects. Follow up regularly for signs of skin atrophy.

DYSHIDROTIC ECZEMA

Dyshidrotic eczema (pompholyx) is a vesicular, recurring rash of the hand or foot. The precise cause is not known.

Chief Complaint

Patient reports recurring, itchy vesicles on the fingers of the left hand.

Clinical Manifestations

- Lesions tend to be small, approximately 1 to 5 mm in size, and *filled with clear fluid.* They are *located on the hands or feet,* usually localized to the fingers, palms, and soles (Figure 2.8, see color insert following page 170).
- *Onset is sudden,* and erythema is usually absent in the early stages of disease.
- Vesicles may develop early in the course of the illness and are usually grouped in clusters. Approximately 80% of the vesicles are found in the hands, localized to the lateral aspects of the fingers.
- Bullae may also occur.
- Later in course of illness, erythema, papules, scaling, and lichenification can occur. Lesions may be painful as a result of fissuring of the skin or secondary bacterial infection.

Epidemiology

Age

Dyshidrotic eczema most often occurs in patients under 40 years of age.

Sex

Distribution among men and women is equal.

Seasonal Factors

Vesicular eruptions often occur in hot, humid weather.

Risk Factors

- Some patients have a history of atopy.
- Affected individuals often have associated allergies to nickel, chromate, and cobalt.
- Stress may be a precipitating factor.

PATHOLOGY

Despite the name dyshidrosis, there are no abnormalities of the sweat glands in the hands or feet, even though these patients have higher perspiration volumes.

Diagnosis

Differential Diagnosis

Bacterial infections, dermatophytosis, atopic dermatitis, id reactions, and scabies are differential diagnoses for dyshidrotic eczema (Table 2.14).

TABLE 2.14. **Dyshidrotic Eczema: Differential Diagnosis**

Dermatophytosis	KOH preparation is positive.
Atopic dermatitis	Distribution of lesions differs from that of atopic dermatitis.
Bacterial infections	Bacterial infections are characterized by a honey-colored crust; culture is positive.
Scabies	Scabies is associated with an itchy, vesicular rash with burrowing; symptoms intensify at night.
"Id" reactions	There is a generalized inflammatory rash secondary to a fungal infection, located at a site away from the fungal infection.
	The rash can appear the same as a dyshidrotic rash. Distant fungal infections (e.g., in feet or groin) should be sought.

KOH, potassium hydroxide.

Diagnostic Tests

- *Bacterial or fungal culture* may be necessary to eliminate *S. aureus* infection or dermatophytosis as an origin. If the diagnosis is unclear or if uncertain, biopsy of the lesion or bacterial/fungal culture is warranted.
- Some patients have a positive test result for nickel allergy.

Referral

The treatment of dyshidrotic eczema can be frustrating because the treatments are not very effective, and when the primary care physician reaches his or her frustration point, referral may be warranted.

Management

Because this disease is chronic, *management of symptoms is paramount.*

Medications

See Table 2.15.

Other Treatment Modalities

Physical

- Some patients respond to PUVA therapy; however, this treatment option may be best left to the dermatologist.
- For patients with moderate disease, soaking hands and feet in cold water every 30 to 60 minutes, followed by application of topical steroid cream covered by damp cotton gloves or socks, may be helpful.
- Patients should use mild cleansers (Dove, Cetaphil, Eucerin) for bathing, followed by application of a fragrance- and lanolin-free emollient, such as Neutrogena, Aquaphor, Eucerin, or Lubriderm.
- Patients should wear gloves if hands are constantly in water.
- For secondary infections involving *S. aureus,* use an appropriate antibiotic as follows:
  - *Cephalexin,* 500 to 1,000 mg 2 times daily for 10 days;
  - *Dicloxacillin,* 250 mg 4 times daily for 10 days;
  - *or*
  - *Erythromycin,* 250 mg 4 times daily for 10 days.

T ABLE 2.15.   Medical Treatment of Dyshidrotic Eczema

Topical medium- to high-potency corticosteroids
Administration:	Apply 2 to 3 times daily.
Duration of use:	Use until pruritus and vesicles resolve.
Side effects:	Long-term use can cause skin atrophy and inhibition of the pituitary-adrenal axis.

Burow solution (dressings of aluminum acetate)
Administration:	Apply gauze soaked in solution 2 to 3 times daily.
Duration of use:	Remove after 15 to 20 minutes; remove before excessive drying and cracking occur.
Side effects:	Burow solution can cause skin drying or fissuring.
Comments:	Mix solution per manufacturer's guidelines. Apply saturated gauze pad until dry, then remove.

Intralesional triamcinolone acetonide
Administration:	1 to 2 mL of a 3-mg/mL solution.
Duration of use:	Once.
Side effects:	Long-term use can cause skin atrophy and inhibition of the pituitary-adrenal axis.
Comments:	Good for small areas of involvement.

Prednisone
Administration:	60 mg daily, tapered 10 to 20 mg every 2 days.
Duration of use:	3 to 4 weeks.
Side effects:	Can cause systemic side effects.
Comments:	For moderate or severe disease or large areas of involvement.

Diphenhydramine (Benadryl), hydroxyzine (Atarax)
Administration:	25 to 50 mg every 6 hours.
Duration of use:	Use until pruritis resolves.
Side effects:	These agents can cause sedation and drowsiness.
Comments:	Patients should not drive or operate hazardous machinery. Alcohol should be avoided while using medication.

Loratadine (Claritin), cetirizine (Zyrtec)
Administration:	10 mg once daily.
Duration of use:	Use until pruritus resolves.
Comments:	These agents are less sedating than diphenhydramine and hydroxyzine.

Environmental

Precipitating and aggravating substances should be avoided or eliminated.

Psychological

Patients who have exacerbations under stressful conditions may find behavior modification or stress reduction techniques to be of benefit.

Follow-up

The patient should be followed up in 1 to 2 weeks to assess response to therapy and to determine whether there is any indication of a secondary infection.

Patient Education
Compliance
• It is important for the patient to keep the lesions clean and dry to avoid secondary infection.
• Because secondary infection or dermatophytosis can occur, patients should be cautioned to keep hands clean but avoid excessive hand washing.
• Patients must keep feet dry and clean and change socks several times daily. Shoes made with synthetic materials should not be worn, and sandals should be worn when possible.

Family and Community Support
• Family and friends should know that dyshidrotic eczema is not contagious.
• There are a number of aspects to dyshidrotic eczema that may cause patients profound distress. The intense pruritus, limited efficacy of treatments, and recurrent nature of this disease may cause patients to be noncompliant. For these reasons, psychological support from the physician, in addition to the appropriate treatment, can be of great benefit.
• Family and patients should be educated about signs and symptoms of bacterial infection and dermatophytosis, such as erythema, skin warmth, and lymphadenitis.

BIBLIOGRAPHY

Danby FW, Maddin WS, Margesson LJ, Rosenthal D. A randomized, double-blind, placebo-controlled trial of ketoconazole 2% shampoo versus selenium sulfide 2.5% shampoo in the treatment of moderate to severe dandruff. *J Am Acad Dermatol* 1993;29(6):1008-1012.

Faergemann J, Jones TC, Hettler O, Loria Y. Pityrosporum ovale *(Malassezia furfur)* as the causative agent of seborrheic dermatitis: New treatment options. *Br J Dermatol* 1996;134[Suppl 46]:12-15.

Hanifin JM, Rajka G. Diagnostic features of atopic dermatitis. *Acta Derm Venereol Suppl (Stockh)* 1980;92:44-47.

Janniger CK, Schwartz R. Seborrheic dermatitis. *Am Fam Physician* 1995;52(1):149-155.

Juckett G. Plant dermatitis: possible culprits go far beyond poison ivy. *Postgrad Med* 1996;100(3):159-171.

Kellum RE. Dyshidrotic hand eczema: a psychotherapeutic approach. *Cutis* 1975;16:875-878.

Rebora A, Rongioletti F. The red face: seborrheic dermatitis. *Clin Dermatol* 1993;11:243-251.

Zug K, McKay M. Eczematous dermatitis: a practical review. *Am Fam Physician* 1996;54(4):1243-1250.

CHAPTER 3

....

Psoriasis and Related Disorders

PSORIASIS VULGARIS

Psoriasis vulgaris is a common, troubling, and difficult-to-treat disorder, which causes significant physical and psychological distress.

Chief Complaint
Patients complain of thick, scaly, often pruritic patches or plaques.

Clinical Manifestations
- The classic lesion is an elevated, thick, scaling plaque, which is silver-white and has sharply demarcated borders (Figures 3.1 and 3.2, see color insert following page 170).
- Lesions may be localized or generalized.
- There may be acute or chronic pruritus.
- There is a predilection for the extensor surface of the elbows and knees as well as the sacral and scalp areas. However, the face is usually spared.
- A thickened plaque, possibly with scales, may appear on the skin of the penis or in the perineal or perianal areas.
- Trauma to the skin, such as scratching, rubbing, or sunburn, may cause psoriatic lesions (Köebner phenomenon).
- Removal of a plaque causes pinpoint bleeding from capillaries close to the skin surface (Auspitz sign).
- Pitting and separation of the distal nail plate from the nail bed (onycholysis) can occur.
- Psoriatic arthritis can occur in 5% to 10% of psoriasis patients. The classic presentation involves the fingers or toes symmetrically.

Epidemiology
Population
Psoriasis affects approximately 1% of the United States population.

Family History
Psoriasis is hereditary (30% of psoriasis patients have a positive family history).

Age
Age of onset varies, and the disease can occur at any time.

Sex
Incidence is equal for men and women.

Risk Factors
- Stress, infections, and medications (e.g., antimalarial agents, systemic interferon, β-blockers, lithium), as well as a family history of the condition, can be risk factors.

- Immunologic factors [e.g., human immunodeficiency virus (HIV)] can be associated with a sudden extreme presentation of psoriasis.

PATHOLOGY

Psoriasis is an epidermal hyperplasia secondary to an accelerated rate of growth (28 times the rate of normal growth) and turnover of cells. There is debate whether the abnormality is within the keratinocytes or is solely T-cell mediated.

Diagnosis
Differential Diagnosis
See Table 3.1.

Diagnostic Tests
Diagnosis can usually be made clinically.

T ABLE 3.1. Psoriasis Vulgaris: Differential Diagnosis

Variants of psoriasis	
Guttate psoriasis	Secondary to streptococcal infections and seen primarily in children and young adults. Initially, small, droplike, and usually nonpruritic lesions appear abruptly and do not last more than 3 months, with treatment directed at the positive throat culture.
	Chronic lesions can occur many years after the initial lesions and are unrelated to streptococcus; therefore they should be treated in the same manner as psoriasis vulgaris.
Acute pustular psoriasis (Von Zumbusch psoriasis)	Lesions are similar to those of psoriasis vulgaris but are milky white and filled with purulent matter. Patients are typically very ill, with fever and leukocytosis, and are possibly septic. Treatment with systemic antibiotics and oral retinoids.
Nonpsoriatic diagnoses	
Seborrheic dermatitis	Early seborrheic dermatitis with thick scale can be indistinguishable from psoriasis; however, the thick silvery scales and nail pitting are absent. Biopsy is helpful to differentiate.
Drug eruptions	Certain medications (e.g., β-blockers, lithium, oral gold) can cause a psoriasis-like drug eruption. The rash should disappear after cessation of medication.
Candidiasis	Candidiasis can cause scales, but lesions are not silver. Satellite lesions are present. No nail pitting is evident. KOH examination shows pseudohyphae and/or yeast.
Secondary syphilis	Serologic testing is positive for syphilis. Mucous membranes may be involved. There is no scaling.

KOH, potassium hydroxide.

Referral

In general, if the physician does not feel comfortable with the extensiveness of the psoriasis and its systemic treatment, referral is indicated. The systemic treatments have side effects that require experience and close follow-up. A patient with acute pustular psoriasis is acutely ill; consultation may be helpful.

Management

The treatment outlined is for psoriasis vulgaris, not for the variants mentioned in the Differential Diagnosis section.

Medications

See Table 3.2.
- When less than 20% of the body is involved, topical treatment is preferred.
- Systemic treatment is recommended when lesions cover more than 20% of the body.
- Alternative treatments for extensive cases are as follows:
  - Phototherapy with ultraviolet B-range (UVB) and psoralen plus ultraviolet A-range (PUVA) radiation.
  - Etretinate (Tegison).
  - Methotrexate (Rheumatrex).
  - Cyclosporine (Neoral).

Other Treatment Modalities

Physical
- Physical trauma to skin, such as kneeling and leaning, should be avoided.

Environmental
- Because psoriasis can be irritated by dry, cold weather, protective clothing and skin lubrication should be suggested.
- Excessive sunlight should be avoided, and sunscreen should be used on exposed skin.

Psychological
- If stress exacerbates the patient's psoriasis, appropriate stress reduction techniques (e.g., biofeedback and exercise) should be advised.

Follow-up

- Patients undergoing topical treatment should be followed every 2 to 3 weeks. If no progress is made, increasing the strength of the topical steroid or changing to a different therapy is warranted.
- Once lesions are stable, patients should be monitored every 2 to 3 months to check on treatment toxicity (e.g., skin atrophy associated with topical steroids).
- Patients undergoing systemic treatment should be followed more closely, depending on the regimen.

Patient Education

Compliance

Some of the treatments are cumbersome, malodorous, and time-consuming. Every effort should be made to get the disease under control using the least medication possible and then stressing avoidance of triggering factors (i.e., stress, infection, medications). Patients need to learn that psoriasis is not curable and it needs to be controlled. Often, they can regulate their own medication within predetermined guidelines.

T **ABLE 3.2.**   **Topical Treatment of Psoriasis Vulgaris**

Moisturizers

Emollients (such as Lubriderm, Eucerin, Moisturel)

Administration:	Apply under occlusive plastic dressing overnight to help hydrate, soften, and loosen plaques.
Duration of use:	Use until plaques resolve.

Keratolytic agents

P & S Lotion is salicylic acid, 2% to 10%, in a petrolatum base.

Administration:	*Scalp:* apply at night and rinse out the next morning.
	Body and extremities: apply once or twice daily to the scales.
Duration of use:	Use until thick scales resolve.
Side effects:	Agents can cause skin dryness or irritation.
Comments:	Use keratolytic agents in conjunction with topical corticosteroids, tar, or anthralin. They are useful adjunctive therapy to remove thick scale and help penetration of other topical agents.

Topical steroids

Administration:	Apply topically 2 or 3 times daily. Use under occlusive plastic wrap overnight.
Duration of use:	Limiting treatment to 1 to 2 weeks is best initially. If there are no results, use a higher-potency agent.
Side effects:	Prolonged use of topical steroids can cause skin atrophy, striae, and telangiectasias.
Comments:	This is a first-line treatment. Remember to use a low-potency agent for face and groin lesions. Medium-potency ointments are preferred over creams because of better skin penetration. Use in conjunction with emollients and keratolytic agents.

Topical vitamin D$_3$

Calcipotriene ointment 0.005% (Dovonex)

Administration:	Use twice daily only on the plaque. Do not use on the face.
Duration of use:	Safety and effectiveness has been shown for up to 8 weeks of treatment.
Side effects:	If used in excess, these agents can cause systemic effects such as hypercalcemia. Most common side effects are skin burning and pruritus.
Comments:	Agents are useful when patients are not responsive to topical steroids. Patients with hypercalcemia or vitamin D toxicity should not use.

Tar preparations

Coal tar (Fototar cream, Zetar emulsion, Estar)

Administration:	Apply up to 4 times daily.
Duration of use:	Use until skin is smooth and free of plaques.
Side effects:	Can cause photosensitivity; patients should avoid direct sun exposure when using.
Comments:	Helpful but unsightly and malodorous; therefore compliance is a problem. Used in conjunction with topical steroids or anthralin.

continued

TABLE 3.2. *continued.* **Topical Treatment of Psoriasis Vulgaris**

Anthralin (Drithocreme 0.1% to 1%)

Administration:	Apply topically once daily, starting with 0.1%; increase strength as tolerated. Initially, leave on for 15 minutes before rinsing off; gradually increase the time left on the plaques to 1 hour.
Duration of use:	Use until skin is smooth and free of plaques.
Side effects:	Skin and nail discoloration can occur. Anthalin also causes skin irritation and burning.
Comments:	Do not use on face or on acutely inflamed lesions. Consult *Physicians' Desk Reference* before using.

Intralesional injections

Triamcinolone acetonide (5 to 10 mg/mL)

Administration:	Inject 2 to 3 mL intralesionally.
Duration of use:	Small, chronic lesions can stay in remission for months with one injection.
Side effects:	Dark-skinned patients can develop hypopigmentation. Long-term use of corticosteroids can cause skin atrophy and telangiectasias.
Comments:	Injections are only useful for small, isolated lesions.

Lifestyle Changes

- Visible lesions can be covered by clothing and makeup. Lesions can be vigorously treated by topical agents, and the use of skin lotions and scale removers helps the lesions be less noticeable.
- Exposure to sun is beneficial in controlling psoriasis. Sunscreens should be used to avoid sunburn.

Family and Community Support

- The psychosocial aspect of this disfiguring disease must not be underestimated. Emotional distress related to psoriasis should be treated aggressively through counseling to lessen the social impact of the disease on the patient. Patients can be referred to the National Psoriasis Foundation for support (telephone number: 503-244-7404).
- Patients and family members should be assured that psoriasis is not a contagious disease.
- However, they need to know that 30% of patients with psoriasis have a positive family history of psoriasis.

ICHTHYOSIS VULGARIS

Ichthyosis is an inherited dominant disorder, which generally presents after the third month of life. Clinical presentation may range from a tendency toward dry skin to actual fine scaling.

Chief Complaint

A young boy is brought to your office with the appearance of fish skin on his face.

Clinical Manifestations

- A fine fish-scale–like rash with rectangular scales is the most common presentation, although scaling can be larger and coarser (Figure 3.3, see color insert following page 170).

- Ichthyosis has a predilection for the face in children. In adults, the thighs, arms, heels, forehead, and back are affected, and the anticubital and popliteal fossae (flexor areas) are spared.
- There is dryness, scaling, and exfoliation of skin.
- The lesions can be pruritic and cause severe discomfort.
- Ichthyosis is worse in dry, cold weather.

Epidemiology

Family History

Ichthyosis vulgaris is *autosomal dominant.*

Age

- Age of onset usually occurs within the first year of life (onset can occur up to age 4 years).
- If acquired later in age (over the age of 20 years), ichthyosis may be associated with a paraneoplastic syndrome associated with lymphoma or HIV.

Sex

Incidence is equal between the sexes.

Risk Factors

- Family history of ichthyosis.
- Association with atopic dermatitis.

PATHOLOGY

The stratum corneum of the dermis is abnormal in that there is increased adhesiveness and normal cell separation does not occur. Therefore the skin is thickened and becomes dry and cracked. Hyperkeratosis is present.

Diagnosis

Diagnosis is made on the basis of clinical presentation.

Differential Diagnosis

See Table 3.3.

Diagnostic Tests

Generally, no diagnostic tests are needed.

Referral

This disease is self-limited, and symptoms can be controlled. If there is concern of lymphoma or other malignancy, further evaluation is indicated.

Management

- The management of this disease is directed toward the stratum corneum. Symptoms generally can be controlled.
- Systemic retinoids [isotretinoin (Accutane), etretinate (Tegison), or acitretin (Soriatane)] can be useful in severe disease or in cases that are resistant to emollients and keratolytic agents. The primary care physician must be familiar with the toxic side effects of systemic retinoids before administering them.

TABLE 3.3. Ichthyosis Vulgaris: Differential Diagnosis

Ichthyosis secondary to other disorders (e.g., Hodgkin disease, leprosy, HIV, other malignancies)	There is evidence of the primary disorder and an absence of precipitating factors.
Psoriasis	There is nail involvement; psoriasis responds to sunlight.
Generalized dermatitis	Onset is recent, and generalized dermatitis is more transient.
Drug induced [nicotinic acid, cimetidine (Tagamet), retinoids]	There is a history of medication use with the absence of other precipitating factors.

HIV, human immunodeficiency virus.

Medications
See Table 3.4.

Other Treatment Modalities

Environmental

- Avoidance of cold, dry weather and application of appropriate skin moisturizers (Lubriderm, Eucerin, Moisturel) can help control symptoms.
- Home humidifiers can be helpful in situations in which the home environment is dry.

Follow-up

- The patient should be seen in a follow-up visit 2 to 4 weeks after the initiation of treatment.
- Then the patient should be seen on an as-needed basis, depending on the symptoms.

Patient Education

Compliance

Patient education should center around control of symptoms; avoidance of cold, dry environments; psychological support; and compliance with medications.

TABLE 3.4. Medical Treatment of Mild to Moderate Ichthyosis

Emollients (Lubriderm, Eucerin, Moisturel)

Administration:	Apply daily after bathing.
Duration of use:	Use until scales are gone.

Keratolytic creams

Lactic acid (5% to 12%) (Lac-Hydrin lotion)

Urea (2% to 20%)

Glycolic acid

Salicylic acid (6%)

Administration:	Apply nightly to wet skin (right after bathing); wash off in the morning. Occlusive dressing after application may also help. Decrease frequency as the condition improves.
Duration of use:	Use until scales are gone.
Side effects:	Can cause transient stinging, burning, erythema, and skin peeling.

Family and Community Support

The rash can be disfiguring and have social and psychological impact for the patient. Every effort should be made to keep the disorder under control. Patients can be referred to the Foundation for Ichthyosis and Related Skin Types, Inc. (telephone number: 800-545-3286).

KERATOSIS PILARIS

Keratosis pilaris is a common hereditary disorder of the keratin layer of the skin, causing multiple rough papules at the orifice of hair follicles.

Chief Complaint

Your patient exhibits a bumpy, usually nonpruritic rash on the upper arms and thighs (Figure 3.4, see color insert following page 170).

Clinical Manifestations

- A fine papular rash associated with hair follicles piercing the papules appears gradually over the upper arms, thighs, buttocks, and trunk. It may be slightly red or have scales.
- A rough sensation is felt when palpating the affected skin.
- Although the rash is usually nonpruritic, it can be pruritic or painful, or both, in cases of inflammatory keratosis.

Epidemiology

Family History

The disorder is hereditary.

Age

The rash can occur at any age.

Sex

The incidence is equal in men and women.

Risk Factors

- Keratosis pilaris may be associated with ichthyosis or atopic dermatitis.
- Tight clothes can aggravate the rash.

PATHOLOGY

The stratum corneum is normal in this condition, unless it is associated with ichthyosis. However, keratin is retained in the hair follicle, causing the raised appearance. The follicular orifice is dilated and plugged with keratin.

Diagnosis

Diagnosis is made on the basis of clinical presentation.

Differential Diagnosis

See Table 3.5.

TABLE 3.5. **Keratosis Pilaris: Differential Diagnosis**

Acne vulgaris	Inflammatory papules and/or pustules associated with acne can involve hair follicles on the shoulders and upper back, whereas keratosis pilaris involves the upper arms and lower back.
Miliaria	The rash involves the sweat glands and not the hair follicles; therefore the hair shaft is not seen protruding from the follicle. Onset of miliaria is acute; keratosis pilaris is a chronic disorder.
Drug eruption	Acute papular rash associated with precedent history of medication use; keratosis pilaris is a chronic rash without associated history of drug use.

Diagnostic Tests

Generally, no diagnostic tests are needed.

Referral

Referral is not indicated, and most primary care physicians can control this disorder.

Management

Medications

The treatment goal is to unplug the hair follicles and remove keratin debris (Tables 3.6 and 3.7).

Other Treatment Modalities

Environmental

- Avoidance of cold, dry environments helps significantly.
- A home humidifier helps to improve a dry environment.
- Hot baths and wool clothing should be avoided.

Follow-up

Follow-up with patients should occur 6 to 8 weeks after initiating treatment to monitor the response to treatment.

TABLE 3.6. **Medical Treatment of Keratosis Pilaris**

Keratolytic creams

Lactic acid (5% to 12%) (Lac-Hydrin lotion)

Urea (2% to 20%)

Glycolic acid

Salicylic acid (6%)

Administration:	Apply nightly to wet skin (right after bathing); wash off in the morning. Occlusive dressing after application may also help.
Duration of use:	Use until improvement is noted, which may take 6 to 8 weeks.
Side effects:	These agents can cause transient stinging, burning, erythema, and skin peeling.

Tretinoin (0.05% to 0.1% cream) (Renova)

Administration:	Apply topically to the rash at bedtime.
Duration of use:	Use until improvement is noted, which may take 6 to 8 weeks.
Side effects:	These agents can cause stinging, erythema, and photosensitivity.

T ABLE 3.7. Medical Treatment of Inflammatory Keratosis Pilaris

Oral antibiotics

Tetracycline (500 mg)

Erythromycin (500 mg)

Doxycycline (100 mg)

Administration:	Use tetracycline and erythromycin twice daily; use doxycycline daily. Use oral antibiotics in conjunction with keratolytics.
Duration of use:	Use daily for 2 months, then taper to lowest dose that controls symptoms.
Comments:	Tetracycline should be taken on an empty stomach; otherwise, absorption is impaired. Avoid tetracycline, doxycycline, and erythromycin estolate in children under 12 years of age and in pregnant women.

Patient Education

The patient should be reminded that the rash can be controlled, but not cured.

BIBLIOGRAPHY

Kirsner RS, Federman D. Treatment of psoriasis: role of calcipotriene. *Am Fam Phys* 1995;52(1):237-240.

Two new retinoids for psoriasis. *Med Lett* 1997;39(1013):105-106.

CHAPTER 4

Oral Mucosal Disorders

APHTHOUS ULCER

Aphthous ulcers (AU, canker sores) are recurrent, painful, and discrete superficial ulcers of the oral mucosa.

Chief Complaint

The patient presents with a sudden occurrence of painful sores in the mouth.

Clinical Manifestations

- Aphthous ulcers occur most commonly on the buccal and labial mucosa. They are also seen on other oral mucosa not bound to the periosteum (nonkeratinized mucosa) such as maxillary mucosa, mandibular sulci, floor of the mouth, ventral surface of the tongue, soft palate, and tonsillar fauces, as well as in the anogenital region and any site in the gastrointestinal tract (Figure 4.1, see color insert following page 170).
- The lesions are idiopathic and occur as single ulcers or in multiples. Recurrent aphthous ulcers (RAUs) may have a gray-white pseudomembranous cover. There may be associated burning or tingling, especially following ingestion of acidic liquids, or pain severe enough to impair nutrition and cause weight loss.
- *Three clinical forms* are noted: RAU minor, RAU major, and herpetiform RAU.
- *RAU minor* lesions (comprising approximately 80% of all RAUs) are small, painful, round or oval, shallow ulcers surrounded by a red halo; the ulcer itself is less than 1 cm in diameter. These lesions heal spontaneously in 1 to 2 weeks.
- *RAU major* lesions (approximately 10% of all RAUs) are large, painful ulcers greater than 1 cm in diameter. They can sometimes persist for weeks to months. RAU major may be associated with human immunodeficiency virus (HIV).
- *RAU herpetiform* (approximately 7% to 10% of all RAUs) consists of numerous small (1- to 3-mm) ulcers, which may coalesce into clusters of up to approximately 100 lesions. The lesions heal spontaneously within 1 to 2 weeks.
- *Behçet syndrome* consists of recurrent oral aphthous ulcers with at least two of the following characteristics: recurrent genital ulcers, uveitis, erythema nodosum, arthritis, and vasculitis.

Epidemiology

Family History

Aphthous ulcers are hereditary; approximately 50% of first-degree relatives of patients with recurrent lesions also have this condition.

Age

While aphthous ulcers can occur at any age, first occurrence is often in the second decade of life, with recurrences persisting into adulthood.

Sex

Aphthous ulcers are more prevalent in women.

Risk Factors

- *Minor injury* to the oral mucosa.
- *Smoking.* Several reports have suggested a negative association (reduced incidence) between RAUs and smoking.
- *Allergies.* Approximately 25% to 75% of patients with RAUs exhibit allergies to a variety of foods, dyes, and food preservatives.
- *Diet.* More recurrent and severe ulcerations are associated with gluten-sensitive enteropathies, regional enteritis, and iron or vitamin B_{12} deficiency.

PATHOLOGY

The etiology of recurrent aphthous ulcers is unclear; however, it is probably an immune-mediated destruction of tissue.

Diagnosis

The diagnosis of aphthous ulcers is usually based on clinical findings accompanied by a complete history. The physician should check for any oral manifestation of a systemic disease. Ocular symptoms, genital lesions, and gastrointestinal tract disease, plus an allergy history, are facets of the patient's history that are essential to an accurate diagnosis.

Differential Diagnosis

Uncertainties in the diagnosis can be eliminated by a biopsy of the lesion or conducting laboratory tests such as the Venereal Disease Research Laboratory (VDRL) or fluorescent treponemal antibody, absorbed (FTA-ABS) test (Table 4.1).

Diagnostic Tests

- Complete blood cell count and serum ferritin, folate, and vitamin B_{12} levels should be sufficient to eliminate common systemic conditions associated with recurrent lesions.
- It is important to note that major aphthous ulcers can be associated with HIV disease. If clinical evidence suggests the presence of HIV, appropriate testing should be considered.

Referral

When the diagnosis is unclear or the treatment modalities used are not effective, referral may be warranted.

Management

Controlling the symptoms of aphthous ulcers is the goal of treatment. Prescribed medications do not prevent recurrences.

Medications

See Table 4.2.

Other Treatment Modalities

Hospitalization may be necessary if hydration or calorie intake is severely impaired, especially in children.

T ABLE 4.1. Aphthous Ulcers: Differential Diagnosis

Herpetic gingivostomatitis	Herpetic gingivostomatitis can occur on any skin site; oral mucosa is the most common site. Aphthous ulcers are more commonly seen on the buccal and labial mucosa.
	It is commonly seen as the primary HSV infection.
	Recurrent herpetic disease occurs mainly on the lips, face, and fingertips.
Herpangina	Lesions are confined to inner oral mucosa and tonsillar pillars and are not recurrent.
Hand-foot-and-mouth disease	Lesions occur most commonly in the mouth and acral areas, but may also involve the legs, arms, and face. Aphthous ulcers are commonly seen on the buccal and labial mucosa.
	Lesions are not recurrent.
Bullous diseases	Bullous diseases can have oral involvement, which leads to bullae formation.
	Target lesions (erythema multiforme) will form elsewhere on the body.
Oral lichen planus	Lesions, usually white and "lacelike," occur on the buccal mucosa.
	There are no ulcerations.
Squamous cell carcinoma	There is persistent erosion or ulceration in the oral mucosa.
	It can be differentiated from aphthous ulcer by biopsy.
Syphilis	There are usually gray erosions on mucous membranes.
	VDRL and FTA-ABS tests are useful in diagnosing syphilis.
Nongenital herpes simplex	Lesions occur mainly on lips, fingers (Whitlow), and face (nose, cheeks, and periorally).
	Lesions can be recurrent.

HSV, herpes simplex virus; VDRL, Venereal Disease Research Laboratory test for syphilis; FTA-ABS, fluorescent treponemal antibody, absorbed (test).

Patient Education

- Patients should be informed that aphthous ulcers are recurrent, sometimes occurring as many as four times per year. Although treatment eradicates the symptoms, it does not usually hasten the disappearance of the ulcer. The ulcers occur less frequently as the patient gets older.
- Recurrent aphthous ulcers are not contagious.
- When ulcers are present, topical analgesics should be applied about 20 to 30 minutes before meals so that the patient may eat more comfortably. Patients should refrain from mouthwashes and salty, spicy, and acidic foods. Cool, bland liquids such as milk are less irritating and are more soothing.

Follow-up
Monitoring Disease Course

Close follow-up of ulcers is usually unnecessary because the ulcers regress spontaneously.

Potential Problems and Complications

Large ulcerations or those that cause pain should be monitored every 2 to 3 days, since they may be sufficient to impair nutrition. In these cases the physician should be alert for dehydration and nutritional deficiencies.

TABLE 4.2. Medical Treatment of Aphthous Ulcers

Topical corticosteroids
Triamcinolone acetonide 0.1% (Kenalog in Orabase); clobetasol propionate (Temovate), fluocinonide 0.05% (Lidex)

Administration:	Apply small amounts topically to ulcer 3 to 4 times daily.
Duration of use:	Use until lesions heal or symptoms dissipate.
Comments:	Probably first choice for treating symptomatic aphthous ulcers. These agents can be used concurrently with topical anesthetic agents. Adrenal suppression is unlikely with topical preparations.

Tetracycline
Mouthwash (one 250-mg tetracycline capsule suspended in 10 to 15 mL water)

Administration:	Rinse 10 to 15 mL in mouth for approximately 2 to 3 minutes and expectorate.
Duration of use:	14 days.
Side effects:	Should not be used in pregnant women and children under 12 years of age. If swallowed, can cause gastrointestinal tract upset and possibly interfere with the efficacy of oral birth control pills.
Comments:	Useful in larger lesions, as seen in recurrent aphthous ulcer major and herpetiform ulcerations; may reduce lesion size, duration, and pain.

Sulcralfate (Carafate) suspension; 1 g/10 mL

Administration:	10 mL swished and expectorated or painted on the lesion by a cotton-tipped applicator 4 times daily.
Duration of use:	Use until lesions are gone.
Side effects:	Constipation is the most common side effect if swallowed.
Comments:	Prompt relief of pain, reduction in healing time, and increased time between recurrences are reported.

Topical analgesics
Viscous lidocaine (Xylocaine) 2% solution

Administration:	*Adults:* 15 mL held in the mouth for 1 minute, then expectorated.
	Children over 2 years of age: 1 to 2 mL, held in the mouth for 1 minute, then expectorated. Use cotton-tipped applicator to paint each ulcer in uncooperative children.
	Use just before meals or every 3 hours (maximum of 8 doses daily).
Duration of use:	Use until lesions are healed.
Side effects:	Prescription-strength medication can cause arrhythmias, confusion, seizures, and death if large amounts are absorbed through irritated mucosal surfaces. May impair the gag reflex if swallowed.
Comments:	Suggest using over-the-counter topical analgesics first. For temporary pain relief. Not recommended for children under 2 years of age.

continued

T ABLE 4.2. *continued.*   **Medical Treatment of Aphthous Ulcers**

Over-the-counter diphenhydramine (Benadryl allergy liquid), liquid over-the-counter
   antacid containing aluminum hydroxide and magnesium hydroxide (Maalox), and benzocaine (Anbesol)

Administration:	*Diphenhydramine/Maalox:* 30 minutes before eating a meal, mix equal proportions of each, rinse mouth for 5 to 10 minutes, and expectorate. Use cotton-tipped applicator to paint on ulcers in uncooperative children.
	Benzocaine: Follow package directions.
Duration of use:	Use until lesions are healed.
Side effects:	If swallowed, sedation, fatigue, and diarrhea may occur.
Comments:	Provides temporary pain relief; probably first-line treatment in patients with minimal symptoms.

Dexamethasone (elixir; 0.5 mg/5 mL); prednisone

Administration:	*Dexamethasone:* 5 to 10 mL held in mouth for 2 minutes, then expectorated; repeat 4 times daily.
	Prednisone: 60 mg per day orally for 2 days initially, then tapered by 5 to 10 mg every 2 days.
Duration of use:	*Dexamethasone:* Should clear the lesions in 7 to 10 days. Restart if lesions recur.
	Prednisone: Use until lesions are gone.
Side effects:	Prolonged use can inhibit the adrenal-pituitary axis, causing severe systemic problems. Consult an internal medicine text or *Physicians' Desk Reference* for specific details.
Comments:	Either regimen especially useful for large lesions seen in recurrent aphthous ulcer major or herpetiform ulcerations. Either regimen best when used concomitantly with tetracycline.

Silver nitrate sticks

Administration:	Cauterize ulcers by painting silver nitrate stick over the lesion.
Duration of use:	Use one time only.
Side effects:	May cause minimal burning or stinging.
Comments:	May help accelerate the healing process. Useful in single, large ulcerations.

Intralesional corticosteroids (triamcinolone acetonide 3 to 10 mg/mL)

Administration:	1 to 2 mL injected directly into each ulcer.
Duration of use:	Use one time only.
Side effects:	None.

NONGENITAL HERPES SIMPLEX VIRUS

Nongenital herpes simplex virus (HSV) infection (herpes labialis, herpes gingivo-stomatitis) is characterized by grouped, painful vesicles on an erythematous base in the oral mucosa or the outer portion of the lips. These lesions have been commonly called cold sores or fever blisters.

Chief Complaint

A young man comes to you complaining of a painful, blistering, sore on the skin bordering his lip.

Clinical Manifestations

Oral HSV has an average 6-day incubation period and can be either asymptomatic or symptomatic, with minor, major, or systemic symptoms.

- Erythematous halos surround grouped, umbilicated vesicles, some of which develop into pustules. Lesions eventually enlarge to erosions that can be moist or crusted. Infections usually heal in 2 to 4 weeks; however, there may be residual postinflammatory hypopigmentation or hyperpigmentation.
- Herpes labialis occurs mainly on the lips (90% of cases) and perioral area (10% of cases) (Figure 4.2, see color insert following page 170).
- HSV associated with gingivostomatitis (1% of HSV) can cause painful erosions on the buccal mucosa, hard and soft palate, gingiva, lips, and tongue. Systemic symptoms associated with gingivostomatitis are fever, malaise, loss of appetite, dehydration, and lymphadenopathy. The illness may be present for weeks; however, fever usually lasts 3 to 5 days.
- Recurrent HSV infection of the oral mucosa may have a prodrome 45% to 60% of the time. The infection consists of tingling or burning preceding any visible mucosal changes by 24 hours.

Epidemiology

Family History

Studies indicate that patients with at least one or more first-degree family members who have had herpes labialis are more likely to develop this disease.

Age

- Herpes labialis is commonly seen in young adults; however, patient age can range from infancy to old age.
- Gingivostomatitis commonly occurs in children ranging in age from 6 months to 6 years.

Risk Factors

- Patients in an immunocompromised state (e.g., those with HIV or a malignancy or those who have undergone transplantation) and patients undergoing chemotherapeutic or systemic corticosteroid treatment are predisposed to HSV.
- Approximately 50% of patients who develop primary HSV will develop a recurrence. Precipitating factors for recurrence include emotional stress, illness, ultraviolet radiation to the skin or mucosa, trauma, fatigue, menstruation, fever, and altered immune states.
- Transmission of nongenital herpetic infections usually occurs from skin-to-skin or skin-to-mucous membrane contact.

PATHOLOGY

Recurrent herpetic infection is caused by viral reactivation from latent sites in neural ganglia.
HSV type 1 (HSV-1) and HSV type 2 (HSV-2) are DNA viruses.

- HSV-1 is the etiologic agent of nongenital herpes simplex infections in 80% to 90% of cases. HSV-1 is susceptible to drying and disinfectants, thereby making transmission from an inanimate object to a human uncommon.
- HSV-2 is the etiologic agent in the remainder of the nongenital herpes cases, typically in association with oral-genital sexual practices. Recurrent nongenital herpetic infections caused by HSV-2 are rare.
- Recurrent erythema multiforme is commonly due to recurrent HSV-1 disease of the orolabial region.

Diagnosis

Nongenital HSV infections are diagnosed by clinical examination.

Differential Diagnosis

See Table 4.3.

Diagnostic Tests

- *Tzanck smear* may be performed fairly rapidly by unroofing a vesicle to expose the fluid beneath. The lesion is then scraped with a scalpel blade, and the results are placed on a glass slide, which should be sprayed with a cytology fixative and air dried. Microscopic examination should reveal multinucleated giant cells. It is important to note, however, that Tzanck smear is nonspecific, since both HSV and varicella-zoster virus may produce a positive test result.

T ABLE 4.3. **Nongenital Herpes Simplex: Differential Diagnosis**

Aphthous stomatitis	Lesions are more shallow than HSV infection and appear mainly on the buccal and labial mucosa. HSV lesions usually appear on the epithelial surface of the lips and perioral region.
	Aphthous stomatitis can be indistinguishable from herpes gingivostomatitis. Viral culture helps differentiate the two.
Hand-foot-and-mouth disease	Oral lesions are scattered, not grouped.
	Lesions also occur on the palms and soles; they do not appear in these locations in HSV infection.
Herpangina	Lesions are more shallow than those of HSV and are usually noted on the inner oral mucosa.
	Viral culture can distinguish between herpangina and herpetic gingivostomatitis.
Herpes zoster	Distribution is unilateral and dermatomal.
	Viral culture is helpful in differentiating herpes zoster from HSV.
Erythema multiforme	Oral lesions evolve as bullae and then progress to erosions. Target lesions, unlike HSV lesions, can be found elsewhere on the body.
	Erythema multiforme can occur secondary to recurrent HSV disease.
Bacterial infection (impetigo)	Impetigo, with its crustule, can be indistinguishable from HSV infection.
	Viral and bacterial cultures are helpful in differentiating bacterial and herpes simplex infections.

HSV, herpes simplex virus.

- *Direct fluorescent antibody (DFA) testing* is more specific, and results are available in several hours. A smear of the lesion is placed on a slide and allowed to air dry. The slide is then sent to the laboratory for testing.
- *Viral cultures* are also more specific than Tzanck smear. Results are available in 2 to 3 days. A Dacron swab is rubbed over the lesions and inoculated into a culture media. Specific virus identification can be expected from a culture.
- *HSV-1 antibody test results (serologic testing)* are positive in 85% of all adult patients worldwide whether they have active infection or not. While a positive test indicates that the patient has been infected with the HSV-1 virus, it is important to note that the lesion in question may have been caused by HSV-2 or another virus. For this reason, the HSV-1 antibody test is not useful in making a diagnosis of HSV-1 infection.

Referral

If the diagnosis is in question or the condition is unresponsive to treatment, referral to a dermatologist is warranted. Referral may also be warranted in cases of severe herpetic disease in and around the eye, genital disease in pregnant women, and infection in neonates.

Management

For patients who have 6 to 12 recurrences per year, suppressive therapy may be indicated.

Medications

See Table 4.4.

T ABLE 4.4.   Intermittent Treatment of Nongenital Herpes Simplex

For herpetic gingivostomatitis

Acyclovir (Zovirax)

Administration:	*Adults:* 200 mg orally every 4 hours, 5 times daily for 5 days; or 400 mg 3 times daily for 5 days. *Children over 2 years of age:* 5 mg/kg per day in 5 divided doses for 7 days. Available as a suspension, 200 mg/5 cc. *For hospitalized adults:* 5 mg/kg per dose intravenously every 8 hours for 5 to 7 days or until clinical resolution occurs.
Duration of use:	Begin treatment during prodrome or within 2 days after onset of visible lesions; continue for 5 days.
Side effects:	Short-term side effects include nausea, vomiting (2.7%), headache (0.6%), and diarrhea (0.3%).
Comments:	Adjust dosage in patients with renal impairment (see package insert or PDR for details). Patients may require hospitalization in the presence of severe disease or impaired nutrition or dehydration.

Valacyclovir (Valtrex)

Administration:	*Adults:* 500 to 1000 mg orally twice daily for 5 days.
Duration of use:	Begin treatment during prodrome or within 2 days after the onset of visible lesions; continue for 5 days.

continued

T ABLE 4.4.   *continued.* **Intermittent Treatment of Nongenital Herpes Simplex**

Side effects:	Nausea (6%), headache (17%), and diarrhea (4%). Thrombotic thrombocytopenic purpura and hemolytic-uremic syndrome can be seen in 3% of immunocompromised patients (those with HIV or who have had transplantation), resulting in death. This has not been seen in immunocompetent patients.
Comments:	Reduce dosage in patients with renal impairment (see package insert or PDR for details).

Famciclovir (Famvir)

Administration:	*Adults:* 125 to 250 mg orally twice daily.
Duration of use:	Begin treatment during prodrome or within 2 days after the onset of visible lesions; continue for 5 days.
Side effects:	Headache (23.6%), nausea (10%), fatigue (6.3%), and diarrhea (4.5%) are commonly seen.
Comments:	Reduce dosage in patients with renal impairment (see package insert or PDR for details).

For herpes labialis

Topical penciclovir (Denavir) 1% cream

Administration:	While awake, apply topically every 2 hours for 4 days.
Duration of use:	As with the oral agents, begin treatment during prodrome or at onset of visible lesions. Treat until lesions disappear or symptoms resolve.
Side effects:	Minimal side effects, with site irritation, hypesthesia, and paresthesia all reported less in clinical trials than in the placebo control group.
Comments:	Studies suggest faster healing and pain resolution than in control group. Not recommended for mucosal lesions. Topical medications shorten and reduce the severity of the eruption, but do not prevent recurrences.

Suppressive therapy for frequent recurrences (approximately 6 to 12 per year)

Oral acyclovir

Administration:	*Adults:* 400 mg orally twice daily, or 200 mg orally 3 times daily.
Duration of use:	Discontinue after 1 year to evaluate need for continued therapy.
Side effects:	Short-term side effects include vomiting, headache, and diarrhea.
Comments:	A substantial reduction in recurrences may be seen after 1 year of treatment: Daily suppressive treatment may reduce the frequency of recurrence by at least 85%, while 20% of patients will have no further recurrences. Suppressive doses of acyclovir will also prevent recurring erythema multiforme.

PDR, *Physicians' Desk Reference;* HIV, human immunodeficiency virus.

Other Treatment Modalities

- For patients with gingivostomatitis, pain control may be achieved with acetaminophen (with or without codeine); by drinking or eating cold liquids, such as iced water or popsicles; and by use of topical anesthetic agents, such as viscous lidocaine 2% solution (Xylocaine) or a 1:1 mixture of an over-the-counter diphenhydramine (Benadryl) and an over-the-counter liquid antacid such as Maalox.
- Patients with systemic symptoms or patients who are immunocompromised may require intravenous antiviral agents such acyclovir (Zovirax) or *foscarnet (Foscavir).*

Follow-up

Monitoring Disease Course

Immunocompetent patients do not have major complications from the disease, and therefore do not need close follow-up.

Potential Problems and Complications

HSV infections can become more aggressive in immunocompromised patients, causing painful ulcerations that can occur on the face, oral mucosa, eye, oropharynx, esophagus, and anorectal area. Nutritional problems may develop. Such patients should be followed closely and referred to the appropriate specialist if necessary.

Patient Education

Patients should be advised that ultraviolet radiation, menstruation, fever, and the common cold can cause recurrences of HSV. Up to 50% of patients have recurrences of HSV; they should be counseled on treatment. Recurrences usually decrease as one gets older.

Compliance

Compliance with the treatment regimen should be emphasized because patients who have few recurrences tend to be less compliant than those who have several occurrences per year.

Lifestyle Changes

- Prolonged and repetitive sun or tanning-light exposure should be avoided. Protective lip balm with sunblock is necessary in patients with lesions triggered by sun exposure.
- Patients should be instructed in appropriate hygiene, including the importance of frequent, thorough hand washing.
- Stress is a precipitating factor for many patients. The physician should counsel the patient with stress-induced HSV to consider stress reduction techniques and other strategies to reduce the impact of situations that may trigger an HSV recurrence.
- Patients are infectious only when they have lesions, and should be advised that skin-to-skin or skin-to-mucous membrane contact should be avoided to prevent the spread of infection to themselves or to others. Certain contact sports, such as wrestling, can also lead to transmission of HSV infections from one participant to another.

HERPANGINA

Herpangina is an infectious exanthem. This is an example of a viral illness with almost exclusively oral manifestations.

Chief Complaint

A young child is brought to your office with a sudden onset of fever, headache, myalgia, and shallow, painful ulcers in the roof of her mouth.

Clinical Manifestations

- Prodromal symptoms, lasting 1 to 4 days, include a sudden onset of fever, headaches, and myalgias; then, ulcerations appear lasting between 7 and 10 days. Incubation period is usually 4 days.
- Multiple small vesicles, erosions, and ulcers are seen on the soft palate and tonsillar pillars. Erythematous halos may be observed around the ulcerations.
- The shallow, 1- to 2-mm lesions may cause a sore throat and pain significant enough to impair nutrition and hydration.
- Taste buds on the posterior tongue may also be inflamed and prominent.

Epidemiology

Age
Herpangina commonly affects children and young adults.

Seasonal Factors
The condition is seen in summer and early fall.

Risk Factors
• Primarily seen in patients under 20 years of age.

PATHOLOGY

Herpangina is caused primarily by the enterovirus coxsackievirus A, which can be transmitted by the respiratory route or by food ingestion. Different antigenic strains of the coxsackievirus may cause patients to have more than one episode of herpangina.

Diagnosis
The diagnosis is usually made by history and physical examination.

Differential Diagnosis
See Table 4.5.

Diagnostic Tests
Acute and convalescent titers of the coxsackievirus A may be helpful to confirm or eliminate the diagnosis.

Referral
If the diagnosis is in question, or if the patient develops pain severe enough to affect nutritional status, referral may be warranted.

T ABLE 4.5. Herpangina: Differential Diagnosis[a]

Aphthous ulcers	Although lesions are similar to those of herpangina, they are usually located on nonkeratinized mucosal surfaces.
	Aphthous ulcers are associated with a strong history of recurrences.
Herpes simplex gingivostomatitis	The prodrome is more severe than that of herpangina.
	Tzanck smears or direct viral culture helps differentiate this disease from herpangina.
Hand-foot-and-mouth disease	Oval, gray papulovesicular lesions occur in the mouth as well as on the palms and soles. Herpangina lesions do not occur outside the oral mucosa.
Herpes zoster	Unilateral distribution of vesicular lesions usually differentiates this illness from herpangina, which is bilateral.

[a]Viral cultures seeking evidence of coxsackie A or acute and convalescent viral titers are helpful in determining the origins of these illnesses.

Management

Herpangina usually resolves spontaneously in approximately 10 days. The primary goal of treatment is to avoid or reduce the pain that is sometimes associated with eating or drinking by advising the patient to take acetaminophen (Tylenol) or ibuprofen (Motrin) or to apply topical analgesics before mealtimes.

Medications

See Table 4.6.

Follow-up
Monitoring Disease Course

Herpangina usually resolves within 7 to 10 days. However, large ulcerations or those that cause pain sufficient to impair nutrition should be monitored closely.

Potential Problems and Complications

The physician should be alert for dehydration and nutritional deficiencies in affected individuals, especially young children.

TABLE 4.6.   Medical Treatment of Herpangina

Over-the-counter liquid diphenhydramine (Benadryl) and over-the-counter liquid antacid containing aluminum dyroxide and magnesium dyroxide (Maalox)

Administration:	Mix equal proportions (1:1) of liquid diphenhydramine and liquid Maalox; use as a gargle 30 minutes before meals. Younger children or those who cannot gargle may have lesions painted with a cotton swab soaked in the mixture 30 minutes before meals.
Duration of use:	Continue use until lesions are not painful.
Side effects:	Sedation, fatigue, and diarrhea can occur if significant amounts are swallowed.

For more severe symptoms
Viscous lidocaine (Xylocaine) 2% solution

Administration:	*Adults:* 15 mL held in the mouth for 1 minute, then expectorated. Use just before meals or every 3 hours, up to 8 doses daily.
	Children over 2 years of age: 1 to 2 mL painted on lesions with a cotton swab soaked in solution. Apply just before meals.
Duration of use:	Continue to use until lesions are no longer painful.
Side effects:	Can be absorbed by nonintact mucosal surfaces present in mouth or esophagus (esophagitis), which may lead to toxic levels, causing arrhythmias, confusion, seizures, and death.
Comments:	Provides temporary pain relief. Use over-the-counter topical analgesics first. Not recommended for children under 2 years of age. Avoid swallowing, as lidocaine may impair gag reflex.

Patient Education

Patients should be cautioned that this virus can be transmitted by the respiratory route or by ingesting food contaminated with the virus. They should be cautioned to cover mouths and noses when they sneeze and to wash hands thoroughly before eating.

BIBLIOGRAPHY

Dover JS, Arndt KA. Dermatology. *JAMA* 1997;277(23):1848-1850.

Hay KD, Reade PC. The use of an elimination diet in the treatment of recurrent aphthous ulceration of the oral cavity. *Oral Surg* 1984;57:504-507.

Miller MF, Garfunkel AA, Ram CA, et al. The inheritance of recurrent aphthous stomatitis. *Oral Surg* 1980;49:409-412.

Nahass GT, Goldstein BA, Zhu WY, Serfling U, Penneys NS, Leonardi CL. Comparison of Tzanck smear, viral culture, and DNA diagnostic methods in detection of herpes simplex and varicella-zoster infection. *JAMA* 1992;268(18):2541-2544.

Peterson M, Baughman RA. Recurrent aphthous stomatitis: primary care management. *Nurse Pract* 1996;21(5):36-47.

Rattan J, Schneider M, Arber N, Gorsky M, Dayan D. Sucralfate suspension as a treatment of recurrent aphthous stomatitis. *J Intern Med* 1994;236:341-343.

Rogers RS III. Common lesions of the oral mucosa. *Postgrad Med* 1992;9(6):141-153.

Spruance SL. The natural history of recurrent oral-facial herpes simplex virus infection. *Semin Dermatol* 1992;11(3):200-208.

Spruance SL, Rea TL, Thorning C, Tucker R, Saltzman R, Boon R. Penciclovir cream for the treatment of herpes simplex labialis. *JAMA* 1997;277(17):1374-1379.

Topical penciclovir for herpes labialis. *Med Lett* 1997;39:57-58.

Tyring SK, Sadovsky R. Management of herpesvirus infections. *Am Fam Physician* (monograph) 1996;2:1-24.

Vincent SD, Lilly GE. Clinical, historic, and therapeutic features of aphthous stomatitis: literature review and open clinical trial employing steroids. *Oral Surg Oral Med Oral Pathol* 1992;74:79-86.

Woo SB, Sonis ST. Recurrent aphthous ulcers: a review of diagnosis and treatment. *J Am Dent Assoc* 1996;127:1202-1212.

CHAPTER 5

....

Benign Neoplasia

MELANOCYTIC NEVI

Melanocytic nevi, more commonly called moles, are small, circumscribed pigmented macules or papules that are located in the epidermis, dermis, and, sometimes, subcutaneous tissue. Nevi are generally benign, although the potential for malignancy does exist.

Chief Complaint

A patient comes into your office complaining of a black, round, large mole on her cheek that occasionally itches and has recently changed in size.

Clinical Manifestations

Melanocytic nevi are usually asymptomatic. These moles fall into three categories, as follows:

Junctional Nevi

• Lesions are usually macular or very slightly raised and less than 1 cm in diameter. They are also a uniform color of tan, brown, or darker brown with smooth, regular borders (Figure 5.1, see color insert following page 170).
• They may be scattered over the body but usually occur on the face, trunk, and upper and lower extremities.

Compound Nevi

• Lesions are usually papules or nodules (Figure 5.2, see color insert following page 170). They are dark brown or, sometimes, black and are associated with terminal hairs.
• Distribution is on the face, scalp, trunk, and extremities.

Dermal Nevi

• Lesions are usually round or dome-shaped papules or nodules, which are skin-colored to tannish brown.
• They are commonly seen on the face and neck but sometimes occur on the trunk and extremities.

Dysplastic (atypical) nevi are usually papular or nodular with variations of color within the nevi and are usually larger than the typical melanocytic nevi. The borders of dysplastic nevi are irregular and blend into the surrounding skin. The trunk and upper extremities are most commonly affected.

Epidemiology

Age

• Melanocytic nevi appear in early childhood, reach their maximal number in young adulthood, and begin to decrease in number at approximately age 60 years.
• Dermal nevi usually present in the second or third decade of life.

Race

Most white adults have approximately 20 nevi that are new growths during their lifetime. Nevi are less often seen in African Americans and other people with darkly pigmented skin.

Risk Factors

- *Congenital nevi.* There is a 3% to 6% chance of congenital nevi developing into a melanoma. If the lesion itches persistently or is tender, it should be followed carefully, since pruritus may be an early indication of malignant change.
- *Fair-skinned individuals* and *those with a large number of nevi* (more than 50) should be followed closely for skin malignancy.
- *Race.* The risk of melanocytic nevi developing into malignant melanoma over a lifetime is 1% in white people.
- *Family history.* Individuals with first-degree relatives with melanoma should be followed closely for skin malignancy.
- A familial syndrome exists in which certain individuals in high-risk families have as many as 75 to 100 dysplastic lesions, varying widely in size, shape, and color. The risk for these people of developing melanoma is between 6% and 10%.

PATHOLOGY

A nevus arises from melanocytic cells (nevus cells) that multiply in the dermis and epidermis. Melanocytic nevi are classified according to the location of the nevus cell clusters within the skin: The junctional melanocytic nevi have their nevus cells at the dermal epidermal junction, the compound nevi combine the histologic features of both the junctional and dermal nevi, and the dermal nevi have their nevus cells located exclusively in the dermis.

Diagnosis

The physician's principal concern in diagnosing melanocytic nevi is to determine whether there is sufficient cause for excisional biopsy. The following mnemonic, *ABCDE,* is helpful in establishing an indication for removal of suspicious moles:

A Asymmetry of the mole

B Border irregularity

C Color change and variegation

D Diameter greater than 6 mm

E Elevation of a previously flat lesion

Differential Diagnosis

See Table 5.1.

Diagnostic Tests

- *Surgical excision* and *histopathologic evaluation* should be considered when the diagnosis is uncertain or the clinical findings are atypical in accordance with the *ABCDE* mnemonic. Removal is also recommended for patients whose pigmented moles were present at birth, for moles greater than 1 cm in diameter, and for moles located on the plantar or palmar surface, on mucous membranes, or in the anal genital area.

T ABLE 5.1.   Melanocytic Nevi: Differential Diagnosis

Solar lentigo	Uniform hyperpigmentation in an oval, flat macule occurs in an older patient.
Lentigo maligna	Lesions have variable pigmentation and irregular borders.
Seborrheic keratosis	Scaly, "stuck-on" appearance contrasts with nevi, which are confluent with surrounding tissue.
Basal cell carcinoma	A pigmented basal cell can be confused with a dermal nevus because of its nodular shape with irregular borders and variegated color pattern. Biopsy can help differentiate the two.
Nodular melanoma	Appearance can be similar to that of a compound nevus. Biopsy can help differentiate the two.

- *Excisional biopsy* is performed by making an elliptic incision using a No. 15 scalpel, excising the lesion down to the subcutaneous tissue. A 1- to 2-mm margin of normal skin around the lesion is considered appropriate. Primary closure of the wound is made, and the lesion is sent in the appropriate transfer medium to a laboratory for pathologic examination. Refer to Appendix B for details on removing skin lesions.

Referral

If the diagnosis of melanocytic nevi is uncertain or if the clinical findings are atypical, the mole should be excised by the physician. If the physician does not feel comfortable performing the excision, referral is warranted.

Management
Medications
Medications are not indicated for the management of melanocytic nevi.

Follow-up

Patients with a history of melanoma or dysplastic syndrome, or with a first-degree relative with melanoma, should have a skin assessment at least every 6 months.

Patient Education

- Patients should be reassured that *melanocytic nevi are not potentially malignant.* However, in cases of doubt or when these moles develop suspect changes, excisional biopsy is warranted.
- Patients should be educated about the signs and symptoms of melanoma and instructed on how to determine suspect signs or changes via the *ABCDE* examination.

Lifestyle Changes
While there are no specific lifestyle changes to reduce the risk of melanocytic nevi, patients can minimize the chance of developing malignant skin disease by limiting sun exposure and using sunblock.

BLUE NEVUS

A blue nevus is a benign, dark blue to gray-black papule or nodule in the skin. The lesion *rarely develops into malignant melanoma* but can be confused with melanoma because of its dark color.

Chief Complaint

Patient complains of a long-standing blue-black papule and expresses concern that it is malignant.

Clinical Manifestations

- The patient is usually asymptomatic.
- Lesions appear gradually (Figure 5.3, see color insert following page 170).
- They do not blanch upon compression.
- Papules or nodules are usually less than 10 mm in diameter, rounded with slightly ill-defined borders, and are either blue, blue-gray, or blue-black. Larger lesions may contain hairs.
- Papules or nodules are most commonly seen on the dorsum of the hands or feet but may occur in any skin surface.

Epidemiology

Age

Blue nevus occurs in late adolescence.

Sex

There is an equal male and female distribution.

PATHOLOGY

Ectopic areas of melanocytes develop in the dermis during their migration from the neural crest to the epidermis.

Diagnosis

Diagnosis is *based on clinical findings.*

Differential Diagnosis

See Table 5.2.

T ABLE 5.2. Blue Nevi: Differential Diagnosis

Dermatofibroma	Lesions dimple when pinched, whereas blue nevi do not.
	Dermatofibroma is usually firmer than nevi are.
Nodular melanoma	Nodular melanoma can be similar in appearance to a blue nevus but usually does not contain hairs.
	Lesions can be differentiated by excisional biopsy.
Venous lake	Blue pigment disappears under compression, in contrast to a blue nevus, which maintains its color.
	Venous lake can occur on the face.

Diagnostic Tests

An *excisional biopsy* is recommended if the nevus developed suddenly, if any signs of malignancy are observed, or if there is a sudden change in its appearance. See Appendix B for description of an excisional biopsy.

Referral

If the physician is uncertain of the diagnosis or if the clinical features are atypical, a surgical excision may be performed by the physician. If the physician is uncomfortable performing the excisional biopsy, the patient may be referred to a dermatologist for the procedure.

Management
Medications

Medications are not indicated.

Patient Education

While a blue nevus rarely becomes malignant, if the appearance changes (alteration of its borders or loss of hair), it should be examined by the physician. Likewise, a blue nevus that has developed suddenly should be examined by the physician. Patients should be taught the *ABCDE* mnemonic to check blue nevi for signs of possible malignancy.

Lifestyle Changes

Lifestyle changes will neither prevent nor eliminate blue nevi. Patients should be instructed to avoid prolonged exposure to ultraviolet radiation and to wear a sunblock during outdoor activities.

MONGOLIAN SPOT

A mongolian spot is a congenital gray-blue lesion usually located in the lumbosacral area but occasionally located on the scalp.

Chief Complaint

The parents of a newborn report a large blue spot on the infant's lower back area and express concern that the lesion is malignant.

Clinical Manifestations

- A single, asymptomatic macular lesion is round or oval and is usually located in the lumbosacral area. However, it can also occur on the scalp (Figure 5.4).
- The lesion is usually gray, blue, or black; however, the pigmentation usually fades as the infant becomes older.

Epidemiology
Age

A mongolian spot occurs at birth.

Race

It is usually found in infants of Asian origin but has also been reported in African American and white infants.

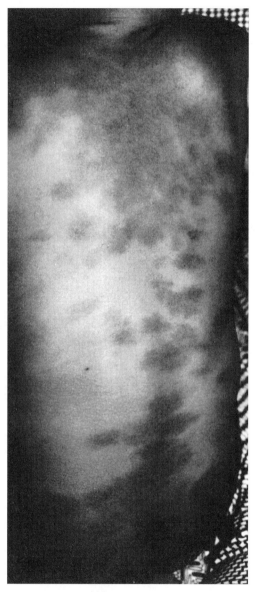

FIGURE 5.4. Mongolian spot. From Roenigk HH. Psoriasis. In Roenigk HH, ed. *Office dermatology.* Baltimore: Williams & Wilkins, 1981:31, Fig. 3-8, with permission.

Risk Factors
- Asian ancestry is most common.
- Mongolian spot is not associated with any systemic disease.

PATHOLOGY
The mongolian spot has elongated melanocytes nestled among the collagen.

Diagnosis
Diagnosis is *based on clinical findings.*

Referral
Since the mongolian spot usually disappears in early childhood, there is no need to refer patients to a specialist.

Management
These spots are *completely benign* and usually regress spontaneously in early childhood.

Medications
Medications are not indicated.

Patient Education
Reassure parents that the mongolian spot will disappear in early childhood and that there is no permanence or malignancy involved with these lesions. Stress that the spot does not herald any systemic disease.

SEBORRHEIC KERATOSIS
Seborrheic keratosis is a common, benign epidermal tumor.

Chief Complaint
Patient presents with numerous large, pigmented moles and is concerned that they may be malignant.

Clinical Manifestations
- Seborrheic keratosis begins as a skin-colored or light tan macule, which becomes more pigmented in time. It usually has a "stuck-on" appearance in the form of a plaque (Figure 5.5, see color insert following page 170). The surface can appear "warty" or waxy and is sometimes scaly. Eventually, the lesions can become nodular and large (up to 6 cm in diameter). They can form cutaneous horns (horn cysts).
- Lesions are usually about 1 to 3 mm in diameter. They increase in number over time, and can range from a few scattered lesions to hundreds in some elderly patients.
- Lesions are commonly seen on the face, trunk, and upper extremities.
- Seborrheic keratosis is rarely pruritic and is usually asymptomatic, unless irritated or secondarily infected. In the latter case, lesions can become tender or bleed. Scraped lesions rarely bleed.

Epidemiology

Family History

Occurrence can be familial, and inheritance may be autosomal dominant.

Age

Occurrence is after age 30 years.

Sex

The lesions are slightly more common in men.

Risk Factors

Family history is the main risk factor.

PATHOLOGY

Seborrheic keratosis is a benign hyperplasia of keratinocytes and melanocytes.

Diagnosis

Diagnosis is *based on clinical findings.*

Differential Diagnosis

See Table 5.3.

T ABLE 5.3.   Seborrheic Keratosis: Differential Diagnosis

Solar lentigo	Uniform hyperpigmentation in an oval, flat macule occurs in an older patient. Biopsy can be used to differentiate, if necessary.
Lentigo maligna	Variable pigmentation and irregular borders are characteristic. Scale and a warty appearance can distinguish mature seborrheic keratosis lesions from those of lentigo maligna. Biopsy can be used to differentiate the two.
Pigmented basal cell carcinoma	This is a slowly changing lesion with a waxy appearance. It contains dilated blood vessels and has a central ulceration. Biopsy is necessary to determine the diagnosis because of the destructive potential of the carcinoma.
Melanoma	Melanoma usually does not have a "stuck-on" appearance; borders are typically irregular and confluent with surrounding skin. Biopsy is necessary to differentiate melanoma from seborrheic keratosis.
Verruca vulgaris	Can be confused with a mature seborrheic keratotic lesion, which has a warty surface; however, verruca vulgaris lesions are not pigmented.
Dry skin	Scales associated with xerosis may initially confuse the diagnosis with that of seborrheic keratosis; however, seborrheic keratotic lesions can be differentiated once the scales are shed and the pigmented, warty surface of the lesion becomes apparent.

Diagnostic Tests

- *Excisional biopsy* is recommended for cases of uncertain diagnosis or if malignancy is suspected.
- An excisional biopsy ensures that the histopathologic features of the seborrheic keratotic lesion are preserved. The base of the lesion must be cauterized to prevent recurrence.

Referral

Seborrheic keratosis can usually be diagnosed by the physician. In cases of uncertain diagnosis, the physician should remove the lesions for histopathologic diagnosis. Very rarely would a patient with seborrheic keratosis be referred to a dermatologist or surgeon unless the lesion was large and needing a rotational flap or graft.

Management

Medications

Medications are not indicated.

Other Treatment Modalities

- *No treatment is necessary for most lesions* unless lesions are symptomatic or cosmetically problematic.
- *Shave biopsy.* While excisional biopsy is recommended for cases of uncertain diagnosis or suspected malignancy, shave biopsy can be used when the lesion is being removed for symptomatic or cosmetic reasons and no malignancy is suspected. However, the biopsy specimen should always be sent for pathologic examination. The base of the lesion should be cauterized. See Appendix B for complete details on removing skin lesions.
- Although *light electrocautery* of the lesion is possible, the histopathologic features are usually not preserved. Therefore the procedure is not recommended.
- *Cryosurgery with liquid nitrogen and curettage* is a procedure in which the pathologic characteristics can be preserved; in experienced hands, this technique is recommended.

Follow-up

Patients should be asked to monitor any new lesions that develop, especially those with variations of color and those that enlarge, and consult the physician promptly if changes occur.

Patient Education

Patients should be reassured that seborrheic keratosis is rarely malignant. These lesions can occur at sites of sun exposure or skin friction, although ultraviolet radiation and trauma have not been scientifically proved to cause seborrheic keratosis. There is no established association between seborrheic keratosis and environmental allergies or oily skin. For these reasons, no specific preventive strategies are recommended.

KERATOACANTHOMA

Keratoacanthoma occurs as an isolated nodule with a central crater. It can mimic squamous cell carcinoma. Lesions occur usually on the face. They grow rapidly and usually remit spontaneously over a period of several months.

Chief Complaint

The patient reports that the mole on his face is craterlike, and he is worried that it has become malignant.

Clinical Manifestations

- Keratoacanthoma occurs as a nodular, dome-shaped lesion with a central crater that can become plugged with keratin (Figure 5.6, see color insert following page 170). It can be found on the cheeks, nose, ears, forearms, and dorsum of the hand (usually *sun-exposed areas* of the skin).
- The lesion is usually skin-colored or slightly red to tannish brown. Fine telangiectasias may be present.
- Lesions may grow up to 2.5 cm over a period of several weeks. They are *asymptomatic;* however, they may occasionally become tender. They are firm but not hard on palpation.
- Lesions are of cosmetic concern because of their size and appearance.
- Rarely, a single lesion may multiply or progress to squamous cell carcinoma.

Epidemiology

Age

Keratoacanthoma may appear in patients older than age 50 years; rarely is the lesion seen in persons younger than 20 years of age.

Race

Rarely seen in Asians and African Americans, the lesion is most notable in whites.

Sex

The lesion is three times more common in men.

Risk Factors

- Keratoacanthoma can be seen in patients exposed to tar.
- Immunosuppression is also a factor in the development of the lesion.
- Chronic ultraviolet light exposure and trauma may be predisposing factors.

PATHOLOGY

Keratoacanthomas are derived from hair follicles in which the epithelium at the periphery undergoes hyperplasia.

Diagnosis

The diagnosis of keratoacanthoma can be made clinically but should be confirmed by pathologic examination to distinguish it from squamous cell carcinoma.

Differential Diagnosis

See Table 5.4.

Diagnostic Tests

Surgical excision is recommended to remove a keratoacanthoma, since the main differential diagnostic consideration is squamous cell carcinoma. Histopathologic diagnosis should always be performed to confirm the benign nature of this lesion. A complete excision down to the subcutaneous tissue with a primary closure is the recommended technique. See Appendix B for details.

TABLE 5.4.   Keratoacanthoma: Differential Diagnosis

Squamous cell carcinoma	Keratoacanthoma is faster growing than squamous cell carcinoma and does not have a central crater.
	Excisional biopsy can confirm the nonmalignant nature of the keratoacanthoma.
Verruca vulgaris	Keratoacanthoma is faster growing than verruca vulgaris, which distinguishes the two. Lesions may have a central crater.
	A biopsy is warranted if the diagnosis cannot be made clinically.

Referral

The physician can easily perform the excisional biopsy in the office. However, referral is indicated for patients with lesions bordering the lip or another structure where closure of the excision would prove difficult.

Management

Medications

Medications are not indicated.

Other Treatment Modalities

The physician can manage the keratoacanthoma with excisional biopsy and histologic diagnosis. Although spontaneous regression may occur in several months, these lesions can heal with a hypopigmented scar that may be cosmetically disfiguring, so *complete removal is recommended.*

Patient Education

- Patients should be reassured that the lesion is benign, with rare malignant potential. However, excision and histologic examination to confirm nonmalignancy are recommended.
- Patients should be advised that new keratoacanthomas can develop in different locations, especially in areas of trauma or chronic sun exposure.
- Surgical removal of the lesion creates a scar; however, allowing it to regress spontaneously results in a scar of greater cosmetic concern than that resulting from a surgical incision.

Lifestyle Changes

Patients should be always advised to maintain healthy skin by avoiding chronic ultraviolet radiation. If they must be out in the sun, patients should use sunscreen to help prevent development of new lesions.

DERMATOFIBROMA

Dermatofibroma is a common nodule, usually appearing in the extremities. It is sometimes mistaken for other lesions, such as malignant melanoma.

Chief Complaint

Patient reports a nodule on her calf, which has been there for months.

Clinical Manifestations

- Dome-shaped papular or nodular lesions, usually appearing on the extremities (only rarely on the head, palms, or soles), reach a size of up to 10 mm in diameter (Figure 5.7, see color insert following page 170). Crusting or scarring may occur as a result of scratching or shaving.
- Colors vary from pink to brownish tan. Borders are ill-defined and fade into the normal skin.
- Pinching the lesion between two fingers causes a dimple or depression in the center.
- Lesions are usually solitary and scattered; however, clusters of up to 10 have been reported.
- Generally, no symptoms are associated with the lesions, although they can occasionally become pruritic.

Epidemiology

Age

Dermatofibroma occurs in adults over 18 years of age.

Sex

Women are affected more often than men.

Risk Factors

This condition is usually idiopathic but can result from trauma or insect bites.

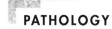

PATHOLOGY

Dermatofibroma consists of collections of spindle cells with small amounts of cytoplasm and an overlying hyperplastic epidermis. Rarely, dermatofibroma can develop into a dermatofibrosarcoma.

Diagnosis

The dimple formed when the lesion is pinched is one diagnostic indicator.

Differential Diagnosis

See Table 5.5.

Referral

Most dermatofibromas can be diagnosed and excised by the family physician, making referral generally unnecessary.

Management

Medications

Medications are not indicated.

Other Treatment Modalities

- *Surgical removal* is usually unnecessary unless the diagnosis is unclear or the lesion is irritated from repeated trauma. Excisional biopsy or shave biopsy with pathologic determination is the usual method of removing the lesion.

T ABLE 5.5.   **Dermatofibroma: Differential Diagnosis**

Malignant melanoma	Lesions usually have a changing size or shape. They may have irregular borders and variegated color patterns.
	Biopsy can determine the diagnosis.
Metastatic carcinoma with a distant primary site	Usually, there is vertical growth, in contrast to dermatofibroma, which remains a stable size.
	Biopsy can determine the diagnosis.
Nevus	Nevi are usually not as firm as dermatofibromas, nor do they exhibit the "dimple" sign.
	Biopsy can determine the diagnosis.

- *Cryosurgery* is also an effective alternative treatment and can produce a cosmetically acceptable scar.

Patient Education

- Patients should be reassured that the dermatofibroma is a benign lesion and rarely becomes malignant.
- The dermatofibroma, if left untreated, will remain the same size and shape. The lesion may be removed for cosmetic reasons or if it is repeatedly traumatized by routine daily activities. Patients should be reminded that the lesions can recur after removal and a scar will replace the lesion.

SKIN TAG

The skin tag, or acrochordon, is a soft, skin-colored to tannish to dark brown lesion, usually pedunculated, varying from less than 1 mm up to 10 mm in size.

Chief Complaint

Patient reports numerous growths around her neck, which occasionally bleed when irritated by her necklace.

Clinical Manifestations

- Skin tags generally range in size from less than 1 mm to 10 mm, and they can be skin-colored, tan, or dark brown. They are usually pedunculated, round, soft papules and nodules (Figure 5.8, see color insert following page 170).
- Generally, they occur at sites of friction, usually the neck, axilla, groin, inframammary area, and eyelids.
- Skin tags tend to become more numerous over time but are usually asymptomatic. However, occasionally they become tender or bleed following trauma or torsion of the stalk.

Epidemiology

Family History

There is a familial tendency to develop skin tags.

Age

Up to 25% of adults of middle age or older are affected.

Sex
The lesions are more common in women.

Risk Factors
Obesity and family history are risk factors.

PATHOLOGY

Acrochordon is an outgrowth of normal skin consisting of a thin epidermal layer with a loose fibrous tissue stroma.

Diagnosis
The skin tag is diagnosed clinically. Diagnosis may be confirmed pathologically if the skin tag is deeply pigmented or firm.

Differential Diagnosis
See Table 5.6.

Diagnostic Tests
If the diagnosis is uncertain or the skin tag is deeply pigmented or firm, histopathologic diagnosis via excisional biopsy is recommended.

Referral
Skin tags close to a mucosal border or with a thin stalk can be managed by the physician in the ambulatory setting; these lesions rarely warrant referral to a dermatologist. When the stalk has a broad base, a determination should be made before excision whether the physician can primarily close the lesion. If this cannot be accomplished or is outside the physician's clinical experience, the patient should be referred to a dermatologist.

Management
Medications
Medications are not indicated.

T ABLE 5.6.   Skin Tag: Differential Diagnosis

Seborrheic keratosis	Seborrheic keratosis has a firm, warty surface on a broad stalk.
Melanocytic nevi	Melanocytic nevi can appear identical to skin tags but are usually firmer. Biopsy is often needed to differentiate the two.
Molluscum contagiosum	Molluscum contagiosum has a central umbilication and is usually vesicular without a stalk.
Neurofibromas	Neurofibromas are large and firmer than skin tags. Biopsy can differentiate the two.

Other Treatment Modalities

The skin tag can be removed either with a simple scissor excision under local anesthesia with 1% lidocaine or removed by cryosurgery. Hemostasis can be achieved by electrocautery or silver nitrate sticks.

Patient Education

- Patients should be reassured that skin tags are *not malignant.*
- Patients should be told that skin tags which bleed or are irritated by clothes or jewelry and are cosmetically problematic should be removed.
- They should also be advised that skin tags can return, especially in the presence of increased friction caused by opposing skin surfaces.

LIPOMA

Lipomas are benign, usually asymptomatic, subcutaneous tumors that are movable against the overlying skin.

Chief Complaint

Your patient presents with a soft, nontender mass under the skin; she is concerned that the mass may be malignant.

Clinical Manifestations

- There is a soft, movable lump beneath the overlying skin (Figure 5.9, see color insert following page 170). The lesion may be single or occur in multiples. It is rounded or sometimes lobulated and is usually less than 6 cm but can reach to 12 cm in size.
- The *neck* and *trunk* are usually affected, although lipoma may occur sometimes in the extremities.
- Lipomas are asymptomatic and rarely painful.

Epidemiology

Occurrence is usually in the fifth or sixth decade of life.

Risk Factors

Familial lipoma syndrome is an autosomal dominant trait. It is characterized by hundreds of slow-growing lesions.

PATHOLOGY

Lipomas consist of well-circumscribed adipose tissue with a connective tissue framework located in the subcutaneous layer.

Diagnosis

The diagnosis is commonly the result of clinical findings, but confirmation can be made by histopathologic diagnosis.

Differential Diagnosis

Metastatic lesions or solitary tumors that have malignant potential should be considered in the differential. Malignant lesions often grow rapidly and have a firm texture; they are not easily moveable. Lipomas are soft and move easily.

Diagnostic Tests

If the lesion is firm and immovable rather than soft, excisional biopsy is indicated.

Referral

Most lipomas can be removed by the physician in an office setting. However, lesions larger than 6 cm may warrant referral.

Management

Medications

Medications are not indicated.

Other Treatment Modalities

- *Excisional biopsy* easily removes lipomas of less than 6 cm in diameter.
- *Subcutaneous and skin sutures* are necessary to close wounds in larger lipomas, since undermining the subcutaneous tissue to free the epidermis is necessary to facilitate closure. In addition to ensuring proper closure of large wounds, placement of subcutaneous sutures will decrease the tension on the epidermal layer, allowing for a smaller, thinner scar.

Patient Education

- Patients should be reassured that lipomas are *not malignant.*
- Patients should be told that in instances when the diagnosis is uncertain or the lipoma is causing irritation or is cosmetically disfiguring, excision of the lesion can be undertaken easily in an outpatient setting.

BIBLIOGRAPHY

Kang S, Barnhill RL, Mihm MC Jr. Melanoma risk in individuals with clinically atypical nevi. *Arch Dermatol* 1994;130:999-1001.

NIH Consensus Development Panel on early melanoma. Diagnosis and treatment of early melanoma. *JAMA* 1992;268:1314-1319.

Schwartz RA. Keratoacanthoma. *J Am Acad Dermatol* 1994;30:1-19.

Tucker MA, Halpern A, Holly EA, et al. Clinically recognized dysplastic nevi: a central risk factor for cutaneous melanoma. *JAMA* 1997;277(18):1439-1444.

Disorders of Blood Vessels

CAPILLARY HEMANGIOMA

Capillary hemangiomas, also known as strawberry marks, are red lesions observed at birth or within the first 2 months of life. The lesions may be solitary or in clusters.

Chief Complaint
Parents report a red lesion on an infant and express concern that it may be malignant.

Clinical Manifestations
- *Hemangiomas* are bright, red lesions appearing over a patch of skin that at first was pale or slightly erythematous (Figure 6.1, see color insert following page 170).
- These lesions are superficial, undergoing a period of rapid expansion during the first year of life, followed by a stationary period and then a spontaneous regression or involution phase usually beginning by 15 months of age.
- The lesions are most commonly found on the face, scalp, back, and chest, with 50% occurring on the head and neck.
- Hemangiomas have sharply demarcated, raised borders and irregular, rough, compressible surfaces.
- These lesions do not blanche completely with compression.
- Posthemangioma resolution residua show hypopigmentation, telangiectasias, fatty deposits, and scarring.
- Ulcerations can occur if hemangioma resolves or regresses rapidly and may become secondarily infected.
- Multiple hemangiomas can be associated with hemangiomas of the central nervous system and gastrointestinal tract.
- Hemangiomas can cause airway obstruction or visual obstruction if they occur on the face.
- In more than 50% of children, the lesion resolves by age 5 years; nearly all lesions resolve by 9 years of age.

Epidemiology
Age
Capillary hemangioma is seen in infants from birth to 2 months of age.

Sex
Girls are more affected than boys with an incidence of 1% to 2%.

Risk Factors
Low birth weight is a risk factor.

PATHOLOGY

Capillary hemangioma is a localized proliferation of angioblastic mesenchymal tissue.

Diagnosis
Differential Diagnosis
See Table 6.1.

Referral

Hemangiomas can cause complications such as airway or visual obstruction, high-output cardiac failure, or consumption coagulopathy, or expand rapidly. Referral to a specialist experienced in their removal is necessary when faced with these complications.

Management

Uncomplicated hemangiomas, except those on the face or in the groin, do not need to be treated because they usually resolve spontaneously. In the rare case that a lesion exists late into childhood, excision may be helpful for cosmetic reasons. However, it should be stressed to patients and their parents that surgery can cause scarring, making it advisable to wait for the lesion to resolve spontaneously.

Medications
See Table 6.2.

Other Treatment Modalities

Other treatment modalities such as the use of a pulsed-dye vascular laser or interferon alfa-2a can be used for facial or groin hemangiomas or any lesions causing consumptive coagulopathy, visual or airway obstruction, or high-output cardiac failure.

Follow-up
Monitoring Disease Course

It is helpful to measure the child's lesion at yearly checkups. This may be reassuring to the parents when it is demonstrated that the hemangioma is not growing and in fact may be shrinking.

Potential Problems and Complications

Occasionally, hemangiomas ulcerate, bleed, or become infected. Treating the infections with antibiotics (see Chapter 16, Table 16.9) resolves this problem.

Patient Education

Parents should be reassured that the lesions will eventually resolve by the age of 5 years and have no risk of becoming malignant.

T ABLE 6.1. Capillary Hemangioma: Differential Diagnosis

Deep (cavernous) hemangioma	Deep hemangioma is a soft, purplish, globular tumor, often described as a "bag of worms."
	It can be associated with arteriovenous malformations, platelet entrapment, and thrombocytopenia.

TABLE 6.2. **Medical Treatment of Capillary Hemangioma**

Prednisone

Administration:	1 to 6 mg/kg per day orally.
Duration of use:	4 to 8 weeks or until lesions resolve.
Comments:	For facial or groin hemangiomas; best started before the rapid-growth phase. Long-term use of corticosteroids inhibits the pituitary-adrenal axis; consult *Physicians' Desk Reference* for details.

CAMPBELL-DE MORGAN SPOT (ALSO CALLED CHERRY ANGIOMA)

The Campbell-De Morgan spot, also called cherry angioma, is a small angioma of common cosmetic annoyance occurring after age 30 to 40 years.

Chief Complaint

Patients report numerous red papules that are unsightly and express concern that they may also be malignant.

Clinical Manifestations

- Cherry angiomas are red, dome-shaped papules first noted in young adults (Figure 6.2, see color insert following page 170).
- These lesions are usually located on the trunk, arms, and scalp.
- Initially, few lesions are present, but numbers increase over time.
- These lesions may bleed after trauma.
- Lesions are usually 1 to 4 mm in size, with sharply demarcated borders.
- Cherry hemangiomas always blanche with compression.

Epidemiology

- Cherry angiomas are very common.
- *Age.* They usually occur in young adults of approximately 30 years of age and then may become more numerous in middle-aged and older adults.
- *Sex.* There is an equal incidence in men and women.

Diagnosis
Differential Diagnosis
See Table 6.3.

PATHOLOGY

Cherry angiomas are small, dilated blood vessels in the superficial dermis covered by a flattened epithelium.

T ABLE 6.3.   Campbell–De Morgan Spot (Cherry Angioma): Differential Diagnosis

Nodular melanoma	Lesions are black to purplish nodules, do not blanche, and have one or more signs of the **ABCDE** mnemonic (see Chapter 5). Angiomas are smaller nodules that blanche under pressure and have sharp borders.

Management
No treatment is necessary in most circumstances.

Other Treatment Modalities
- Electrocautery or shave excision may be performed with 1% lidocaine local anesthetic if these lesions are cosmetically unpleasant or bleed when irritated (see Appendix B).
- Pulsed-dye vascular laser can also be used by physicians experienced in its use.

Patient Education
- Patients should be advised that cherry angiomas are completely benign.
- Since cherry angiomas can bleed if irritated or traumatized, patients may be advised to apply cold compresses to the lesion to halt bleeding.
- Patients may develop as many as 100 cherry angiomas, the development of which cannot be prevented.

SPIDER ANGIOMA

This common collection of very superficial blood vessels can occur in various locations.

Chief Complaint
Patients report a red, unsightly lesion, which may be new or old, that is increasing in size.

Clinical Manifestations
- Spider angiomas (nevi) may develop suddenly, or an established nevus may increase in size (Figure 6.3, see color insert following page 170).
- Lesions consist of a center of redness (arteriole) with an expanding network of dilated capillaries surrounding the center.
- Spider angiomas are usually solitary and can be up to 1.5 cm in diameter.
- The capillaries disappear under compression and reappear on release of pressure.
- These lesions are commonly seen on the face, arms, and hands.

Epidemiology
Age
Spider angiomas can occur in children without any associated diseases.

Sex
Women are more commonly affected.

Risk Factors
- Spider angioma is more common in patients who are long-term, heavy alcohol drinkers.

- Spider angioma is associated with high-estrogen states, such as occur during pregnancy or when taking oral contraceptives.
- It is also associated with chronic or acute liver disease.

PATHOLOGY

Spider angiomas are superficial capillaries covered with a thin layer of epidermis.

Diagnosis

Differential Diagnosis

See Table 6.4.

Diagnostic Tests

If liver disease is suspected, liver function tests should be performed.

Management

No treatment is necessary, although these lesions may be removed for cosmetic reasons.

Other Treatment Modalities

Laser treatment or electrocautery is the most common treatment, but cryotherapy has also been used.

Follow-up

Follow-up is necessary only if spider angiomas are associated with liver disease or if the patient desires removal of the lesions for cosmetic reasons.

T ABLE 6.4. Spider Angioma: Differential Diagnosis

Cherry angiomas	Lesions are red and dome-shaped and are located on the trunk.
Hereditary hemorrhagic telangiectasia (Osler-Weber-Rendu syndrome)	Hereditary hemorrhagic telangiectasia are matlike telangiectasias with no radiation of capillaries, and are located on face, lips, tongue, hands, feet. They can be accompanied by gastrointestinal and genitourinary tract bleeding.
	Large arteriovenous malformations lead to high-output cardiac failure.
Ataxia-telangiectasia	Lesions occur as telangiectasias of the bulbar conjunctiva, nose, ears, forearms, and neck; associated with ataxia and recurrent sinopulmonary infections.
Systemic scleroderma	Systemic scleroderma is a connective tissue disorder associated with sclerodactyly and Reynaud phenomenon. There are matlike telangiectasias of the face, nose, tongue, palms, lips, and periungual region.
	The two are differentiated by location and appearance of telangiectasias and a negative ANA test result.

ANA, antinuclear antibody.

Patient Education

Patients should be advised that these lesions frequently resolve spontaneously if they developed during childhood, during pregnancy, or while taking oral contraceptives. In rare cases the lesions grow.

PYOGENIC GRANULOMA

Pyogenic granuloma, a collection of granulation tissue that forms at a site of trauma, can grow rapidly and bleed easily if irritated.

Chief Complaint

Patients complain of a bleeding bump on the finger or other area where trauma occurred.

Clinical Manifestations

- Pyogenic granuloma appears as a smooth nodule with sharply demarcated borders, is less than 1.5 cm in size, and may have a superficial crust (Figure 6.4, see color insert following page 170).
- Lesions are benign and are usually solitary with color varying from red to brown or black (although not within the same lesion).
- There is a predilection for the fingers, toes, lips, mouth, and trunk. Lesions develop over a few days to a few weeks and may be present for months.
- They are not pruritic but may bleed easily (friable).

Epidemiology
Age
Pyogenic granuloma typically appears in young adults less than 30 years of age and is more common in children.

Sex
There is an equal incidence between men and women; however, the condition is more frequent in pregnant women (especially on the gingiva).

Risk Factors
Pyogenic granuloma usually occurs in an area of previous minor trauma.

PATHOLOGY
Pyogenic granulomas are a lobular proliferation of capillaries with an overlying epithelium.

Diagnosis
Differential Diagnosis
See Table 6.5.

Diagnostic Tests
Biopsy may be indicated if diagnosis is uncertain.

TABLE 6.5. Pyogenic Granuloma: Differential Diagnosis

Amelanotic melanoma	Amelanotic melanoma is clinically indistinguishable from pyogenic granuloma except for its rapid growth. Biopsy is useful to differentiate the two.

Referral

Plastic surgery or dermatologic referral may be indicated if biopsy is needed in a highly visible area.

Management

The lesion can be surgically removed via *shave biopsy* and *the base destroyed by electrocautery,* removed by *laser surgery* or *cryosurgery.* Total excision is needed to avoid recurrences (see Appendix B).

Follow-up

Advise patients to return to the office if they observe satellite recurrences around the original lesion site. Satellite lesions should be treated similarly to the original lesion.

Patient Education

Patients should be reassured that pyogenic granulomas are totally benign.

BIBLIOGRAPHY

Ezekowitz RAB, Mulliken JB, Folkman J. Interferon alfa-2a therapy for life-threatening hemangiomas of infancy. *N Engl J Med* 1992;326:1456–1463.

Hurwitz S. *Clinical pediatric dermatology,* 2nd ed. Philadelphia:WB Saunders, 1993.

CHAPTER 7

··

Mucocutaneous Cysts

MILIA

Milia are small, firm, keratin-filled mucocutaneous cysts commonly found at sites of pilosebaceous follicles or healing dermal trauma.

Chief Complaint

Patients report painless small papules, usually located in the nasolabial folds or around the eyes. Parents of newborns may complain of small papules noted primarily on the face and cheeks of the otherwise healthy infant.

Clinical Manifestations

- Milia are white to yellow pigmented papules 1 to 2 mm in size.
- These lesions are distributed on the face, particularly around the eyes and the nasolabial folds.
- Milia are firm and nontender to palpation, with no central punctum or visible opening to the epidermis.
- The lesions have no erythema or other evidence of inflammation, as is the case in pustular miliaria.
- Milia are generally idiopathic and may be present at birth.
- Milia may be seen during the healing process following dermal trauma such as dermabrasion therapy, following certain dermatoses such as acute contact dermatitis or severe acne with scarring, or during the healing phase of porphyria cutanea tarda.

Epidemiology

Age

- Milia are present in 40% to 50% of all normal healthy newborns within the first 4 weeks of life.
- Milia may persist into the second or third month of life, but generally resolve spontaneously in 3 to 4 weeks.
- Despite the high incidence in newborn infants, any age may be affected.

Race and Sex

There is no specific predilection toward race or gender.

PATHOLOGY

Milia are subepidermal keratin cysts that are covered by squamous epithelium.

Diagnosis

Diagnosis of milia is based on clinical findings and patient history. No diagnostic testing is necessary.

T ABLE 7.1. Milia: Differential Diagnosis

Pustular milia (neonatal pustulosis)	Small pustules forming on an erythematous base.
Folliculitis	Involvement of pustules on the hair shaft and follicle.
Erythema toxicum neonatorum	Plugging of the pilosebaceous unit resulting in red macules, pustules, or vesicles on the trunk and face.

Differential Diagnosis

See Table 7.1.

Management

Since milia resolve spontaneously, no medical treatment is necessary.

Other Treatment Modalities

Milia may be removed for cosmetic purposes with a simple incision and expression of the keratin content. This procedure is performed using an 18-gauge needle or a No. 11 scalpel blade, which is used to "unroof" the cysts. Expression of the contents may be accomplished by the use of a Schomberg extractor. Electrodesiccation is another means of removing milia.

Follow-up

Follow-up is not usually needed given the self-limited and benign nature of this disorder, unless surgical removal was required.

Patient Education

Patients should be reassured that milia are benign and will eventually shed or resolve spontaneously in both adult and newborn patients.

EPIDERMOID CYSTS

The epidermoid cyst is the most common of the mucocutaneous cysts; it is also called an epidermal cyst, wen, or infundibular cyst.

Chief Complaint

Patients report a severely painful, inflamed cyst with an unpleasant appearance.

Clinical Manifestations

- *Epidermoid cysts* are usually solitary lesions, but multiple cysts have been reported (Figure 7.1, see color insert following page 170).
- These cysts generally feel like a dermal or subcutaneous nodule or tumor and vary from 0.5 to 5 cm in diameter. They can remain small for years or progressively develop over a short time, forming a much larger mass.
- While typically found in the face, neck, back, base of ears, chest, and scrotum, epidermoid cysts may occur on virtually any part of the body.
- The cysts are generally soft and freely movable but may demonstrate calcification, particularly in scrotal lesions.
- Narrow, keratin-filled pores or channels (called central punctum) may exude keratinaceous material upon application of firm pressure.
- Because the cysts are relatively thin-walled, rupture of these cysts is a common occurrence, causing the contents to be released in the dermal or subcutaneous

regions, thereby initiating an intense inflammatory reaction. The resulting inflammatory mass is often much larger than the original cyst, with accompanying surface erythema and tenderness to palpation.

- Epidermoid cysts and their contents can become infected. A ruptured epidermoid cyst generally creates a sterile inflammatory process and is often misdiagnosed as an infection.
- If the cyst wall is destroyed during the active inflammatory process created by epidermoid cyst rupture, the lesion will not recur.

Epidemiology

Age

- Epidermal cysts usually occur in young to middle-aged adults, but all ages may be affected.
- Rarely do they occur before puberty.

Race and Sex

There is no significant predilection to race or gender.

PATHOLOGY

Histopathologic study reveals a cyst with an epidermoid wall with stratified squamous epithelium and a well-formed granular layer capable of producing keratin.

Diagnosis

Diagnosis is generally based on clinical findings and physical examination. Examination should reveal a subcutaneous nodule or tumor at typical sites with the hallmark of epidermoid communication.

Diagnostic Tests

Diagnosis may be confirmed by gross and histopathologic examination following removal of the lesion.

Differential Diagnosis

See Table 7.2.

Management

- The goal of treatment is to remove the cyst, with particular attention given to removing as much of the cyst wall as possible to reduce the chance of recurrence. Inflamed or flocculent cysts should be drained and evacuated properly via surgical

T ABLE 7.2. Epidermoid Cysts: Differential Diagnosis

Epidermal inclusion cyst	The cyst appears on the palms and soles as a dermal nodule secondary to traumatic implantation of epidermis within the dermis.
Pilar (trichilemmal) cysts	Pilar cysts occur on the scalp and face and are derived from the hair root sheath. There is no communication to the epidermis.

incision. With larger cysts, excision is the treatment of choice. Depending on the size of the incision, closure with sutures may be necessary with appropriate follow-up for suture removal (see Appendix B, Cyst Excision).
- Evidence of bacterial infection is an indication for treatment with an oral antibiotic. Antibiotic selection should cover *Staphylococcus aureas, Streptococcus* species, *Escherichia coli, Peptostreptococcus* species, and *Bacteroides* species. A practitioner may elect to initially incise and drain an infected epidermoid cyst. Complete removal of the cystic structure, including the cyst wall, should be performed after the infection resolves.

Follow-up
Monitoring Disease Course
In cases of ruptured or infected cysts, patients should be followed from a few days to 1 week for a recheck. For patients who received surgical treatment and suturing, follow-up for suture removal and wound check is appropriate.

Patient Education
Patients should be reassured that the nodules or tumors are benign and have no pre-malignant tendencies. However, the patient should also be cautioned that incision and draining do not preclude the possibility of recurrence, even if the entire cyst is excised.

TRICHILEMMAL CYST

Trichilemmal cyst, also known as a pilar or sebaceous cyst, are a common type of cutaneous cyst.

Chief Complaint
Patients report a painless nodule, usually on the scalp, which may be traumatized when combing or brushing their hair (Figure 7.2, see color insert following page 170).

Clinical Manifestations
- Trichilemmal cysts are generally smooth, firm, dome-shaped nodules or tumors that range from 0.5 to 5 cm in diameter.
- About 90% of these cysts are located on the scalp.
- Although there is usually no associated alopecia, there may be some thinning of the hair in larger lesions.
- Trichilemmal cysts are not connected to the epidermis and have no central punctum or connection to the surface.
- Although the cyst is usually a solitary lesion, it is not uncommon to find multiple lesions or a small cluster of lesions.
- When small, they are generally firm, but may be noted to be soft or even flocculent if larger.
- Although not typically, a pilar cyst may rupture and demonstrate tenderness and erythema upon examination.
- Trichilemmal cysts are essentially painless subcutaneous nodules, although they can become painful with bumping or repeated rubbing.
- These cysts do not usually drain; however, subcutaneous rupture can occur, causing the cyst to become infected and present as a tender nodule or mass.
- A trichilemmal cyst usually demonstrates a thick wall composed of stratified squamous epithelium.
- These cysts contain keratin and keratin breakdown products, which may become calcified.

Epidemiology

Family History
Often familial, trichilemmal cysts demonstrate an autosomal dominant pattern.

Age
The cyst is most often seen in middle-aged persons.

Sex
Trichilemmal cysts occur predominantly in females.

Risk Factors
A family history of trichilemmal cysts is a risk factor.

PATHOLOGY

Histopathology reveals a stratified squamous epithelial wall with an outer layer resembling the outer root sheath of a hair follicle. The inner layer of the cyst lacks a granular layer.

Diagnosis
Diagnosis is based on clinical findings and appearance.

Diagnostic Tests
Diagnosis may be confirmed with gross and histopathologic examination of the excised lesion.

Differential Diagnosis
See Table 7.3.

Referral
Trichilemmal cysts can be treated in the office setting, making referral usually unnecessary.

Management
- Removal of pilar cysts is recommended when cysts occur in areas subjected to repeated trauma, such as that imposed by combing or brushing hair. These cysts may also be removed for cosmetic reasons.
- Standard treatment is surgical removal via incision, excision, or curettage, with a focus on removing all components of the cyst. Typically the skin above the cyst is incised with care given not to incise into the cyst. The cyst is then dissected, and attempt is made to remove the cyst intact. If the cyst does rupture, care should be given to remove as much of the cyst wall as possible. Cysts may regrow following surgical removal, particularly if removal of the cyst sac was incomplete. The wound is usually thoroughly irrigated, and larger incisions closed with sutures.

T ABLE 7.3. Trichilemmal Cysts: Differential Diagnosis

Epidermoid cysts	There is communication to the epidermis or surface of the skin through a central punctum.

Other Treatment Modalities

If evidence of infection exists, oral antibiotics, such as cephalexin (Keflex) 250 mg four times daily for 7 to 10 days, should be used to cover staphylococci and strepto-cocci.

Follow-up

Follow-up in approximately 1 week is recommended after surgical removal of trichi-lemmal cysts for removal of sutures and to check the wound site for signs of infection.

Patient Education

- Patients should be reassured that trichilemmal cysts are benign. However, patients should also be advised that the cysts may reappear despite treatment, especially if any portion of the cyst wall is not removed.
- Patients should be cautioned that pilar cysts can occasionally become infected and that these cysts can rupture, generating a painful inflammatory reaction in the sur-rounding tissue.

BIBLIOGRAPHY

Brook I. Microbiology of infected epidermal cysts. *Arch Dermatol* 1989;125: 1658-1661.

Smirniotopoulos JG, Chiechi MV. Teratomas, dermoids, and epidermoids of the head and neck. *Radiographics* 1995;15:1437-1455.

Wolfe SF, Gurevitch AW. Eruptive milia. *Cutis* 1997;60:183-184.

Carcinoma of the Skin

In this chapter we consider premalignant (actinic keratosis and oral leukoplakia) and malignant (squamous cell, basal cell, and melanoma) carcinomas.

PREMALIGNANT ACTINIC KERATOSIS

Actinic keratosis, also called solar keratosis, is a single or multiple scaly, premalignant lesion usually seen on the sun-exposed skin of adults. Progression to squamous cell carcinoma is possible.

Chief Complaint

Patients report a red, scaly lesion located on the forehead, and express concern that the lesion is not healing.

Clinical Manifestations

- Round or oval erythematous macules or papules with coarse scales and less than 1 cm in size are present (Figure 8.1, see color insert following page 170).
- Lesions are skin-colored, yellow-brown, brown to red in color and have a sandpaper texture.
- Actinic keratosis lesions are distributed on the face, ears, neck, forearms, hands, or shins (sun-exposed surfaces).
- They can occur on the orolabial area as a form of cheilitis; these lesions have a higher malignant potential.
- Lesions can have a stinging or "sticking" sensation and can be pruritic.

Epidemiology

Age

The condition usually affects middle-aged to older adults but can occur in persons under 30 years of age living in areas such as Australia, where greater sun exposure is likely.

Race

The condition usually is not seen in darker-skinned individuals.

Sex

It is more common in men.

Malignancy Potential

Malignancy potential of an untreated lesion is 1:10 to1:1000 per year.

Skin Phototypes

The condition is more common in fair-skinned individuals such as redheads, blondes, and those with a tendency to freckle [skin phenotypes 1 and 2 (SPT 1 and SPT 2)] (see Chapter 9, Table 9.1 for details).

Risk Factors

Environmental
Chronic, cumulative sun exposure.

Occupational
Occupations such as farming or ranching.

Recreational
Outdoor sports or hobbies.

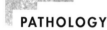

PATHOLOGY
Atypical epidermal keratinocytes are the characteristic histologic changes seen in actinic keratosis.

Diagnosis
Diagnosis is usually based on a history of a sticking or stinging sensation of a papular, scaly lesion with a sandpaper texture.

Differential Diagnosis
See Table 8.1.

Diagnostic Tests
Tests are usually unnecessary.

Referral
Referral may be appropriate if diagnosis is unclear or the lesion is located in an area that makes removal difficult. Patients with cheilitis should be referred to a dermatologist familiar with laser surgery techniques for removal of these lesions.

Management
- Large papular and nodular lesions should be removed by the physician via excisional biopsy and sent for histologic diagnosis (see Appendix B).

TABLE 8.1.   Actinic Keratosis: Differential Diagnosis

Discoid lupus erythematosus	The flat red lesions of discoid lupus erythematosus may be indistinguishable from actinic keratosis.
	Biopsy is useful to differentiate the two.
Squamous cell carcinoma	Papular lesions are present.
	Biopsy is useful to differentiate the two.
Seborrheic keratosis	Lesions appear "stuck on" and may be pigmented.
	Biopsy is useful to differentiate the two.
Nummular eczema	Large, erythematous, pruritic scaling lesions appear on the trunk and extremities.
	Biopsy is useful to differentiate the two.

- Any ulcerated, bleeding, or recurrent lesion should be removed by excisional biopsy and examined pathologically, since these lesions could be malignant.

Medications
See Table 8.2.

Other Treatment Modalities
Cheilitis lesions are best removed surgically via carbon dioxide laser.

Follow-up
Patients should be followed up at least every 6 months to examine for new lesions.

Patient Education
Compliance
- Patients should be advised that actinic keratosis is premalignant, with a 1:1000 to 1:10 per year chance for developing a squamous cell carcinoma of the skin, making immediate treatment essential.
- Because of the high potential for malignancy, any ulcerated, bleeding, or nonhealing lesions that occur following treatment for actinic keratosis should be reported immediately.

Lifestyle Changes
- Prevention of future occurrences is the best treatment. Sunscreens with a skin protection factor (SPF) 15 or higher, covering both ultraviolet B-range (UVB) and ultraviolet A-range (UVA) radiation, should be applied daily to face, ears, and other

TABLE 8.2. Medical Treatment of Actinic Keratosis

5-Fluorouracil	[(Efudex, Fluoroplex) 1%, 2%, or 5% solution; 1% or 5% cream]
Availability:	Prescription
Dosage:	Applied topically to lesion *twice daily.*
Duration:	Use for 2 to 8 weeks.
	Complete healing may occur 1 to 2 months following end of treatment.
Side effects:	5% Preparation causes initial erythema followed by necrosis of lesion.
	Can cause photosensitivity; advise patients to avoid sun exposure or use protective measures (clothing, sunscreens).
Comments:	Use 1% or 2% preparations for short duration; use 5% preparations on extremities for longer duration.

Topical liquid nitrogen (cryosurgery)	
Dosage:	Apply to lesion with a cotton-tipped applicator for 10 to 20 seconds, remove, repeat (procedure listed in Appendix B).
Duration:	Usually 1 time only; may repeat if lesion is recurrent.
Side effects:	Hypopigmentation or erythema. Scarring can occur after aggressive freezing.
Comments:	Thin skin, such as facial skin, may require only 1 "freeze-thaw" cycle; thicker skin or lesions on extremities may require 2.

exposed skin surfaces before individuals go out in the sun. If patients cannot avoid exposure, they should be instructed to wear protective clothing, eyewear, gloves, and hats.

- Patients should be warned that sunscreen should be worn even on cloudy days because ultraviolet radiation is probably more intense and still able to damage the sun-exposed skin surfaces. Patients should also be reminded that sun exposure during the period from 11:00 A.M. to 3:00 P.M. should be avoided, since this is the time of maximum ultraviolet radiation. Parents should be advised to apply sunscreens even to infants and young children before taking them outdoors. There are several such products available specifically for use on infants and small children.

Family and Community Support
Patients should be cautioned about the typical side effects of 5-fluorouracil (5-FU); patient education brochures can be obtained from the manufacturer.

ORAL LEUKOPLAKIA

Oral leukoplakia is a white, sharply defined, macular lesion with irregular margins that occurs on the inner side of the cheek, tongue, or the vermilion border of the lips. The lesions cannot be removed by rubbing or scratching because they are firmly adherent to the underlying mucosa.

Chief Complaint
Patients report white plaques on the sides of the tongue or inner side of the cheek. Some patients may complain that the plaques cause a burning sensation.

Clinical Manifestations
- Raised, firmly adherent lesions that do not scrape off and can vary in size from 2 to 4 cm are present.
- The surface of the lesion is rough or leathery in appearance.
- Lesions are plaquelike but can sometimes be macular.
- They are usually homogeneously white to gray-white; however, speckled areas of red can be found within the lesion.
- Sometimes ulcerations can be present.
- Lesions can be found on the buccal mucosa, hard palate, gingiva, central portion of the tongue, and the vermilion border of the lips.
- They can also be found on the penile mucosa and vulva.
- Oral hairy leukoplakia involves the lateral portions of the tongue.

Epidemiology
- This premalignant condition progresses to squamous cell carcinoma in about 10% of cases.
- Oral hairy leukoplakia is related to immunodeficiency, whereas oral leukoplakia is not.
- Oral leukoplakia is premalignant, whereas hairy leukoplakia is generally benign.

Age
Adults from 40 to 70 years of age.

Sex
More likely in males, with a 2:1 ratio of predominance.

Risk Factors
Long-term exposure to irritants such as tobacco smoke, smokeless tobacco, alcohol, and irritation from dentures or teeth are risk factors.

PATHOLOGY

Epstein-Barr virus or herpesvirus is the etiologic agent for hairy leukoplakia, a benign disease associated with human immunodeficiency virus (HIV)–induced immunodeficiency or other immunodeficient states.

Human papillomavirus (HPV) is the etiologic agent for oral leukoplakia.

Syphilis can be an infectious etiologic agent for leukoplakia in the tongue.

Biopsy specimens of lesions reveal dysplasia of keratinocytes with abnormal mitoses.

Diagnosis

The diagnosis of leukoplakia is a clinical one, but biopsy should be performed. The frequency of malignant lesions is related to the site of oral leukoplakia. Leukoplakia on the floor of the mouth or the central surface of the tongue is associated with a higher risk for frank malignancy or in situ carcinoma. Oral leukoplakia on the buccal mucosa, however, is usually benign. Therefore biopsy of lesions on the floor of the mouth or central portion of the tongue, or those with speckled areas within the white plaque, should be performed to rule out malignancy. Biopsy of other sites can be performed if the diagnosis is uncertain.

Differential Diagnosis

See Table 8.3.

Diagnostic Tests

Oral hairy leukoplakia is a generally benign disease related to immunodeficient states. A leukoplakia workup should include an HIV determination and immune status testing if the lesion involves the tongue (especially if the lesion is on the lateral portions of the tongue).

Referral

Referral may be indicated for patients with extensive lesions, when the diagnosis is not evident, or if malignancy is suspected.

Management

Biopsy of leukoplakia should be performed to discern the malignant potential. Lesions that are frank carcinomas, carcinoma in situ, or dysplasias may need treatment

T ABLE 8.3. Oral Leukoplakia: Differential Diagnosis

Lichen planus and condyloma acuminatum	There is no history of prolonged exposure to irritants such as tobacco or alcohol. Both cause white oral lesions that are indistinguishable from leukoplakia. Biopsy is useful to differentiate the two.
Candida	Candida may be clinically indistinquishable from oral leukoplakia. A KOH preparation or biopsy is useful to differentiate the two.
Oral hairy leukoplakia	White lesions occur on lateral tongue margins that do not scrape off. Patient's immune and HIV status should be determined. Biopsy is useful to differentiate the two.

KOH, potassium hydroxide; HIV, human immunodeficiency virus.

by a specialist, since lesions that show in situ carcinoma or invasive carcinoma must be completely excised surgically with clear margins. Patients should also be tested for an immune-compromising condition such as HIV.

Other Treatment Modalities

Recent studies show that synthetic retinoids and possibly oral beta-carotene may cause some regression of leukoplakia, but these agents are *not recommended* at this time.

Follow-up

Close, periodic follow-up, at least every 4 to 6 months, is essential to monitor existing lesions and examine for newly developing dysplastic lesions. Prompt treatment is essential to prevent these lesions from advancement to disfiguring carcinoma.

Patient Education

Compliance

Patients should be cautioned to perform regular self-examinations and seek immediate biopsy and treatment for new lesions or expanding old lesions.

Lifestyle Changes

- Prevention is a key factor in reducing the incidence of oral leukoplakia. Patients should be counseled against smoking and the use of smokeless tobacco (snuff) and advised to decrease their intake of alcohol. In patients with a positive history of these irritant exposures, a careful scrutiny of the oral cavity should be performed periodically by the physician.
- Patients should be informed that these may be precancerous lesions which can proceed to very serious carcinomas of the oral mucosa, causing significant disfigurement if left untreated.

MALIGNANT SQUAMOUS CELL CARCINOMA

Squamous cell carcinoma, a tumor of malignant keratinocytes, is the second most common skin malignancy in the United States.

Chief Complaint

Patients report an isolated, crusted papule or nodule that will not heal.

Clinical Manifestations

- Slow-growing indurated papule, plaque, or nodule whose shape is either round, oval, or umbilicated is present.
- Sometimes, lesions have adherent keratotic scales or central crusting and can appear ulcerated.
- Lesions are erythematous or pearly in color and are hard to palpation.
- They are usually isolated but can occur as multiple lesions.
- Lesions are usually located on sun-exposed areas such as the face, tips of ears, scalp, dorsum of the hand, forearms, trunk, and shins (Figure 8.2, see color insert following page 170).

Bowen Disease

The clinical manifestations of Bowen disease are as follows:
- In situ (noninvasive) squamous cell carcinoma.
- Can be red or pigmented.
- Usually solitary scaly plaques, and either solitary or multiple lesions.
- Can be found on both sun-exposed and non–sun-exposed areas.

Erythroplasia of Queyrat

The clinical manifestations of Erythroplasia of Queyrat are as follows:
• Specific in situ squamous carcinoma of the glans penis or inner surface of the prepuce.
• Erythematous plaques usually lack scales.

Epidemiology

Second most common skin carcinoma in the United States.

Age

Generally seen in patients over 55 years of age in the United States; however, in areas of high sun exposure such as Australia, patients can be in their early 20s or 30s.

Race

The disease usually occurs in white or light-skinned individuals.

Sex

It occurs more often in men.

Risk Factors

Occupational

• Exposure to chemical carcinogens, such as aromatic hydrocarbons, nitrous ureas, arsenic, or tar.
• Occasionally psoralen ultraviolet A-range (PUVA) photochemotherapy.
• Ionizing radiation exposure such as x-rays or grenz rays.

Lifestyle

• Smoking.
• Excessive and chronic sun exposure.

Health

• Actinic keratosis.
• Lip and ear tumors have higher risk for metastasis than other sites.
• Regional lymphadenopathy can occur as a result of metastatic lesions.
• *SPT 1 or SPT 2* skin type, with skin resistant to tanning.

Family history

History or family history of skin cancer.

PATHOLOGY

Invasive squamous carcinoma involves atypical keratinocytes extending into the dermis in an irregular manner. Squamous carcinoma in situ (Bowen disease) is characterized by atypical epidermal lesions without dermal invasion.

Diagnosis

The diagnosis of squamous cell carcinoma is made by biopsy and histopathologic investigation.

Differential Diagnoses
See Table 8.4.

Diagnostic Tests
Shave or punch biopsy may be performed to confirm diagnosis.

Referral
Smaller lesions can be removed surgically by a knowledgeable physician (see Appendix B). Referral is indicated for patients with extensive lesions requiring a larger excision with or without grafting, and those needing microsurgery or irradiation.

Management
Management of squamous cell carcinoma depends on location and surface area of the lesions, and depth of invasion.

Medications
See Table 8.5.

Other Treatment Modalities
- *A shave or punch biopsy* is recommended before treatment to plan the best removal technique. Complete healing following a biopsy does not alleviate the need for definitive therapy.
- *Excisional surgery* may be performed by the physician for removal and primary closure of small lesions. The excision area should extend to a minimum margin of 5 mm surrounding the lesion. Histopathologic investigation should always be conducted (see Appendix B).
- *Mohs microsurgery* can be useful to remove squamous cell carcinomas in high-risk areas of the body. Mohs surgery is also useful in poorly differentiated lesions, longstanding or large lesions, and lesions with ill-defined margins and at sites such as the nasolabial fold, nose, eyes, and postauricular areas, where deep extension is possible. However, this type of surgery should be performed only by physicians trained and experienced in the technique.

T ABLE 8.4.   Squamous Cell Carcinoma: Differential Diagnosis

Nummular eczema	Lesions may be indistinguishable if elevated or indurated but respond to topical corticosteroids.
	Biopsy may be useful to differentiate the two.
Psoriasis	Lesions may be indistinguishable.
	Biopsy may be useful to differentiate the two.
Paget disease of the breast	Lesions may be indistinguishable.
	Biopsy may be useful to differentiate the two.
Basal cell carcinoma	Lesions may be indistinguishable.
	Biopsy may be useful to differentiate the two.
Keratoacanthoma	Lesions present a classically rapid growth; otherwise, they are indistinguishable from squamous cell carcinoma.
	A biopsy is recommended to differentiate the two.
Actinic keratosis	Lesions may be indistinguishable.
	Biopsy is necessary to differentiate the two.

T ABLE 8.5. Medical Treatment of Squamous Cell Carcinoma

5-Fluorouracil 5% cream (Efudex)

Availability:	Prescription.
Dosage:	Applied topically twice per day.
Duration:	4 weeks.
Comments:	Useful for lesions arising from actinic keratosis or *in situ* lesions as determined by skin biopsy; see section on actinic keratosis.

- *Radiation therapy* can also be performed on extensive squamous cell carcinomas in areas that are not amenable to surgical excision or if lymphatic involvement is considered. These patients should be referred to a radiation oncologist.
- *Electrodesiccation* is recommended for carcinomas arising from actinic keratosis or in situ lesions, as determined by biopsy.
- *Lymphadenopathy* should be evaluated in the patients with the following:
  - Large lesions.
  - Lesions involving the lip, mucous membranes, or ear.
  - Lesions in sites previously exposed to ionizing radiation or old burns.
  - Lesions subject to chronic inflammation.

Follow-up

Patients should be examined every 6 months for the first year and yearly thereafter, for any recurrent or new lesions. Suspect, recurrent lesions are identified by new, scaly, nonhealing lesions located near the original site.

Patient Education

Compliance

- Patients should be informed that with early treatment, including complete excision, there is only a 3% to 5% chance of a metastasic incident. Recurrence may be seen as new, scaly, nonhealing lesions close to where the initial lesion was removed, making frequent self-examination and regular check-ups essential. In particular, patients should be educated about the signs of lymphadenopathy and advised to report any such signs to the physician as soon as possible because they may identify metastatic disease.
- Adult patients with a familial history of skin cancer should be advised to return for screening every 6 months, especially if these patients are at high risk, such as those with chronic sun exposure, old burn scars, or exposure to ionizing radiation or those of SPT 1 or SPT 2.

Lifestyle Changes

Patients whose occupations or recreational pursuits necessitate extensive exposure to sun should be reminded to use sunscreens of SPF 15 or higher and to avoid sun between 11:00 A.M. and 3:00 P.M. as much as possible.

Family and Community Support

Parents should teach children about the harmful effects of sun exposure and the use of sunscreens to help prevent damage to the skin.

BASAL CELL CARCINOMA

Basal cell carcinoma is a skin malignancy of the basal cells in the epidermis and the most common type of all cancer in the United States. Several types of basal cell carcinoma are classified by histologic appearance, including nodular, infiltrative, pigmented, superficial, morpheaform, and fibroepithelioma types. The nodular type is the most common.

Chief Complaint

Patients report a growing red skin lesion with telangiectasia.

Clinical Manifestations

- Basal cell carcinoma can take the form of an erythematous plaque, nodule, or ulcer with prominent telangiectasia that grows gradually over several months to several years.
- Lesions are usually hard, firm, and oval with an umbilicated center (Figure 8.3, see color insert following page 170).
- They usually appear as isolated lesions, but occasionally, multiple lesions are seen.
- They are generally asymptomatic, although ulcerated lesions can bleed.
- Papular or nodular lesions are often referred to as pearly or translucent but can also be skin-colored, pink, or red.
- Pigmented basal cell carcinomas also are seen (brown, black, or blue).
- Lesions have a rolled border and are commonly called "rodent-type" ulcers because of their chewed appearance.
- More than 80% of the lesions occur on the head or neck, but they can occur on any hair-bearing skin, the nose being the most common site.
- Lesions rarely metastasize but can cause significant patient morbidity.

Epidemiology

- Most common skin cancer in the United States.

Age
Usually seen in adults 40 to 80 years of age.

Race
Occurs almost exclusively in whites or light-skinned individuals.

Sex
Occurs more often among men.

Risk Factors

- Exposure to arsenic, ionizing radiation, or thermal burns.
- Prolonged sun exposure in individuals with poor tanning ability.

PATHOLOGY

Basal cell carcinoma is an atypical proliferation of basal cells in the dermal layer of the skin.

Diagnosis

Diagnosis of basal cell carcinoma is made by histologic examination of the excised lesion. While the initial biopsy site may appear to have healed completely, basal cell tumors that were not entirely excised may reside under the skin, causing extensive destruction before reaching the skin's surface. Therefore it is important to ensure that the margins of excised tumors are free of malignancy. Careful documentation of the lesion's exact location is essential in the event that excision of residual carcinoma becomes necessary.

Differential Diagnosis

See Table 8.6.

Diagnostic Tests

- A preliminary *punch biopsy* specimen can be examined to determine the diagnosis.
- Definitive treatment can be conducted by a total *excisional biopsy* of the remaining tumor with histopathologic evaluation.

Referral

Tumors larger than 2 cm in diameter, tumors located in the nasolabial fold or medial canthus, tumors with poorly visualized margins, and recurrent tumors require special consideration when choosing the appropriate treatment because these areas are predisposed to subclinical extension and recurrence. In these cases referral to a dermatologist or plastic surgeon is recommended. All patients with lesions requiring skin flaps or grafting should also be referred to the appropriate specialist.

Management

- For basal cell carcinomas less than 1 cm in diameter, which are in regions of the body amenable to easy removal, total excision with primary closure is recommended (see Appendix B).
- All specimens should be removed and sent for histologic diagnosis.

Other Treatment Modalities

- *Cryosurgery is not recommended* for removal of basal cell carcinoma because the specimen is not preserved for histopathologic examination, making it difficult to confirm that the entire carcinoma was removed.
- *Electrodesiccation and curettage* can be used for superficial spreading lesions. However, hypertrophic scarring can develop after electrodessication.

T ABLE 8.6. **Basal Cell Carcinoma: Differential Diagnosis**

Melanoma	Lesions may be indistinguishable from pigmented basal cell carcinoma. A biopsy is necessary to differentiate the two.
Keratoacanthoma	Keratoacanthoma usually has rapid growth and a central keratin plug.
Scars	Lesion is stable and nongrowing, and there is a history of trauma. Morpheaform basal cell can arise from minor trauma.
Eczema	Lesions are scaly, have regular borders, and are lacking in telangiectasia.
Squamous cell carcinoma	Lesions have regular borders and are lacking telangiectasia. Since they may occasionally appear similar to basal cell carcinoma, a biopsy may be necessary to differentiate the two.

- *Mohs microsurgery* is sometimes used for removal of basal cell carcinoma, particularly in delicate areas such as the nasolabial area, around the eyes, and in the ear canal. This technique is also the preferred method of treatment for morpheaform and recurrent lesions (see Appendix B).
- Pathology reports from excised basal cell carcinoma often reveal that some carcinoma remains within the margins, a common occurrence because of the aggressive and invasive nature of basal cell carcinoma. In these cases the outward appearance of the tumor is smaller than the actual tumor involvement under the skin. If the pathology report reveals more extensive involvement, referral to a dermatologist or surgeon for removal of the remains of the tumor is recommended.
- *Radiation therapy* is an option in older or debilitated patients who are unable to undergo excision; in these cases, referral to a radiation oncologist is recommended.

Follow-up
Monitoring Disease Course
- Patients should be followed up every 6 months for the first year and yearly thereafter, to examine for recurrences of the old lesion or new lesions. The physician should be suspicious of any elevated, ulcerated, or indurated lesions on sun-exposed skin, including the trunk.
- The physician should instruct the patient and parents of infants about the dangers of sun exposure at an early age. Parents should be advised that young children receiving ongoing unprotected sun exposure at an early age will be predisposed to skin cancers and other sun exposure–related lesions.

Potential Problems and Complications
Patients should be informed that excisional surgery, and occasionally electrodesiccation, can lead to hypertrophic scarring.

Patient Education
Compliance
- Patients should be assured that total removal of the lesion is usually curative and that these lesions rarely become metastatic. However, 40% to 50% of patients develop a new basal cell carcinoma within 3 to 5 years, making self-examination of the skin and regular follow-up visits to the physician essential.
- Because large ulcerative or nodular-type lesions can lead to considerable disfigurement if left untreated, it should be stressed that any elevated lesions or lesions that do not disappear within 6 to 8 weeks should be reported to the physician immediately.
- Patients should also be taught to watch for recurrences at the old scar site. Changes, such as elevation, ulcerations, or induration, should be reported immediately.

Lifestyle Changes
These patients should be advised to limit their exposure to the sun, use sunscreen of SPF 15 or higher, and avoid the sun from 11:00 A.M. to 3:00 P.M.

MELANOMA

Clinical types of melanomas ("black tumor") include the superficial spreading melanoma, nodular melanoma, acral lentiginous melanoma, and lentigo maligna. The superficial spreading melanoma is the most common, accounting for 75% of melanomas; nodular melanoma is next in frequency, accounting for 15% of melanomas. The lentigo maligna accounts for only 5% of all melanomas, and the acral lentiginous melanoma accounts for 5%. Melanomas are potentially fatal (Figures 8.4 and 8.5, see color insert following page 170).

Chief Complaint

Patients report a lesion, usually asymptomatic, with a suspect or ominous appearance. These lesions are sometimes found serendipitously during a physical examination.

Clinical Manifestations

- Bleeding or ulcerated lesions that may be painful or pruritic and over 6 mm in size are present.
- They have an asymmetric shape and irregular borders.
- There is a seeping of pigment from lesion into the surrounding skin.
- There is a variety of colors within a lesion.
- Usually isolated lesions are on sun-exposed areas such as the forehead, nose, face, neck, forearms, and dorsum of the hands.

Superficial Spreading Melanoma
(approximately 75% of all melanomas)

- A flattened papule has a diameter of 8 to 12 mm.
- Older lesions may be as large as 10 to 25 mm.
- Lesions have an asymmetric shape and irregular borders.
- They are dark brown to black but may be variegated with colors including yellow, tan, brown, black, red, and blue.
- Lesions are usually isolated and occur on the face, back, legs, and anterior trunk.
- Regional lymph nodes may be enlarged.

Nodular Melanoma (approximately 15% of all melanomas)

- Elevated, nodular (blueberry nodule) lesion that sometimes appears ulcerated or polypoid.
- Oval or round lesions with smoothly defined borders range from 1 to 3 cm in diameter.
- Lesions are usually uniformly dark blue or black, but can be gray on a background of brown to black.
- They are usually seen in sun-exposed areas but can occur at any location including subungual areas.
- Test results for regional lymph nodes also can be positive.

Acral Lentiginous Melanoma
(approximately 5% of all melanomas)

- Lesions are initially macular and then sometimes become papular or nodular.
- They tend to be large (3 to 12 cm) with irregular borders and have marked color variation from brown or black to depigmented areas (called amelanotic areas).
- Lesions can be found on the soles, palms, fingers, toes, subungual areas, and even mucous membranes.

Lentigo Maligna Melanoma (uncommon)

- Lesions are usually flat with focal areas of papules or nodules, have irregular borders, and can vary in size from 3 to 20 cm.
- There is usually a striking variation of color ranging from skin-colored or tan (called amelanotic) to dark brown and black.
- Lesions are usually isolated on sun-exposed areas such as the forehead, nose, face, neck, forearms, and dorsum of the hands.

Epidemiology and Risk Factors

- Melanoma is the seventh most common cancer in the United States and prevalence is increasing steadily.
- Five percent of all skin cancers and 1% to 2% of all cancer deaths in United States are attributed to melanoma.
- Patients often have a history of melanoma in first-degree family members; these patients carry a fourfold to tenfold increased risk of developing melanoma themselves.
- The following phenotypic factors, in descending order of risk, are relative risk factors for developing melanoma: freckles, fair skin, blonde or red hair, sunburns easily, tans poorly, and blue eyes.
- Individuals with SPT 1 and SPT 2 are at higher risk of developing melanoma.
- Those with a history of repeated severe sunburn as a child are at increased risk.
- Patients with a history of pigmented mole at birth (congenital nevi) or a history of dysplastic or other atypical nevi are at risk (see Chapter 5).
- The projected risk for melanoma in the United States by the year 2000 is 1 in 75 individuals.

Superficial Spreading Melanoma

- Risk factors include dysplastic nevi, congenital nevi, family history in first-degree relatives, SPT 1 and SPT 2, excessive sun exposure as a child.
- Disease is usually seen in the fourth through sixth decades of life, but occurs in all age groups.
- Incidence is slightly higher in women.
- Whites are usually at greater risk; however, about 2% of cases are seen in darker-skinned individuals.
- Melanomas are more virulent in pigmented races.

Nodular Melanoma

- Risk factors are the same as for superficial spreading melanoma.
- Median patient age is 50 years.
- Incidence is equal in men and women.
- The disease occurs in all races.

Acral Lentiginous Melanoma

- Median patient age is 65 years.
- There is a 3:1 predisposition of men over women.
- The disease is most often seen in darker-skinned individuals such as Asians, sub-Saharan Africans, and African Americans.

Lentigo Maligna Melanoma

- Risk factors include dysplastic nevi, lentigo maligna, congenital nevi.
- The disease is usually seen in patients over 65 years of age.
- Incidence is equal in men and women.
- Occurrence is rare in darker-skinned individuals.
- Incidence is higher in whites, individuals who tan or burn easily, and individuals who have a great deal of sun exposure.

PATHOLOGY

Melanomas are a malignant proliferation of melanocytes located in the skin.

Diagnosis

The diagnosis of any of the four types of melanomas is made by excisional biopsy with histopathologic investigation.

Differential Diagnosis

See Table 8.7.

Referral

Referral to a specialist in the treatment of melanoma should be considered for excision of these lesions.

Management

- There are two classification systems for grading melanomas: the *Breslow system*, based on tumor thickness; and the *Clark system*, based on the location of the melanoma (Table 8.7A).
- Five-year survival is based on tumor thickness (Table 8.7B).

Other Treatment Modalities

- Melanomas that have not spread beyond the site at which they developed are highly curable. The recommended definitive treatment of melanoma is total excision of the lesion and the appropriate surgical margins based on tumor thickness (see Appendix B). The physician should perform an elliptic excision around the

T ABLE 8.7. Melanoma: Differential Diagnosis

Melanocytic nevus	Melanocytic nevi are usually less than 6 mm in diameter, symmetric, and have regular borders.
	Changes in lesions indicate a need for excision and histopathologic examination.
Seborrheic keratosis	Lesions have sharp borders, a "stuck-on" appearance, and a scaly surface.
	A biopsy may be useful to differentiate the two.
Solar lentigo	Solar lentigo lesions have an irregular shape and appear on sun-exposed surfaces of older patients.
	A biopsy may be useful to differentiate the two.
Dysplastic nevi	Lesions have irregular borders.
	With multiple lesions, there is an increased risk for melanoma.
	A biopsy may be useful to differentiate the two.
Hemangioma	A blood vessel tumor that blanches under pressure.
	A biopsy may be useful to differentiate the two.
Pyogenic granuloma	Red, glistening, friable lesion; resembles amelanotic melanoma.
	A biopsy is recommended to differentiate the two.
Pigmented basal cell carcinoma	Lesions have a waxy surface and telangiectasia, and may occasionally resemble melanoma.
	A biopsy may be useful to differentiate the two.
Subungal hematoma	Lesion is preceded by a history of nail trauma and grows as the nail grows.
	A biopsy may be useful to differentiate the two.

Changes in any lesions or unclear diagnosis warrants biopsy.

T ABLE 8.7A. Classification of Melanomas

Breslow classification	Clark classification
No evidence of primary tumor	I Tumor confined to epidermis (not considered invasive)
Tumor thickness less than 0.76 mm	II Melanoma cells in papillary dermis
Tumor thickness 0.76 to 1.5 mm	III Melanoma cells entirely filling papillary dermis
Tumor thickness 1.51 to 3.0 mm	IV Melanoma cells in reticular dermis
Tumor thickness 3.01 to 4.0 mm	IV Melanoma cells in subcutaneous fat
Tumor thickness larger than 4.0 mm	

entire pigmented lesion, down to the level of subcutaneous fat. All removed specimens must be sent for *histopathologic examination*. When the lesion is confirmed as a melanoma, referral for wider excision with appropriate margins depending on the tumor size is recommended. Do not attempt initial removal of suspect lesions or margins via a shave biopsy or electrodesiccation. These procedures can inadequately remove the lesion or destroy the staging criteria, thus interfering with correct diagnosis and choice of appropriate adjuvant treatment.

- The treatment of lesions less than 1 mm deep is total surgical excision of the primary lesion with 1-cm margins around the entire lesion.
- Melanomas ranging from 0.76 to 4.0 mm should be removed with surgical margins no larger than 2 cm. No statistical difference was noted in local recurrence rates, distant metastasis, or overall 6-year survival when compared with 4-cm surgical margins.
- Melanomas larger than 4 mm must be totally excised with 3-cm surgical margins and regional dissection of the clinically involved lymph nodes. Adjuvant therapy with interferon alfa-2b appears to prolong survival when compared with patients who receive no adjuvant therapy.
- Melanomas that have spread to regional lymph nodes may be curable with wider excision (2- to 4-cm margins) around the primary tumor, plus removal of the involved regional lymph nodes.
- Distant metastases can occur in adjacent skin, regional lymph nodes draining the primary site, and distant organs such as liver, lung, bone, brain, and viscera. Melanoma metastatic to distant lymph nodes or other organs may be palliated by resection, whereas radiation therapy may provide symptomatic relief to brain, bone, or visceral metastases.

T ABLE 8.7B. Five-Year Survival Rates[a]

Tumor thickness (mm)	Five-year survival (%)
Less than 0.75	99
0.76 to 1.5	94
1.51 to 2.25	83
2.26 to 3.0	72
Larger than 3.0	Less than 50

[a]Based on tumor thickness.

- Advanced melanoma can be resistant to most standard systemic therapy, and these patients should be referred for clinical trials.
- Recurrent or advanced tumors may be responsive to immune-system–enhancing therapy. Referral to cancer specialists experienced in the treatment of melanoma is recommended for these patients. Therapy options include interleukin, interferon, and tumor necrosis factor.
- Vaccine therapy (immunotherapy) is another promising treatment for melanoma that is metastatic to distant sites. Currently there are many clinical trials being sponsored by the National Cancer Institute (NCI) that may be helpful for a specific clinical situation. Contact the NCI or local cancer specialist for more details.

Follow-up

- Patients should be followed up by the physician every 3 to 6 months for 2 years and annually thereafter. Patients with invasive lesions should receive annual chest radiographs and liver testing for 3 to 5 years following treatment. The physician should pay attention to the primary melanoma site and any adjacent adenopathy when examining for recurrent lesions.
- Biopsy of any new pigmented lesions should be performed and specimens sent for histopathologic diagnosis. Any congenital nevi should also be considered for excision. Lesions that appear odd or out of the ordinary should also be evaluated by excision. Survival is based on tumor thickness (Table 8.7B).

Patient Education

Compliance

- Patients should be informed that 3% of melanoma patients develop a second melanoma within 3 years. Early diagnosis and immediate therapy improve survival rates, making a total-body self-examination on a regular basis every 2 to 3 months essential to these patients. Educate the patient on the *ABCDE*s of suspected lesions (see Chapter 5) and stress that any changing mole meeting the *ABCDE* criteria, or any mole that exhibits symptoms such as itching or tenderness for more than 2 weeks, should be examined by the physician.
- First-degree relatives of patients with melanoma are at risk; these family members should be advised to perform self-examinations regularly and see a physician every 6 to 12 months.

Lifestyle Changes

Patients who have been treated for melanomas, those who have a dysplastic nevi, or those with SPT 1 or SPT 2 should be advised to avoid extensive sun exposure. Patients should be instructed to avoid exposure to sunlight, especially between 11:00 A.M. and 3:00 P.M. Sunscreens with SPF greater than 30 should be used in persons with dysplastic nevi or a history of melanoma. Many patients believe that sun beds and sunlamps are innocuous; however, these forms of ultraviolet radiation are just as dangerous as sun exposure. Patients whose occupations require working outdoors should always wear appropriate protective clothing.

Family and Community Support

- Family members should be asked to assist the patient with self-examination.
- Patients diagnosed with malignant melanoma often need extensive psychological support and counseling in dealing with this disease.
- Studies have shown that therapeutic support groups have great value; many patients have experienced strengthening of their immune systems as a result of attending these groups.

• The patient can contact the American Melanoma Foundation (telephone: 619-534-3840) or the National Institutes of Health Cancer Information Service (telephone: 800-422-6237), or use the following excellent Internet Web site for more information on the latest diagnostic and treatment options: http://cancer.med.upenn.edu/disease/melanoma.

BIBLIOGRAPHY

Keller KL, Fenske NA, Glass LF. Cancer of the skin in the older patient. *Clin Geriatr Med* 1997;13(2):339–361.

Kirkwood JM, Strawderman MH, Ernstoff MS, Smith TJ, Borden EC, Blum RH. Interferon alfa-2b adjuvant therapy of high-risk resected cutaneous melanoma: The Eastern Cooperative Oncology Group Trial EST 1684. *J Clin Oncol* 1996;14(1):7–17.

Kopf AW, Salopek TG, Slade J, Marghoob AA, Bart RS. Techniques of cutaneous examination for the detection of skin cancer. *Cancer Suppl* 1995;75(2):684–690.

Le AV, Fenske NA, Glass LF, Messina JL. Malignant melanoma: Differential diagnosis of pigmented lesions. *J Fla Med Assoc* 1997;84(3):166–174.

Marghoob AA. Basal and squamous cell carcinomas: what every primary care physician should know. *Postgrad Med* 1997;102(2):139–159.

Marghoob AA, Slade J, Salopek TG, Kopf AW, Bart R, Rigel DS. Basal cell and squamous cell carcinomas are important risk factors for cutaneous malignant melanoma. *Cancer Suppl* 1995;75(2):707–714.

NIH Consensus Development Panel on Early Melanoma. Diagnosis and treatment of early melanoma. *JAMA* 1992;268(10):1314–1319.

Rigel DS. Identification of those at high risk for developing malignant melanoma. *Adv Dermatol* 1995;10:151–171.

Ringborg U, Anderson R, Eldh J, et al. Resection margins of 2 versus 5 cm for cutaneous malignant melanoma with a tumor thickness of 0.8 to 2.0 mm: a randomized study by the Swedish Melanoma Study Group. *Cancer* 1996;77(9):1809–1814.

Wornom IS III, Soong S, Urist MM, Smith JW, McElvein R, Balch CM. Surgery as palliative treatment for distant metastases of melanoma. *Ann Surg* 1986;204:181–185.

CHAPTER 9

....

Photosensitivity

ACUTE SUN DAMAGE

Acute sun damage, or sunburn, is an intense, delayed, transient inflammatory response of the skin following excessive exposure to the sun's ultraviolet radiation (UVR).

Chief Complaint

Patients report a red, painful, sometimes pruritic rash on the sun-exposed surfaces of the body. The patient's primary concern is usually pain relief.

Clinical Manifestations

- Sunburn is usually erythematous; vesicles and bullae may be seen occasionally.
- Edema of the skin can also occur in moderate to severe exposure.
- Sun-damaged areas can be raised, tender, and sometimes pruritic.
- Sunburned skin rarely causes scarring after healing.
- In patients with severe sunburn, pulse rate may be rapid.
- Constitutional symptoms can include headache, chills, fever, and weakness, especially in cases of severe sunburn.
- Ultraviolet B-range (UVB) erythema develops 12 to 24 hours after exposure and fades within 3 to 5 days.
- Ultraviolet A-range (UVA) erythema peaks about 4 to 16 hours after exposure and fades within 2 to 5 days.

Epidemiology

- Skin phototypes (SPTs) are genetically determined, although SPTs are, to an extent, based on patients' histories of sun exposure and how they react.
- Sunburn occurs most frequently in individuals of skin phototype 1 or 2 (SPT 1 or SPT 2) (Table 9.1), those with light skin and a limited capacity to tan. The

T ABLE 9.1. Skin Phototypes

Phototype	Reactions to sun	Comments
1	Burns easily; never tans	Comprises, with SPT 2, 25% of light-skinned people in the United States
2	Burns easily; tans minimally	Comprises, with SPT 1, 25% of light-skinned people in the United States
3	Burns moderately; tans gradually	
4	Burns minimally; tans always	
5	Burns rarely; tans profusely	Comprises people with brown skin; can sunburn following long exposures to UVR
6	Never burns; deeply pigmented	Comprises people with black skin; can sunburn following long exposures to UVR

SPT, skin phototype; UVR, ultraviolet radiation.

categories of SPT 1 and SPT 2 account for 25% of the light-skinned persons in the United States.

- Individuals with skin phototypes 5 and 6 (SPT 5 and SPT 6) can sunburn following long exposures to UVR.
- The unit of measurement of sunburn, called minimum erythema dose (MED), is the minimum amount of UVR exposure that produces clearly marginated erythema at the irradiated site after a single exposure. Individuals with lighter skin have a lower MED, correlating with the variable sensitivity of human skin to UVR and the capacity to produce and retain melanin.

Risk Factors

- The ability to tan is the skin's capacity to produce melanin after sun exposure. Whites fall into four SPT categories (Table 9.1). Not all people with light skin are SPT 1, nor are all people with moderately pigmented skin SPT 4, since Asians and Hispanics tend to be SPTs 1 and 2, despite darker skin pigmentation.
- Sunburn is less of a problem for populations indigenous to equatorial land and high altitudes and more of a problem for those who come from higher latitudes and low altitudes.
- Outdoor work and outdoor recreational activities are risk factors for sunburn.
- Sunburn from natural sunlight results primarily from the effects of UVB light. The spectrum for UVB is 290 to 320 nm.
- UVA-induced sunburn is becoming more common as the use of tanning salons and home-tanning devices becomes more widespread. The UVA spectrum is 320 to 400 nm.
- Sunburn may also occur after exposure to the incidental radiation caused by the reflection of UVR from bodies of water, white sand, or snow.
- Repeated blistering sunburns in young children are a risk factor for development of malignant melanoma of the skin in later years.

PATHOLOGY

Nucleic acids in the DNA of the epidermal keratinocyte absorb UVR, resulting in the formation of photoproducts, which lead to the inhibition of DNA synthesis. The resultant cell death causes the desquamation of the epidermis.

Diagnosis

Clinical presentation. Acute sunburn is a clinical diagnosis based on the reaction of exposed skin and the history of excessive UVR exposure. There is usually no concomitant ingestion of medication or application of topical agents or cosmetics.

Differential Diagnosis
See Table 9.2.

Diagnostic Tests
Skin biopsy is usually unnecessary to confirm the diagnosis of acute sunburn.

Referral

Acute sunburn damage can be treated successfully by the family physician. In cases of severe sunburn, toxicity may be best managed in a specialized burn unit for parenteral fluid replacement, pain control, and prophylaxis against infection.

T ABLE 9.2. Acute Sun Damage: Differential Diagnosis

Photosensitivity (phototoxic or photoallergic)	Photosensitivity reactions are erythematous rashes on sun-exposed areas specifically caused by the cross-reactions of medications or topical agents and ultraviolet radiation. A history of medication ingestion or topical agent application in association with ultraviolet radiation exposure is diagnostic, since both rashes can appear identical.
Systemic lupus erythematosus (SLE)	Sunburn-type erythema usually occurs on the face and is symmetric. SLE rash is persistent.

Management

- For mild sunburn with erythema or vesicles limited to a small area, cool tap water or saline solution compresses for 20 minutes three or four times daily are helpful in reducing the pain.
- In more extensive sunburn covering a large portion of the skin, use cool baths for 20 minutes three to four times daily; topical fluorinated corticosteroids are helpful as well.
- In vesicular disease, the *vesicle should not be unroofed* and the wound should be covered with bacitracin or silver sulfadiazine if there are no contraindications. Treatment is the same as that used for a second-degree thermal burn.
- Immediate medical attention is necessary for any person who appears toxic after a sunburn. These patients often need hydration, sometimes parenterally, and prophylaxis against infection.

Medications
See Table 9.3.

Follow-up
Patients with mild to moderate sunburn do not need to be closely monitored. However, in patients who appear toxic with an extensive burn and dehydration, follow up in 1 to 2 days to assess hydration status and to determine whether fluid replacement is needed. The sun-damaged areas should also be monitored for infection.

Patient Education

- Patients should be informed that acute sun damage is more easily prevented than treated. Current prevention strategies include the use of sunscreens and avoidance of the sun, which is especially appropriate for those of SPT 1 or SPT 2.
- Sun exposure between 11:00 A.M. and 3:00 P.M. (when UVR exposure is the greatest) should be avoided.
- While most sunscreens are formulated to protect against UVB radiation, some also protect against UVA radiation, albeit at a much less effective rate. It is recommended that a sunscreen which protects against both UVB and UVA, with sun protection factor (SPF) 15 or greater, be used in all cases.
- For recreational exposure, sunscreens of SPF 15 or greater are appropriate.
- Individuals of SPT 1, SPT 2, and SPT 3 should routinely apply a sunscreen of at least SPF 15 before and during exposure.
- For those who want to reduce the adverse risks of UVR, protection of exposed skin with a sunscreen of greater than SPF 15 is recommended.
- Sunscreen should be reapplied immediately after swimming unless a waterproof lotion is used.

T ABLE 9.3.   Medical Treatment of Acute Sun Damage

Topical corticosteroids

Availability:	OTC or prescription.
Dosage:	Applied topically to sun-damaged areas 2 or 3 times daily.
Duration:	Until pain and inflammation resolve.
Comments	Mid- to high-potency agents recommended. Long-term use of topical fluorinated agents can lead to skin atrophy.

NSAIDs, including ibuprofen (Motrin or Advil) and naproxen (Aleve)

Availability:	OTC
Dosage:	See package insert.
Duration:	Use until inflammation and pain resolve.
Comments:	Concomitant use with topical steroids may reduce the pain and erythema in sunburn. NSAIDs can cause severe gastritis and gastrointestinal tract bleeding; use with caution in patients with previous peptic ulcer disease or gastrointestinal tract bleeding. Avoid using NSAIDs in patients with hypersensitivity reactions to these medications.

Diphenhydramine (Benadryl)

Availability:	OTC
Dosage:	*Adults:* 25 to 50 mg orally every 4 to 6 hours, as needed.
	Children: 5 mg/kg per day orally divided every 6 hours, as needed.
Duration:	Use until pruritus resolves.
Comments:	Drowsiness and sedation are common side effects. Driving or using dangerous machinery is to be avoided. Should not be used concomitantly with alcoholic beverages.

Oral prednisone

Availability:	Prescription.
Dosage:	*Adults:* 40 to 60 mg daily, tapered by 10 to 20 mg every 1 to 2 days.
	Children: 1 mg/kg of body weight daily and taper.
Duration:	7 to 10 days
Comments:	For use in cases of extreme sunburn with vesicles or bullae, or sunburn covering a large portion of the body, although studies do not show effectiveness in severe cases. Long-term use of systemic corticosteroids can inhibit the pituitary adrenal axis.

OTC, over the counter; NSAIDs, nonsteroidal antiinflammatory drugs.

- Suntan lotions and oils do not prevent a sunburn because they do not have any SPF.
- In patients whose occupations require sun exposure, sunscreens are essential, as is protective clothing, such as hats with wide brims, long-sleeved shirts, and clothing with a denser weave to prevent UVR penetration.
- Patients who work or sunbathe near water or in areas with white sand should be reminded that UVR can be enhanced by the reflection off these surfaces. Exposure to UVR can also occur under cloudy conditions and at high altitude. Snow-related activities can also lead to UVR exposure. These exposures also require sunscreen use of SPF 15 or greater.
- People with SPT 1 and SPT 2 have increased sun sensitivity and should be warned about increased risk for premalignant and malignant skin disease and photoaging.
- Patients who have thinner, more sensitive skin (infants, children, aging adults) should avoid direct UVR exposure and should wear protective clothing and sunscreens when exposure is necessary.

- Sunglasses with UVR protection should be worn during sun exposure to prevent the development of cataracts.
- Patients should be reminded that chronic sun damage can lead to a variety of problems over time. Photoaging can occur, which creates severe wrinkling of the skin. Actinic keratosis and solar lentigo can also occur over time after chronic sun exposure. Severe blistering of the skin in young adults is a risk factor for the development of malignant melanoma in later years.
- Patients should be reminded that ointments or butter does not help a mild to moderate sunburn and can be painful to wash off.
- First-aid sprays or creams often contain benzocaine, which can sensitize the skin and can lead to an allergic rash.

DRUG-INDUCED PHOTOSENSITIVITY

Two types of reactions occur with drug-induced photosensitivity: *phototoxic reaction,* which is an exaggerated sunburn after the use of certain oral or topical medications, and *photoallergic reaction,* which is an immune response secondary to the interaction between UVR and certain drugs in previously sensitized patients. Table 9.4 lists the common photosensitizing drugs.

Chief Complaint

Patients report an erythematous rash that is painful, possibly pruritic, and possibly blistering. This rash resembles sunburn (Figure 9.1, see color insert following page 170).

Clinical Manifestations

Phototoxic Reaction

- Phototoxic reactions may be immediate or may occur 16 to 24 hours after exposure. Reactions usually occur with the first drug exposure.
- This rash may be pruritic, stinging, or burning; symptoms may worsen if the patient continues to take the medication.

T ABLE 9.4.   Common Photosensitizing Drugs

Phototoxic agents	Photoallergic agents
Antibiotics [griseofulvin (Grisactin), tetracycline, quinolones, and sulfanilamide]	*Topical* Sunscreens (PABA, benzophenones, methoxy cinnamate)
Amiodarone (Cordarone)	
Coal tar	Fragrances (musk)
Chlorpromazine (Thorazine)	*Systemic medication*
Chemotherapeutic agents [vinblastine (Velban), 5-fluorouracil (Efudex), methotrexate (Rheumatrex)]	Benzodiazepines
Diltiazem (Cardizem)	Chlorpromazine
Diuretics [furosemide (Lasix) and hydrochlorthiazide (Esidrix)]	Nifedipine (Procardia)
NSAIDs	NSAIDs
Plant materials (celery, fig, lime, parsnips)	Quinidine
Psoralens	Retinoids
Quinidine	Sulfanilamide
Retinoids	
Tolbutamide (Orinase)	

PABA, para-aminobenzoic acid; NSAIDs, nonsteroidal antiinflammatory drugs.

- The rash is usually located on sun-exposed areas of the body, such as the face, the distal portions of the arms, and the exposed areas of the chest. The rash spares the philtrum (the area beneath the lower lip), the area behind the ears, and the skin creases of the posterior portion of the neck. The rash is erythematous, resembling a sunburn.
- The affected skin may be edematous or contain vesicles; scaling can also develop with repeated exposures.
- The rash blanches when pressure is applied.
- Systemic symptoms such as headache, malaise, and weakness may also be present.

Photoallergic Reaction

- Photoallergic reactions usually do not occur on the first drug exposure.
- The rash may spread to non–sun-exposed skin.
- A photoallergic reaction occurs within 24 to 48 hours of sun exposure, although the rash usually does not become evident until about 48 hours after exposure; the delay is caused by the time taken for the allergic sensitization reaction to develop.
- The rash resembles an eczematous rash or lichen planus type of rash. Scaling is marked and is seen to a greater extent than with phototoxic rashes.
- The rash can cause pruritus.

Epidemiology

Phototoxic Reaction

- The phototoxic reaction is the more common type of photosensitivity reaction.
- This reaction can occur at any age.
- Phototoxic reactions can occur in individuals of any skin color.

Photoallergic Reaction

- Photoallergic reaction is the less common type of photosensitivity reaction.
- It commonly occurs in individuals over 18 years of age.
- Photoallergic reactions can occur in patients of any skin color.
- Sun exposure is unnecessary for the reaction to occur.

Comparison Chart

See Table 9.5.

T ABLE 9.5.   Comparisons Between Phototoxic and Photoallergic Reactions

Reaction	Occurrence	Appearance	Time after sun exposure	Location	Dose-related
Phototoxic	Common	Erythematous rash resembling sunburn.	Within minutes to 24 hours of exposure to UVR; will occur with first exposure.	Usually occurs only on sun-exposed areas of the body.	Sometimes
Photoallergic	Less common	Eczematous or lichen planus–type rash.	Within 24 to 48 hours of exposure to UVR; will occur only after repeated exposure.	Usually occurs first on sun-exposed body surfaces but can spread to nonexposed areas.	No

UVR, ultraviolet radiation.

Risk Factors
Phototoxic Reaction
Concomitant drug and sun exposure is necessary for this reaction to occur (Table 9.4).

Photoallergic Reaction
Topically applied agents are the most commonly implicated drugs; however, photoallergic reactions can occur with ingested agents (Table 9.4).

PATHOLOGY

Phototoxic reactions. There are inflammatory cells in the epidermis, with necrobiosis and vesiculation. There is an absence of eczematous changes.

Photoallergic reactions. These represent a delayed type (type IV) of hypersensitivity reaction. There is lymphocytic infiltration in the epidermis.

Diagnosis
Differential Diagnosis
See Table 9.6.

Diagnostic Tests
- Phototesting can confirm a suspected diagnosis of photosensitivity.
- *Phototoxicity.* In suspected phototoxicity, phototesting is performed before and after administering a therapeutic dose of the suspected agent for 2 or 3 days. Standard skin sites are exposed to increasing amounts of UVA radiation. A positive test result is regarded to be a change in the patient's reactivity, which would be a lower MED than that associated with premedication UVA exposure. In other words, the medication lowers the MED in phototoxic patients, making them more photosensitive.
- Photoallergy. *Photopatch testing* should be conducted in suspected cases of photoallergic reactions.
  On the first day of testing, duplicate sets of suspected allergens are applied to the skin on the patient's back. The threshold of sensitivity to the UVA source is determined with a total exposure of UVA radiation of 1, 5, and 10 J/cm^2 on normal back skin.

T ABLE 9.6.   **Drug-Induced Photosensitivity: Differential Diagnosis**

Phototoxic reaction

Systemic lupus erythematosus	No history of ingestion or application of a sensitizing compound. The rash is not limited to sun-exposed areas of the skin.
	Distinctive facial rash; positive antinuclear antibody (ANA) test titer.
Porphyria	No history of ingestion or application of a sensitizing compound. The rash is not limited to sun-exposed areas of the skin.
Pellagra	No history of ingestion or application of a sensitizing compound. The rash is not limited to sun-exposed areas of the skin.

Photoallergic reaction

Contact dermatitis	Occurs on any body surface, including non–sun-exposed skin.
	Photopatch tests may be necessary to differentiate.

Twenty-four hours later, the results of the first day's exposure are recorded, and only one set of patches is recovered, with opaque paper fixed in place. The two sets of patches are irradiated again with 5 J/cm^2 of UVA radiation.

On the fourth day, the irradiated and "patched" sites are examined again. A positive test result in a photoallergic patient shows a negative reaction in the control patch and a strongly erythematous to bullous reaction in the patch exposed to the UVA radiation. If the results of both patches are positive, a diagnosis of contact irritant dermatitis can be made.

- There are many variables in phototesting and photopatch testing, including concentrations of photoallergens for photopatch testing and UVR sources. Therefore it is recommended that, to achieve reproducible results, someone with the experience and necessary equipment perform these tests. Family physicians, if interested, can learn this technique.

Referral

- Consider referral for photopatch testing to determine the offending medication in either a phototoxic or photoallergic reaction. Experienced primary care physicians with the necessary equipment can perform phototesting and photopatch testing. If persistent photosensitivity affects a patient's activities of daily living, referral to a dermatologist is warranted.
- Referral to a dermatologist is indicated for patients whose photoallergic reactions necessitate immunosuppressive medications such as azathioprine (Imuran) or cyclosporine (Sandimmune).

Management

Identification and elimination of the causative agent are necessary for the successful treatment of both types of photosensitivity reactions.

Medications

See Tables 9.7 and 9.8.

Other Treatment Modalities

Physical

- Cool, moist dressings, bed rest, and oral rehydration are important general constitutional measures in patients with mild to moderate photosensitivity reactions.

Environmental

- *Sun protection* using a broad-spectrum sunscreen with an SPF greater than 15 that provides protection against both UVA and UVB radiation is an important preventive measure.
- *Protective clothing* such as headwear and long-sleeved garments also prevent minimum sun exposure.
- The *offending chemicals, medications, or cosmetics* should be avoided to preclude a repeat reaction (see Table 9.4).

Psychological

- Psychosocial support is important if the patient has severe chronic photoallergic reactions. These reactions are disfiguring and annoying, and can last from months to years, causing interruption of activities of daily living.

Patient Education

- Patients should be informed that it is not the drug alone, but the combination of the drug with sun exposure, that causes the rash.

T ABLE 9.7. Medical Treatment of Drug-Induced Photosensitivity

Hydrocortisone cream 1% (Nutracort), hydrocortisone valerate 0.2% (Westcort), alclometasone dipropionate 0.05% (Aclovate)

Availability:	Over the counter and prescription.
Dosage:	Applied topically to the *face* and *neck* 2 to 3 times daily.
Duration:	Until rash and symptoms resolve.
Comments:	First-line agents for mild symptoms. These are lower-potency agents. Long-term use of topical corticosteroids can cause skin atrophy.

Triamcinolone 0.1% cream (Aristocort)

Availability:	Prescription.
Dosage:	Applied topically 2 to 3 times daily.
Duration:	Use until rash and symptoms resolve.
Comments:	This fluorinated topical agent should be used for mild symptoms occurring on areas other than the face and neck (*i.e., recommended for hands, arms, and chest*). Minimal side effects with short-term use. Long-term use can cause skin atrophy.

Oral corticosteroids

Availability:	Prescription.
Dosage:	60 mg/daily initially orally, then taper by 10 to 20 mg/day every 1 to 2 days.
Duration:	7 to 10 days; expect some results in 48 hours.
Comments:	May be more beneficial for severe or widespread disease. Long-term use can inhibit the pituitary-adrenal axis.

- The medication can be used again, but to avoid a photosensitivity reaction, the patient should avoid sun exposure, wear protective clothing, or use sunscreens when taking the medication.
- In photoallergic reactions, the rash waxes and wanes over time and can occur with sun exposure even if the drug is discontinued.

T ABLE 9.8. Medical Treatment of Pruritus Associated with Drug-Induced Photosensitivity

Hydroxyzine hydrochloride (Atarax)

Availability:	Prescription only.
Dosage:	10 to 50 mg every 4 to 6 hours.
Duration:	As needed.
Comments:	To be used only when pruritus is present. Fatigue is a side effect; should not be used when driving or operating hazardous machinery. Concomitant use with alcohol should be avoided.

Cetirizine (Zyrtec)

Availability:	Prescription only.
Dosage:	10 mg every 24 hours.
Duration:	As needed.
Comments:	To be used only when pruritus is present. More expensive, but less sedating, than hydroxyzine.

- Patients should be informed that, although hypopigmentation may occur occasionally after the healing process, scarring rarely occurs with any sunburn after photosensitivity reactions.
- The photosensitivity reaction does not increase the likelihood for skin cancer; however, repeated exposure to UVR without the use of skin protection can lead to skin cancer.

Follow-up

When using systemic steroids, the patient should be followed at least weekly until treatment stops. Slower steroid weaning may be necessary. As with any systemic steroid use, adrenal suppression is a concern.

POLYMORPHOUS LIGHT ERUPTION

Polymorphous light eruption (PMLE) is an idiopathic, acquired photodermatosis characterized by a wide variety of delayed responses to UVR. This disease is commonly referred to as "sun poisoning."

Chief Complaint

Patients complain of the sudden onset of a pruritic rash on their trunk, arms, and legs.

Clinical Manifestations

- Exposed areas such as the forearms, neck, trunk, and legs are the most common sites; this rash usually spares the face.
- The lesions consist of clusters of confluent pink or red macules, papules, or papulovesicles. The rash may also consist of elevated erythematous lesions.
- This rash develops suddenly, within 24 hours to 3 days of UVR exposure; the rash may last 7 to 10 days.
- The rash is highly pruritic.
- Paresthesia (tingling) can also occur.

Epidemiology

- PMLE is the most common sun-sensitivity rash.
- This rash occurs most commonly in individuals in the third decade of life.
- PMLE can occur in individuals of all SPTs.
- It is more common in women.
- A hereditary (autosoal dominant) form of PMLE called actinic prurigo is commonly seen in Native Americans.

Risk Factors

- PMLE usually occurs with the first sun exposure of the season, in spring or early summer, to an area of the body that has not been previously exposed.
- PMLE usually does not occur at the end of the sun season because of the skin "hardening" to the sun's effect over time.
- Hypersensitivity reaction can be increased with subsequent exposures to sunlight.
- PMLE may also occur in patients who have traveled to a lower latitude or higher altitude where the intensity of the sun is greater.

PATHOLOGY

PMLE appears to be a delayed type (type IV) of hypersensitivity reaction in the skin to an antigen produced by UVR.

T ABLE 9.9. Differential Diagnosis: Polymorphous Light Eruption (PMLE)

Systemic lupus erythematosus (SLE)	Usually a violaceous red papular or plaquelike rash on the face and other sun-exposed areas, which makes SLE indistinguishable from PMLE. Laboratory tests and skin biopsy are useful to differentiate.
	SLE does not disappear in 7 to 10 days.
Contact dermatitis	History of exposure to systemic or topical drugs or cosmetics.
	May be indistinguishable from PMLE; photopatch testing may be useful to differentiate.

Diagnosis

Clinical presentation. The diagnosis is mainly clinical with a characteristic rash that has a delayed onset of eruption and disappears after 7 to 10 days. There is a history of sun exposure.

Differential Diagnosis

See Table 9.9.

Diagnostic Tests

- Appropriate laboratory studies such as antinuclear antibody (ANA), anti-SS-a (Ro), anti-SS-B (La), and anti-DNA titers should be obtained in patients with plaque-type PMLE, since it can be indistinguishable from systemic lupus erythematosus (SLE). Skin biopsy with subsequent histopathologic examination can also be helpful to rule out SLE.
- Results of phototesting, exposing a patient with suspected PMLE to both UVA and UVB radiation, can be positive in up to 50% of patients, thus confirming the diagnosis.

Referral

Depending on the treatment choice for severe cases, dermatologic referral may be very helpful. The patient may be referred to a dermatologist for phototesting if the physician is unfamiliar with this technique or does not have the necessary testing equipment.

Management

Medications

See Tables 9.10 and 9.11.

Other Treatment Modalities

Physical and environmental

- Avoidance of sunlight, especially between 11:00 A.M. and 3:00 P.M., wearing of protective clothing such as hats and long-sleeved shirts, and use of a good sunscreen providing both UVA and UVB coverage (greater than SPF 15) are the best preventive measures.

Psychological

- Because PMLE can be cosmetically disfiguring, psychological support from the physician is important.

T ABLE 9.10.   Medical Treatment of Polymorphous Light Eruption

Topical corticosteroids

Availability:	Over the counter and prescription.
Dosage:	Applied topically 2 to 3 times daily.
Duration:	7 to 10 days, or until rash resolves.
Comments:	Use of least- to mid-potency agents suggested. Not only helpful in treating the rash, but also decreases pruritus. Should not be used on the face or other areas of the skin for long periods (i.e., months). Prolonged use can cause skin atrophy.

Oral prednisone

Availability:	Prescription only.
Dosage:	60 mg daily for 2 to 3 days, then taper by 10 to 20 mg every 1 to 2 days.
Duration:	7 to 10 days.
Comments:	Useful when the rash and symptoms are more severe. Long-term use can cause serious systemic side effects.

T ABLE 9.11.   Treatment for Prevention of Polymorphous Light Eruption

Beta-carotene

Availability:	Over the counter.
Dosage:	180 mg orally daily starting 6 weeks before sun exposure.
Duration:	Begin use approximately 6 weeks before sun exposure and throughout sun exposure.
Comments:	Use before trying antimalarials and PUVA photochemotherapy. Can cause benign skin yellowing that resolves when the drug is stopped.

PUVA

Availability:	Desensitizing with PUVA photochemotherapy should be performed by a dermatologist.
Duration:	Three times per week for 3 to 4 weeks before sun exposure and throughout the spring and summer months.
Comments:	Can cause nausea after ingestion of psoralens; may also cause insomnia, nervousness, and depression. Erythema and pruritus may follow exposure to UVA radiation.

Hydroxychloroquine (an antimalarial) (Plaquenil)

Availability:	Prescription only.
Dosage:	200 mg twice daily.
Duration:	1 day before and each day during exposure to sunlight.
Comments:	For use only during sun exposure. Effective for chronic rashes or when response to steroids or beta-carotene is poor.
Side effects:	Can cause CNS reactions (vertigo and seizures); neuromuscular reactions (eye movement palsies); skeletal muscle weakness, absent deep-tendon reflexes; eye reactions (blurred vision, corneal deposits after 3 to 4 weeks, and muscular problems); skin reactions (pruritus, alopecia, and pigmentation); hematologic reactions (aplastic anemia, thrombocytopenia).
Follow-up:	An ophthalmologic examination should be performed every 3 months to detect development of retinal damage. A CBC should be performed every 4 to 6 weeks to detect hemotologic problems.

PUVA, psoralen plus ultraviolet A radiation; CNS, central nervous system; CBC, complete blood cell count.

Follow-up

Closely monitor patients on regimens of oral and topical steroids, and treat flare-ups accordingly. Encourage patients to think about PMLE each spring and prepare with sunscreens and other protective measures. Patients should be in touch with the physician at the first sign of a flare-up. PMLE usually resolves in 2 weeks and worsens with repeated episodes of sun exposure.

Patient Education

- Patients should be advised to adhere to the prescribed course of steroid treatments, for flare-ups to resolve successfully.
- PMLE is a delayed sensitivity to sun exposure; therefore avoidance of or protection against UVR is the only way to prevent this reaction from recurring. Light, densely woven, opaque clothing is the best protector against UVR exposure when outdoors. Light-colored clothes reflect sunlight better than dark-colored clothes.
- PMLE itself poses no malignant risk. However, repeated exposure to UVR without adequate precautions increases the risk for skin cancer.
- PMLE itself does not "age" skin faster, since it is only a hypersensitivity reaction to sun exposure. However, repeated doses of UVR over long periods without proper skin protection lead to skin aging.
- PMLE is caused by a sensitivity to sun exposure; cosmetics and moisturizers neither prevent nor cause PMLE.
- Patients should be reminded that SLE is an autoimmune disease and is not derived from PMLE.
- PMLE does not lead to any long-term complications.

BIBLIOGRAPHY

Emmett EA. Evaluation of the photosensitive patient. *Dermatol Clin* 1986;4(2): 195-202.

Hughes GS, Francom SF, Means LK, Bohan DF, Caruana C, Holland M. Synergistic effects of oral nonsteroidal drugs and topical corticosteroids in the therapy of sunburn in humans. *Dermatology* 1992;184:54-58.

Lichtenstein J, Flowers F, Sheretz EF. Nonsteroidal anti-inflammatory drugs: their use in dermatology. *Int J Dermatol* 1987;26(2):80-87.

Manders SM. Serious and life-threatening drug eruptions. *Am Fam Physician* 1995;51 (8):1865-1872.

Thompson SC, Jolley D, Marks R. Reduction of solar keratoses by regular sunscreen use. *N Engl J Med* 1993;329(16):1147-1151.

CHAPTER 10

··

Inflammatory Skin Disorders

PITYRIASIS ROSEA

Pityriasis rosea is a relatively common, self-limited inflammatory skin eruption of uncertain origin. It is a benign disorder that usually follows a characteristic, distinctive disease course.

Chief Complaint

Patients report a mildly to severely pruritic, plaque type of rash that is widely distributed over the trunk and proximal extremities. Pruritus is usually the only symptom present.

Clinical Manifestations

- The initial lesion, called the *herald patch,* is a typically singular, but occasionally multiple, erythematous lesion that is approximately 2 to 5 cm in diameter and is usually larger than the numerous individual lesions of the generalized rash. Although named the herald patch, it is often more plaquelike, being slightly raised with a fine scale near its periphery. This lesion occurs in 50% to 80% of patients (Figure 10.1, see color insert following page 170).
- Numerous exanthematous lesions (as many as 100) develop over a course of 1 to 2 weeks after the first presence of the herald patch. In the following 2 to 3 weeks considerable slowing of the exanthematous process is evident. Spontaneous remission within 6 to 12 weeks is typical.
- The lesion is generally a fine, dull pink or salmon-colored, scaly, oval plaque.
- While usually asymptomatic, 50% of patients report pruritis and 25% of patients report that the pruritis is severe.
- Lesions often bear a characteristic *marginal collarette;* that is, the light scale is attached peripherally with its free edge pointed toward the center. The scale is behind the advancing edge of the lesion, not at the advancing edge of the lesion, as seen in tinea.
- *Characteristic distribution* of the lesions demonstrates the long axis of their oval shape oriented along the lines of skin cleavage (called Langer lines). This orientation is most typically seen on the trunk and the proximal aspects of the extremities, creating the "Christmas tree" or "fir tree" pattern of distribution.
- Pityriasis rosea does not generally affect exposed areas such as the face, hands, or feet. In *atypical* pityriasis rosea, however, the rash is found on the face, hands or feet, axilla, groin, or neck. Distribution of the lesions in this atypical form is the same as that found in the more typical lesions.
- Pityriasis rosea may begin with macules or papules, but these always become plaques as the disease progresses. Papular lesions often predominate among dark-skinned individuals, pregnant women, and children.
- After spontaneous resolution of the lesions, there may be postinflammatory hyperpigmentation, especially in dark-skinned individuals.

- In approximately 20% of cases, patients report a recent history of upper respiratory tract infection–like symptoms just before the onset of the rash. Whether there is a clear etiologic association with these symptoms and pityriasis rosea remains unclear.

Epidemiology
Age
Three-fourths of cases occur among patients aged 10 years to 35 years, with a mean age of 23 years.

Sex
The condition is more common in female patients, with a ratio of 1.5:1.

Risk Factors
- Outbreaks are most common in spring and autumn, particularly in temperate climates.
- The condition often occurs among college-age students residing in close proximity, such as in dorm rooms or fraternity/sorority houses.
- Pityriasis rosea outbreaks have been reported at military bases.
- There is little contagious risk to family members, coworkers, or schoolmates.

PATHOLOGY
Dermatopathologic examination demonstrates focal spongiosis and microscopic vesicles of the epidermis with lack of a granular layer and diffuse or localized parakeratosis of the epidermis. The dermis demonstrates edema with lymphocytic and keratocytic infiltration.

Pityriasis rosea targets a specific age group, is seasonal, remits spontaneously, and has a rare recurrence rate; these facts suggest a viral origin. However, no virus has been discovered as a definitive cause for pityriasis rosea.

Diagnosis
Diagnosis is usually based on history and clinical presentation.

Differential Diagnosis
See Table 10.1.

Diagnostic Tests
- Skin biopsy for pityriasis rosea may be indicated in cases of persistent disease.
- A serologic test for syphilis is appropriate in all patients.
- A potassium hydroxide (KOH) smear can eliminate the possibility of fungus. See Chapter 17, Dermatophytosis (diagnostic tests) for a description of this procedure.

Referral
- If pruritus remains unresolved following the standard treatment modalities, referral may be warranted for consideration of ultraviolet B-range (UVB) light treatment.

T ABLE 10.1.   **Pityriasis Rosea: Differential Diagnosis**

Secondary syphilis	A nonpruritic genital rash is present. Serologic testing is useful to differentiate the two.
Drug reaction	Patient has a history of ingestion of captopril (Capoten), barbiturates, gold, metronidazole (Flagyl), bismuth compounds, or clonidine (Catapres).
Dermatophytosis	Hyphae or pseudohyphae are present. Free edge of scale points outward toward the leading edge of the rash. KOH examination is useful to differentiate between the two.
Lichen planus	These are mucous membrane lesions that are more erythematous than violaceous.
Seborrheic dermatitis	Greasy, irregularly shaped lesion.
Psoriasis	There is a different distribution, silver or white scale, and occasional nail involvement. There is no marginal collarette in guttate psoriasis.
Parapsoriasis	Lesions are more chronic than pityriasis rosea.

KOH, potassium hydroxide.

- If the lesions do not demonstrate evidence of spontaneous remission after 12 weeks, the patient may benefit from a referral for a skin biopsy to rule out parapsoriasis.

Management

Pityriasis rosea is a self-limited disease that remits spontaneously. Treatment with medication is indicated primarily to reduce pruritus (Table 10.2).

Other Treatment Modalities

- UVB light therapy over a course of five consecutive exposures is indicated in patients who are unresponsive to more typical treatment modalities.
- Increased exposure to natural sunlight may be of benefit.

Follow-up

In the presence of severe pruritus or pruritis that is unresponsive to initial conservative treatment, or when using long-term corticosteroid therapy, follow-up as often as every 2 weeks is indicated.

Patient Education

- Patients should be informed that, although the initial appearance of pityriasis rosea is somewhat alarming, it is a self-limited disease that should spontaneously remit in 6 to 12 weeks.
- They should also be cautioned that during treatment new lesions may develop, but these newer lesions will regress spontaneously as well.
- Patients may be reassured that lesions do not usually affect the arms or face, nor do the lesions leave scars on remission.
- In general, it is not believed that pityriasis rosea is contagious. Patients may be reassured that the disease is not a blood-borne disease, nor does it affect any internal organs.

T ABLE 10.2.   Medical Treatment of Pityriasis Rosea

Topical

Colloidal oatmeal baths (Aveeno)

Availability:	OTC.
Dosage:	One packet in 6 to 8 inches of bath water; soak 10 to 15 minutes every day or every other day.
Duration:	Until pruritus resolves.
Comments:	Minimal side effects; initial conservative treatment.

Topical calamine lotion

Availability:	OTC.
Dosage:	Apply daily to lesions.
Duration:	Until pruritus resolves.
Comments:	Minimal side effects.

Oral antihistamines

Diphenhydramine (Benadryl)

Availability:	OTC.
Dosage:	*Adults:* 25 to 50 mg 4 times per day as needed.
	Children: 5 mg/kg per day, divided every 6 hours, 12.5 mg/5 mL, as needed.
Duration:	Until pruritus resolves.
Comments:	Can cause drowsiness.

Hydroxyzine (Atarax)

Availability:	Prescription.
Dosage:	*Adults:* 25 to 50 mg 4 times per day as needed.
	Children: 2 to 5 mg/kg per day, divided every 6 hours, 10 mg/5 mL.
Duration of use:	Until pruritus resolves.
Comments:	Can cause drowsiness.

Topical corticosteroids

Triamcinolone 0.1% cream (Aristocort)

Availability:	Prescription.
Dosage:	Apply every night, advancing to twice daily as necessary.
Duration:	Until pruritus resolves.
Comments:	Long-term use can cause skin atrophy or telangiectasia. Use only if pruritus is persistent or severe; starting with lowest effective potency, avoid on face, groin and axilla.

Oral prednisone

Availability:	Prescription.
Dosage:	Up to 20 mg twice daily, taper by 5 mg to 10 mg every 2 to 3 days.
Duration:	7 to 21 days.
Comments:	Long-term use can inhibit the pituitary-adrenal axis. Use only in cases of severe pruritus.

OTC, over the counter.

- Pityriasis rosea has not been shown to have any effect on the fetus of a pregnant woman who is passively exposed or actively affected by the disorder.
- Patients should be advised that pityriasis rosea recurs in approximately 2% of cases.

GRANULOMA ANNULARE

Granuloma annulare is a moderately common granulomatous or focal chronic inflammation that becomes evident by an annular arrangement of self-limited, asymptomatic papules, usually affecting the dermis on the dorsa of the hands, feet, elbows, and knees.

Chief Complaint

- Patients report annular, papular, beaded lesions or subcutaneous nodules causing cosmetic concerns. The lesions are essentially asymptomatic.
- Some patients have a more generalized form consisting of hundreds of erythematous to tan papular lesions throughout the trunk and on the extremities. These lesions may have been present for months to years.

Clinical Manifestations

- Granuloma annulare presents as a nodule on the dorsa of hands, feet, fingers, or extensor aspects of the arms, legs, and trunk, which slowly progresses to an expanding, ringlike lesion (Figure 10.2, see color insert following page 170).
- No scaling or pruritus is usually evident.
- The localized form usually spontaneously regresses after several months to several years.
- The primary skin lesion comprises skin-colored, yellowish, or erythematous papules lacking scales. The lesion coalesces, ultimately assuming an annular form that tends to enlarge in a centrifugal manner. Some lesions, however, may be arciniform.
- These lesions are rarely larger than 5 cm in diameter.
- Granuloma annulare lesions are distributed to the dorsa of the hands, feet, and fingers and extensor aspects of the arms, legs, and trunk. However, in the generalized form, hundreds of circular lesions may be found, particularly on the trunk and extremities.
- Subcutaneous nodules in granuloma annulare may also be found in the palms, legs, scalp, and buttocks.

Epidemiology

Age

- Granuloma annulare primarily affects children and young adults.
- The generalized form often affects older individuals in the fourth to seventh decades of life, whereas the more common localized form usually affects individuals in the first three decades of life.

Sex

Lesions occur more in female patients, with a ratio of approximately 2.5:1.

Risk Factors

- *Recurrences* can develop in 40% of patients.
- *Endocrine.* The generalized form of granuloma annulare appears to have an increased association with diabetes mellitus.

PATHOLOGY

Dermatopathologic examination demonstrates superficial and middermal areas of inflammation and histiocytic infiltration. Connective tissue may be surrounded by histocytes and multinucleic giant cells and have evidence of incomplete and reversible necrobiosis, thereby altering collagen and elastic tissues.

Although localized trauma, immune-complex vasculitis, and cell-mediated immunity have all been proposed as a possible cause, no specific etiologic agent for granuloma annulare is known.

Diagnosis

Diagnosis is primarily based on clinical presentation and history. A biopsy of the lesion should be performed only if the diagnosis is uncertain.

Differential Diagnosis

See Table 10.3.

Referral

- Referral to a dermatologist may be indicated if the diagnosis is uncertain, if the rash does not respond to conventional treatment modalities, or if the patient has diffuse disease with discomfort.
- Referral is also indicated for patients requiring psoralen ultraviolet A-range (PUVA) photochemotherapy.

Management

The medical management of granuloma annulare is located in Table 10.4. Granuloma annulare regresses spontaneously within several years of development.

Other Treatment Modalities

PUVA photochemotherapy may be indicated in some cases of generalized granuloma annulare.

T ABLE 10.3.   Granuloma Annulare: Differential Diagnosis

Tinea corporis	Scales and hyphae are present.
	KOH preparation is useful to differentiate between the two.
Lichen planus	Lesions are distinguished by the presence of symmetric, flat-topped papules, Wickham striae, and associated mucous membrane lesions.
	Biopsy may be useful to differentiate the two.
Secondary syphilis	Serologic testing for syphilis is necessary to differentiate the two.
Rheumatoid arthritis	Morning stiffness, joint pain and deformities, and malaise are present in rheumatoid arthritis.
	Rheumatoid factor test useful to differentiate the two.
Urticaria	Transient rather than lingering lesions are present.
Erythema multiforme	Erythematous, transient lesions are present.

KOH, potassium hydroxide.

TABLE 10.4.   Medical Treatment of Granuloma Annulare

Potent topical steroids

Availability:	Prescription.
Dosage:	Apply topically twice daily, cover with occlusive dressing.
Duration:	Up to several years, until rash regresses.
Comments:	Long-term use may cause skin atrophy or telangiectasia.

Intralesional triamcinolone acetonide (3.0 to 10 mg/mL concentration)

Availability:	Prescription.
Dosage:	Inject 1 to 2 mL intralesionally along the elevated border.
Duration:	Use every 1 to 2 weeks until rash regresses without causing skin atrophy.
Comments:	Treatment can cause skin atrophy. Use for localized lesions.

Liquid nitrogen

Availability:	Prescription.
Dosage:	See Appendix B for administration.
Duration:	May be repeated in 2 to 3 weeks.
Comments:	Skin atrophy may occur.

Follow-up

Granuloma annulare may persist for 1 to 2 years. Follow-up every 2 to 4 weeks is necessary when using potent topical or intralesional corticosteroids, to monitor for skin atrophy (Table 10.4).

Patient Education

- Patients should be reassured that the rash regresses spontaneously in 75% of cases, but may take 1 to 2 years to completely resolve.
- Granuloma annulare is a local skin disorder which does not affect the internal organs or blood.
- Patients should be advised that there is a 40% recurrence rate.
- Patients may be reassured that granuloma annulare is not contagious.

LICHEN PLANUS

Lichen planus is a relatively uncommon, benign inflammatory skin eruption of insidious or acute onset, which can last months to years. It is often characterized as "the disease of the four P's": *P*urple, *P*ruritic, *P*lanar, and *P*olyangular.

Chief Complaint

Patients complain of a flat-topped, pruritic skin eruption usually affecting the wrists, ankles, groin, or genitalia, with or without oral mucous membrane involvement. The rash occasionally may be generalized.

Clinical Manifestations

- Lichen planus begins with a relatively rapid onset of pruritic lesions. Onset may be acute over the course of a few days or more gradual over the course of a few weeks (Figure 10.3, see color insert following page 170).
- Papules and papulosquamous lesions coalesce to form the characteristic planar eruption of lichen planus (Figure 10.4, see color insert following page 170).

- A fine, reticular pattern (known as *Wickham striae*) may be seen on the top of the eruption by rubbing the lesion with an alcohol swipe or oil to enhance the fine, white, polyangular etched lines that are pathognomonic for lichen planus.
- The lesions have a shiny surface with a slight scale.
- Secondary skin findings generally include obvious lichenification, scaling, and excoriation from scratching.
- During the time of active disease, development of typical lichen planus–like lesions in localized areas of minor trauma to the skin (called the *Koebner phenomenon*) may be observed.
- Except for the cutaneous manifestations and the pruritus, patients are usually asymptomatic.
- At the time of the outbreak, or just before the onset of the eruption, patients may describe a period of particular emotional upset or stress.
- Although the lesions of lichen planus are self-limited and spontaneously resolve, there can be residual postinflammatory hyperpigmentation in the affected areas of the skin.
- *Average duration* of the lesions is 9 months; however, a more chronic condition can occur that may persist for years.
- The *distribution of lesions* is often symmetric, generally occurring on the flexural body surfaces, particularly the wrists and ankles. In some cases, however, the rash may be generalized. This rash is rarely seen on palms and soles.
- *Other common presentations* include the oral mucosa and the genitalia. The oral lesions are generally present in the buccal mucosa and demonstrate lacy, white or gray lesions in a reticular pattern. These oral lesions, which occur in up to 75% of all cases of lichen planus, may occasionally ulcerate and become painful.
- Typical eruptions involving the genitalia, particularly the penis, are usually annular lesions with a light-colored border.
- Other physical findings associated with lichen planus include nail involvement. When affected, the nails demonstrate a thin nail plate with longitudinal striation that could lead to total nail loss.

Variations of Lichen Planus

- *Lichen planus actinicus.* Papular lesions occur in sun-exposed areas, such as the dorsum of hands and arms.
- *Follicular lichen planus.* Keratotic, follicular papules and plaques, which may lead to scarring alopecia of the scalp, are present. Typical cutaneous and mucous membrane lesions of lichen planus may accompany this variant.
- *Vesicular lichen planus.* Vesicular or bullous lesions develop within lichen planus lesions or independent of the plaques and papules of lichen planus.
- *Ulcerative lichen planus.* Painful bullae and ulcers, especially on the soles and mucous membranes, are present. This variation can also cause scarring alopecia. The condition may become therapy resistant and necessitate skin grafting.
- *Lichen sclerosis et atrophicus (LSA).* Well-defined, angular, white, mucocutaneous plaques and papules cause a chronic atrophic disorder. These lesions may be non-genital in distribution, affecting the trunk, neck, and axilla while rarely affecting the palms and soles; or genital in distribution, affecting the vulvar perineum and peri-anal regions in female patients and the prepuce and glans penis in male patients.

Epidemiology
Age
Lichen planus commonly occurs in individuals from 30 to 60 years of age; the condition is rare in children.

Sex
It generally affects women more than men.

Risk Factors

- *Drugs.* Certain drugs, such as angiotensin-converting enzyme (ACE) inhibitors [captopril (Capoten)], thiazide diuretics, chlorpropamide (Diabinese), furosemide (Lasix), quinidine, propranolol (Inderal), antimalarial agents, gold, streptomycin, methyldopa (Aldomet), and tetracycline, may induce a lichen planus–like eruption.
- *Family history.* Lichen planus occurs in up to 10% of first-degree relatives of patients affected by the disease.

PATHOLOGY

Pathogenesis of lichen planus is poorly understood at present, but is most likely to be caused by an underlying abnormality in immune response. On histopathologic examination there is a characteristic degeneration of the basal layer of the epidermis with hyperkeratosis, hypergranulosis, and acanthosis of the epidermis. The dermis demonstrates an infiltration of lymphocytes and macrophages.

Although the etiologic agent is largely unknown, emotional stress and upset may cause exacerbation.

Diagnosis

Diagnosis is generally based on clinical presentation and physical finding.

Differential Diagnosis

See Table 10.5.

Diagnostic Tests

- *Deep shave or punch biopsy* of the lesion reveals focal increases in the third cellular (or granular) layer of the epidermis, downward projection of the epidermal layer (rete pegs), and inflammatory infiltrates or lymphocytes beneath the epidermis.
- Coexistent candidal infections may occur in oral or genital lichen planus. Use *KOH preparation* to rule out coexistent infection.

Referral

- Referral may be indicated if diagnosis is uncertain or standard treatment modalities have provided little benefit.
- Referral may also be indicated for patients who require PUVA photochemotherapy.

TABLE 10.5. Lichen Planus: Differential Diagnosis

Lichenoid drug reaction	Reaction is associated with drug ingestion. Biopsy is useful to differentiate the two.
Psoriasis	Lesions appear on the extensor surfaces and have a shinier scale. They are rarely pruritic. Biopsy may be useful to differentiate the two.
Pityriasis rosea	Herald patch is present, and there is a different distribution of lesions. Biopsy is useful to differentiate the two.
Secondary syphilis	Skin eruption is nonpruritic and is present on palms and soles. VDRL is often positive.

VDRL, Venereal Disease Research Laboratory test for syphilis.

TABLE 10.6.   **Medical Treatment of Lichen Planus**

Topical corticosteroids

Availability:	Prescription.
Dosage:	Apply topically twice daily, cover with occlusive dressing.
Duration:	Until lesions resolve.
Comments:	Long-term use can cause skin atrophy and telangiectasia. Use for mild to moderate disease. Start with low to moderate potency, then advance to a higher potency, if needed. Occlusive dressing is the treatment of choice to combat the inflammation and pruritus of localized lesions. If applied to localized lesions of the lower legs, occlusive dressings may aid resolution of untreated lesions elsewhere on the body as the treated lesions improve. See Appendix A for further details.

Triamcinolone acetonide (5 to 10 mg/mL)

Availability:	Prescription.
Dosage:	Inject 0.5 to 1 mL per 2-cm lesion.
Duration:	May be repeated in 2 to 3 weeks.
Comments:	Long-term use can cause skin atrophy and telangiectasia. Use for hypertrophic lesions.

Oral prednisone

Availability:	Prescription.
Dosage:	60 mg daily tapered over 2 to 8 weeks.
Duration:	2 to 8 weeks.
Comments:	Rash may recur when steroids are stopped; taper slowly. For severe symptoms such as pruritus, painful erosions, and cosmetic disfigurement. Long-term use will inhibit the pituitary-adrenal axis and cause serious systemic problems.

Oral antihistamines

Diphenhydramine (Benadryl)

Availability:	Over the counter.
Dosage:	25 to 50 mg every 6 hours as needed.
Duration:	Until pruritus resolves.
Comments:	May cause drowsiness.

Hydroxyzine (Atarax)

Availability:	Prescription.
Dosage:	25 to 50 mg every 6 hours as needed.
Duration:	Until pruritus resolves.
Comments:	May cause drowsiness.

Triamcinolone in orabase (Kenalog in Orabase) or flucinonide (0.05 gel)

Availability:	Prescription.
Dosage:	Apply to mucosal lesions 2 to 3 times daily.
Duration:	Until lesions resolve.
Comments:	Use for mucosal lesions.

Management

Management of lichen planus should be focused on discovery and elimination of all potentially causative medications.

Medications

See Table 10.6.

Other Treatment Modalities

PUVA photochemotherapy may be indicated for generalized lichen planus or in patients for whom standard treatment was ineffective.

Follow-up

Monitoring Disease Course

Follow-up is individualized to the patient, keeping in mind that the disease is largely chronic with a 9-month average duration. Routine follow-up at approximately 2-week intervals to monitor for skin changes and atrophy is advised for patients who may be using potent topical steroids.

Potential Problems and Complications

There have been reported associations of lichen planus and underlying malignancies. These associations are typically described with variants of lichen planus. Lichen planus pemphigoides is associated with stomach cancer, lymphosarcoma, neuroblastoma, and craniopharyngioma, and vesicular lichen planus is associated with pituitary cancer. No cause-and-effect relationship has been clearly identified.

Patient Education

- Patients should be informed that, although medications may provide resolution of the symptoms and spontaneous remissions do occur, lichen planus can be a chronic, recurrent disease.
- They should also be advised to avoid excessive bathing with very hot water and the use of harsh soaps.
- Patients may be reassured that lichen planus is not transmissible to others.
- Because lichen planus may be exacerbated by stress, behavioral modification and stress management techniques may be helpful to some patients.

BIBLIOGRAPHY

Barron DF, Cootauco MH, Cohen BA. Granuloma annulare: a clinical review. *Lippincott's Prim Care Pract* 1997;3(1):33-39.

Boyd AS, Neldner KH. Lichen planus. *J Am Acad Dermatol* 1991;25(4):593-619.

Oliver GF, Winkelmann RK. Treatment of lichen planus. *Drugs* 1993;45(1):56-65.

Shai A, Halevy S. Lichen planus and lichen planus–like eruptions: pathogenesis and associated diseases. *Int J Dermatol* 1992;31(6):379-384.

CHAPTER 11

··

Disorders of Skin Pigment

VITILIGO

Vitiligo is a common skin disorder characterized by depigmented macules that may coalesce as a complete absence of skin melanocytes over an extensive area.

Chief Complaint

Patients report single or multiple white patches of skin located on the face and hands and express concern about the appearance of these *patches* (Figure 11.1, see color insert following page 170).

Clinical Manifestations

- Macules range from 5 mm to 5 cm in diameter.
- These lesions can be completely white or off-white to cream colored.
- The depigmented area can gradually progress to a larger lesion, or new lesions can develop.
- Vitiligo lesions, while usually asymptomatic, can become inflamed where the macule becomes elevated with a red margin and can be pruritic.
- The usual margin is convex and confluent with the normally pigmented surrounding skin.
- The depigmented area is usually symmetric and can be round, oval, or elongated.
- Vitiligo is usually distributed around the eyes and mouth; on the digits, elbows, and knees; and on the low back and genital areas.
- The lesion may slowly progress or remain stable for years.
- Repigmentation can occur spontaneously around hair follicles, causing small islands of pigmented skin in the vitiliginous macule; this occurs in 10% to 20% of patients.

Epidemiology

Age

Vitiligo can occur at any age, but 50% of cases begin between the ages of 10 and 30 years, with occurrences reported in patients up to age 60 years. Vitiligo has also been reported in newborns.

Race

Vitiligo has been observed in patients of all races.

Sex

These lesions occur more often in female patients.

Population

This depigmentation affects approximately 1% to 2% of the population in the United States.

Risk Factors

- Vitiligo appears to be an inherited disease (autosomal dominant with a family history of vitiligo, halo nevi, or premature graying of hair) with 30% of patients reporting a parent or sibling with vitiligo.
- It is associated with thyroid disease, adrenal insufficiency, biliary cirrhosis, rheumatoid arthritis, scleroderma, alopecia areata, pernicious anemia, and diabetes mellitus.
- Patients often report predisposing factors such as physical trauma, concomitant medical illness, sunburn, or considerable emotional stress.

PATHOLOGY

Although the exact etiology is uncertain, vitiligo is most likely an autoimmune disease causing absent and abnormal melanocytes.

Diagnosis

Diagnosis of vitiligo is based on clinical findings and physical examination.

Differential Diagnosis

See Table 11.1.

T ABLE 11.1.   Vitiligo: Differential Diagnosis

Piebaldism	There is an absence of pigmentation on trunk or head, usually seen at birth, and is genetically inherited.
Discoid lupus erythematosis	Lesion is usually asymmetric with postinflammatory hypopigmentation. Biopsy and ANA test may be useful to differentiate the two.
Pityriasis alba	Lesions are off-white, slight scaling with fuzzy margins, and commonly seen on the face. Biopsy may be useful to differentiate the two.
Pityriasis versicolor	Fungal infection, causes skin not to tan at the same rate as unaffected skin. There is a positive KOH prep result.
Leprosy	Hypopigmented areas are usually anesthetic.
Tuberous sclerosis	Lesion is a hypopigmented macule on the trunk or limb, may be in the shape of an ash leaf. It is usually seen on infants. It may be accentuated by Wood's lamp. Biopsy may be useful to differentiate between the two.
Post-inflammatory hypopigmentation	There is hypopigmentation rather than absence of pigment and a history of trauma or inflammation. Biopsy may be useful to differentiate the two.
Morphea (localized sclerodema)	Lesion is an atrophic, hypopigmented plaque with thin skin and a rim of inflammation. Biopsy and ANA test may be useful to differentiate the two.

ANA, antinuclear antibody; KOH, potassium hydroxide.

Diagnostic Tests

- In the event that diagnosis is uncertain, *skin biopsy with histologic investigation* may be indicated.
- Patients with vitiligo have an increased frequency of hyperthyroidism and hypothyroidism, insulin-dependent diabetes mellitus, pernicious anemia, Hashimoto thyroiditis, rheumatoid arthritis, Addison disease, biliary cirrhosis, alopecia areata, multiple endocrinopathies, autoimmune diseases, and gastrointestinal tract cancers. Laboratory studies such as thyroid-simulating hormone and thyroxine levels (T4) tests; erythrocyte sedimentation rate; liver function and Venereal Disease Research Laboratory testing; fasting blood glucose level; complete blood count with indices; antithyroid antibody (thyroglobulin and microsomal), antiparietal cell antibody, and antinuclear antibody tests; and an adrenocorticotropic hormone (ACTH) stimulation test can be performed to eliminate the possibility of systemic illness.
- Chorioretinitis and iritis can be associated in 10% of patients with vitiligo. Therefore a *baseline eye examination* is necessary in these patients and should be repeated periodically.

Referral

Referral to a dermatologist may be indicated for cosmetic camouflage, topical and systemic photochemotherapy, autologous grafting, repigmentation, or depigmentation.

Management

Management of vitiligo is twofold, involving repigmentation or depigmentation of the skin as well as managing any possible concomitant systemic disease.

Medications

See Table 11.2.

Other Treatment Modalities

- Topical or oral photochemotherapy is a repigmentation option when topical corticosteriods are not helpful. Repigmentation is designed to cause a permanent return of the normal melanin pigmentation. This goal can be achieved by the use of topical photochemotherapy with 8-methoxypsoralen or systemic photochemotherapy with trimethylpsoralen or 5-methoxypsoralen. Photochemotherapy [psoralen ultraviolet A-range (PUVA)] should be performed by an experienced physician who is knowledgeable about repigmentation. PUVA photochemotherapy is effective in more than 75% of patients with vitiligo. A baseline eye examination is nec-

T ABLE 11.2. Medical Treatment of Vitiligo

Topical corticosteroids

Availability:	Prescription.
Dosage:	*Adults and children:* Apply daily.
Duration:	*Adults:* 4 to 6 months.
	Children: 4 months.
Side effects:	Long-term use can cause skin atrophy, telangiectasia, or adrenal suppression.
Comments:	Midpotency is first line; 50% success rate. If repigmentation occurs, repeat until no further response is obtained. Follow-up every 4 weeks to watch for side effects; discontinue if side effects develop. See Appendix A for more details.

essary in patients who are considering photochemotherapy and should be repeated in 6 months and then yearly.

- Autologous minigrafting is an option that can be used in conjunction with PUVA photochemotherapy or by itself. Surgical referral is recommended for this technique.
- Cosmetic cover-up or makeup, such as Clinique, Covermark, or Dermablend, is also useful to hide the vitiligo. Agents with dihydroxyacetone such as Vitadye or Chromelin are effective dyes or stains to cover the vitiligo. The dyes last longer than cosmetic cover-ups. These agents can be used alone or in conjunction with medication to camouflage the vitiligo until the medication can take effect.
- Depigmentation therapy, using a bleaching agent with 20% monobenzone, is a process whereby the normal pigmented skin is bleached to more closely resemble the vitiligo. Depigmentation is successful in about 90% of the cases and is particularly efficacious for patients with vitiligo across more than 50% of the body or face and in those patients whose lesions have been resistant to other therapies. Because this is a permanent, irreversible process, referral to a dermatologist is recommended.

Follow-up
Monitoring Disease Course

Follow-up consists primarily of reinforcing compliance with the dermatologist's treatment plan. Patients using topical corticosteriods should be followed up every 4 weeks to keep track of potential skin side effects.

Potential Problems and Complications

Skin cancers arising from vitiligo appear to be rare.

Patient Education

- Patients should be counseled to comply carefully with the treatment of vitiligo.
- Although it is possible for vitiligo depigmentation to spread, patients should be advised that it can also remain stable.
- Vitiligo is an inherited disease in 30% of patients.
- Vitiligo is a chronic disease that cannot be prevented. Up to 20% of patients may report some spontaneous repigmentation, usually in sun-exposed areas. The treatment of vitiligo-associated disease such as thyroid disease or pernicious anemia has no impact on the vitiligo that has already occurred.
- Patients should be cautioned that lesions of vitiligo may be subject to severe sunburn, making avoidance of sun exposure desirable. Sunscreens of skin protection factor (SPF) 30 or higher, protecting against both ultraviolet A-range and ultraviolet B-range (UVA and UVB) radiation, are recommended to minimize tanning. This limits the tanning reaction of normal skin and protects the vitiligo from acute sunburn.
- Vitiligo does not progress to serious illness, but several illnesses such as diabetes, thyroid disease, pernicious anemia, and adrenal disease can be associated with these lesions.
- Patients should be reassured that vitiligo rarely develops into skin cancer.
- Patients with large, obvious patches of vitiligo can often suffer emotional stress resulting from the disfiguring quality of these lesions. The physician should counsel these patients and give them hope about successful treatment options. Patients can also contact the National Vitiligo Foundation (telephone: 903-531-0074).

MELASMA

Melasma, also known as chloasma or the "mask of pregnancy," is a hyperpigmentation occurring in exposed skin surfaces associated with pregnancy or the use of certain medications.

Chief Complaint

Patients, usually pregnant women, report blotchy brown pigmentation on the face.

Clinical Manifestations

- Melasma evolves rapidly over weeks, particularly with a great deal of sun exposure (Figure 11.2).
- Hyperpigmentation usually resolves spontaneously over several months following delivery or after discontinuing medication.
- The macular rash, which is light to dark brown, is arranged symmetrically on the face and may have irregular borders. The color is usually uniform, but can be blotchy.
- The rash is usually seen in the cheeks, forehead, nose, upper lip, and chin and sometimes on the dorsum of the forearm.
- Wood lamp examination can aid in the diagnosis by accentuating the hyperpigmented macules.

Epidemiology

The rash is seen more frequently in individuals of skin phototypes 4, 5, and 6 (SPT 4, SPT 5, and SPT 6) (see Chapter 9, Table 9.1).

Age

Hyperpigmentation occurs most often in young adults.

Sex

Only 10% of patients with melasma are male.

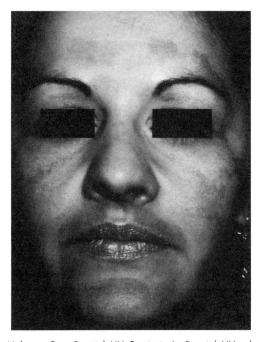

FIGURE 11.2. Melasma. From Roenigk HH. Psoriasis. In: Roenigk HH, ed. *Office dermatology.* Baltimore: Williams & Wilkins, 1981:272, with permission.

Season
Melasma develops most often in the summer months.

Risk Factors
- Melasma is inherited, but the mode of inheritance is unknown.
- Investigators have reported a correlation between thyroid autoimmune disease and melasma.
- Some women have increased levels of leutinizing hormone (LH) and lower levels of estradiol.

PATHOLOGY

Melasma is caused by increased melanin in the epidermis that is exacerbated by sun exposure. The rash has multiple etiologic factors, including pregnancy, cosmetic use, genetic predisposition, use of estrogen-progesterone therapy, intense sun exposure, oral contraceptive use, thyroid dysfunction, or phenytoin (Dilantin) use.

Diagnosis
Diagnosis is based on physical examination and patient history; biopsy is unnecessary.

Differential Diagnosis
See Table 11.3.

Management
- *No medication is recommended during pregnancy.*
- Pregnant women should, however, be counseled to avoid sun exposure.

Medications
See Table 11.4.

Other Treatment Modalities
- Laser treatments have been used with only minimal success.
- The hypopigmentation effect of hydroquinone (Eldoquin Forte) can be enhanced if the agent is used in conjunction with tretinoin. Tretinoin should be added to the hypopigmentation regimen in difficult-to-treat cases starting with the lowest strength and increasing if no additive effect is noted.

T ABLE 11.3. Melasma: Differential Diagnosis

Postinflammatory hyperpigmentation	There is a history of an inflammatory lesion on the face. Lesion does not worsen or spread with sun exposure.
Tar melanosis	There is a history of exposure to tar products or cosmetics on the face causing contact dermatitis and hyperpigmentation.

T ABLE 11.4. Medical Treatment of Melasma

Bleaching agents for nonpregnant patients

Topical hydroquinone 2% (Esoterica)

Availability:	Over the counter.
Dosage:	Apply topically twice daily to reduce pigmentation.
Duration:	Use for 2 to 4 months.
Side effects:	Can cause ochronosis (bluish-black skin pigmentation); mostly associated with the 2% over-the-counter preparation; can cause allergic or irritant dermatitis.
Comments:	Apply to small test area of skin 2 or 3 times before beginning daily therapy to identify any potential allergic or irritant reactions. Use skin protection factor (SPF) 30 sunscreens between treatments to reduce repigmentation.

Topical hydroquinone 3% solution with sunblock (Melanex); 4% cream or gel with sunblock (Solaquin Forte); cream without sunblock (Eldoquin Forte)

Availability:	Prescription.
Dosage:	Apply topically twice daily to reduce pigmentation.
Duration:	Use for 2 to 4 months.
Side effects:	Can cause ochronosis (bluish-black skin pigmentation); mostly associated with the 2% over-the-counter preparation; can cause allergic or irritant dermatitis.
Comments:	Apply to small test area of skin 2 or 3 times before beginning daily therapy to identify any potential allergic or irritant reactions. Use SPF 30 sunscreens between treatments to reduce repigmentation.

Tretinoin 0.05% or 0.1% cream (Retin-A)

Availability:	Prescription.
Dosage:	Apply topically once at bedtime.
Duration:	Use for 4 to 6 months.
Side effects:	Can cause erythema, dryness, or stinging.
Comments:	Apply to small test skin site 2 or 3 times before daily use to see if an irritant dermatitis reaction occurs; can cause postinflammatory hyperpigmentation.

Azelaic acid 20% (Azelex)

Availability:	Prescription.
Administration:	Apply topically twice daily.
Duration of use:	Use until desired hypopigmentation is achieved.
Side effects:	Can cause erythema, burning, scaling, and pruritus.
Comments:	This antiacne cream may cause hypopigmentation by inhibiting overactive melanocytes.

Chemical peel

Glycolic acid (35%, 50%, and 70%)

Dosage:	Remove surface oils from skin with cleanser; apply glycolic acid with sponge or sable brush to hyperpigmented area for 3 to 5 minutes, then neutralize the acid.
Duration:	Repeat weekly, biweekly, or monthly until desired effect is reached.
Side effects:	Can cause burning or scarring of skin if not neutralized or if left on too long. Can cause hypopigmentation in darker-skinned individuals.
Comments:	For moderate to severe disease. Use lower concentrations first; increase strength if unresponsive.

Follow-up

Patients using hydroquinone should be followed up within 1 to 2 weeks after initial therapy to monitor for allergic or irritant dermatitis, then every 4 weeks to check for signs of ochronosis.

Patient Education

- Patients should be advised to avoid sun exposure; patients who must be exposed to sun should use opaque sunblocks of SPF 30 or higher containing titanium dioxide or zinc oxide.
- All patients, including those who are not pregnant, should be reminded about using sunscreens to help prevent further hyperpigmentation.
- Additional measures include wearing protective clothing and avoiding sun exposure from 11:00 A.M. and 3:00 P.M., when UVA and UVB radiation are the most intense.
- Patients may be reassured that melasma usually disappears spontaneously over several months after pregnancy; however, patients whose rash is attributable to oral contraceptives should be made aware that the rash may persist longer following discontinuation of these medications.
- Patients whose rash is caused by oral contraceptives should be advised to cease taking these medications. Although it may not necessarily spread, the rash will continue to persist. If an alternative birth control agent is inadvisable, the physician may recommend bleaching agents to minimize the contrast between the rash and surrounding skin.
- Mild ovarian dysfunction can also lead to hyperpigmentation on the face. Some researchers have also reported a correlation between certain autoimmune thyroid diseases and melasma.

BIBLIOGRAPHY

Grimes PE. Melasma: etiologic and therapeutic considerations. *Arch Dermatol* 1995; 131:1453–1457.

Grimes PE. Vitiligo: an overview of therapeutic approaches. *Dermatol Clin* 1993;11: 325–338.

CHAPTER 12

....

Immune and Autoimmune Disorders

BASICS

Immune Hypersensitivity Types

There are four classically defined types of immune hypersensitivity, or inflammation. Although there is crossover among these types in defining the pathophysiology of some diseases, and while some reactions and disease processes remain poorly understood, the majority of diseases can be explained by one type of inflammation (Table 12.1).

Complement

The complement cascade system comprises more than 20 plasma proteins that interact in two pathways:

- The classic pathway is activated by the binding of C1 to, primarily, antigen antibody immune complexes.
- The alternative pathway can be activated by immunoglobulin A (IgA) immune complexes and also by nonimmunologic substances such as bacterial endotoxins.

The pathways produce components that act as anaphylactic mediators, stimulating histamine release and enhancing phagocytosis of the offending agents. Enhancement of phagocytosis is by opsonization, or coating, of the offending antigen with complement and immunoglobulins for increased recognition by phagocyte cells (Table 12.2).

URTICARIA

Chief Complaint

Patients complain of red, severely pruritic hives of sudden onset. While some patients cannot identify a specific trigger to the event, others may describe a history of urticaria when exposed to certain allergens. The underlying cause of urticaria is identifiable in less than 50% of cases (Table 12.3).

Clinical Manifestations

- Urticaria appears as erythematous, raised circles or wheals ranging from 2 to 8 mm in size (Figure 12.1, see color insert following page 170).
- The lesions may be confluent.
- Initially the lesions are red and papular, with faint white halos. Over time, these lesions assume the appearance of plaques, occasionally with scaling.
- Symptoms include pruritus, burning, pain, wheezing, dyspnea, fever, stridor, flushing, and hoarseness.

T ABLE 12.1.   Immune Hypersensitivity Reactions

Reaction type	Mechanism	Signs and symptoms	Examples
I. Anaphylactic	Immediate reaction (within 30 minutes). IgE mediated Antigens bind with mast cells, causing degranulation of histamine, which causes immediate cellular damage and inflammation.	Pruritic papules, blisters, or wheals of erythema, usually within 30 minutes of exposure	Urticaria Anaphylaxis Angioedema
II. Cytotoxic	Reactions occur within 5 to 12 hours. Antigens on cellular surfaces are destroyed by IgG and IgM antibodies, causing cellular destruction.	Various systemic manifestations within 5 to 12 hours.	Erythroblastosis Goodpasture syndrome Pemphigus vulgaris Bullous pemphigoid Grave's disease
III. Immune complex disease	Reactions occur within 3 to 8 hours following exposure to drug or antigen. Antigen–antibody complexes are formed and activate complement, which enhances recruitment of other inflammatory mediators.	Fever, arthralgias, proteinuria, lymphadenopathy, vasculitis	Arthus reaction Serum sickness SLE Vasculitis Erythema multiforme
IV. Delayed cell-mediated	Reactions occur within 24 to 48 hours following exposure. T cells are sensitized and thereby reactivate when reexposed to the same antigen.	Erythema, induration, blisters	TB skin test Delayed contact dermatitis Erythema nodosum

IgE, immunoglobulin E; IgG, immunoglobulin G; IgM, immunogloblin M; SLE, systemic lupus erythematosus; TB, tuberculosis.

Epidemiology
- Approximately 20% of patients develop urticaria at some time in their lives; of those, 25% develop chronic urticaria.
- Urticaria may occur at any age, and occurrence is equally divided between the sexes.

Risk Factors
Heredity is a possible predisposing factor.

TABLE 12.2. Anaphylactic Mediators

Mediator	Mechanism
Histamine	Increased capillary permeability (erythema).
	Increased contraction of smooth muscle.
	Increased mucous gland secretion.
Slow-reacting substance of anaphylaxis (SRSA); also known as leukotrienes C_4, D_4, and E_4	Slower in onset than histamine, but longer in duration. Increased contraction of smooth muscle.
Eosinophilic chemotactic factor of anaphylaxis (ECFA)	Substance attracts eosinophils to area of inflammation. Also can block further reaction by dampening the immune response.
Platelet activating factor (PAF)	Activates platelets to secrete serotonin, increasing smooth muscle contraction and vascular permeability.
Neutrophil chemotactic factor (NCF)	Attracts neutrophils to the area of inflammation. Neutrophils produce superoxides, which cause direct tissue injury.
Heparin	Causes local anticoagulation.
Basophil kallikrein of anaphylaxis (BKA)	Cleaves kininogen to form bradykinin. Bradykinin increases vascular permeability and smooth muscle contraction more potently than histamine.
Prostaglandin D_2	Potent inhibitor of platelet aggregation.

PATHOPHYSIOLOGY

Urticaria is usually a type I inflammatory reaction, which is immunoglobulin E (IgE) mediated and immediate. Mast cell surface IgE binds with an antigen and then degranulates, releasing histamine into the local area or to a distant site by way of axons. Histamine increases capillary permeability, thereby allowing fluid leakage and local wheal edema.

Diagnosis

A thorough history is important not only to diagnose urticaria, but also, if possible, to establish its cause. The patient should be questioned regarding medications, foods, environment at home and work, and physical trauma to the skin. The physician should also determine whether the urticaria is acute or chronic and whether outbreaks seem to be related to seasonal changes.

Whenever possible, the offending agent should be identified through a thorough history before performing laboratory tests, especially in cases of acute urticaria. The following diagnoses can be made by history:

• *Acute contact urticaria.* Symptoms are immediate in onset, and duration is less than 30 days.
• *Acute delayed urticaria.* Symptoms occur hours later, after exposure to the inciting agent.
• *Chronic urticaria.* Duration is more than 30 days.
• *Cold contact urticaria.* There is a history of cold exposure.

T ABLE 12.3. Etiology of Urticaria

Medications
Antibiotics (most commonly penicillin)
NSAIDs
Aspirin
Narcotic analgesics (morphine, codeine, meperidine)
Radiocontrast dyes

Foods
Shellfish
Nuts
Eggs (whites)
Chocolate
Strawberries
Tomatoes
Cow's milk
Cheese
Yeast
Food additives (BHA, BHT)

Systemic conditions
Thyroid disease
Cancer (lymphoma, leukemia)
Blood products
Sinus infection
Dental infection
Gallbladder infection
Gastrointestinal tract infection
Connective tissue diseases
Rheumatic disease
Serum sickness (horse serum)
Vasculitis
Pregnancy

Inhalants
Pollens
Animal danders
Mold
Dust mites
Aerosols
Volatile chemicals

Infections
Bacterial (streptococci)
Fungal (dermatophytes, *Candida* organisms)
Viral (hepatitis B, childhood viruses)
Parasitic (helminthiasis, amebiasis, giardiasis, malaria)
Spirochetal (syphilis, Lyme disease)

Physical factors
Pressure
Vibration
Cold
Heat
Exercise
Sun exposure
Emotional stress
Bites and stings (bees, fleas, or bedbugs)

Environmental contactants
Chemicals
Perfumes
Dyes
Soaps
Latex

Genetic factors
Hereditary angioedema (C1 esterase inhibitor deficiency)

NSAIDs, nonsteroidal antiinflammatory drugs; BHA, butylated hydroxyanisole; BHT, butylated hydroxytoluene.

Differential Diagnosis
See Table 12.4.

Diagnostic Tests
Although most cases of chronic urticaria are idiopathic, in children, food is the most common factor causing urticaria, followed by medications, and then by physical and contact causes. If tests must be used to determine the origin of chronic disease, history and physical examination indicate what types of tests may be necessary (Table 12.5).

T ABLE 12.4.   Urticaria: Differential Diagnosis

Insect bites	Lesions may have central puncture. They usually occur in unclothed or exposed skin areas. Lesions last longer than urticaria.
Contact dermatitis	There is an associated history of contact with an irritant. Vesicles may form that last longer than urticaria.
Vasculitis	There are bright red papules. Lesions usually last longer than urticaria.
Erythema multiforme	Constitutional symptoms are noted. There are target lesions.

T ABLE 12.5.   Tests for Urticaria

Test	Suspected etiology
CBC with differential	All causes
Multichannel chemistry profile	All causes
Sedimentation rate	Vasculitis
Antinuclear antibody	Vasculitis, connective tissue disease
Thyroid profile	Hyperthyroidism, hypothyroidism
Complement levels	Vasculitis, serum sickness, angioedema
Rheumatoid factor	Rheumatoid arthritis
Cryoglobulins, cold hemolysis	Cold urticaria
VDRL	Syphilis, cold urticaria
Urine or serum HCG	Pregnancy
Urinalysis and culture	Urinary tract infection
Wet mount (vagina)	Vaginal infection (*Candida, Trichomonas*)
Streptococcal throat culture	Streptococcal tonsillitis/pharyngitis
Mononucleosis spot test	Infectious mononucleosis
Hepatitis antigens	Hepatitis
Stool for ova and parasites	Helminth infections
Giardia antigen	Giardiasis
Serum IgE	Parasitic infections
Immediate scratch and intradermal tests	Inhalant allergens, dermatophytes, *Candida*
RAST	All causes
Skin biopsy	Vasculitis
Elimination diets	Food allergies
Food provocation tests	Food allergies
X-rays	
Sinus	Sinusitis
Chest	Pneumonia, lung abscess, cancer
Dental	Dental abscess
Gastrointestinal tract	Cholecystitis, cancer
Genitourinary tract	UTI, cancer

CBC, complete blood cell count; VDRL, Venereal Disease Research Laboratory; HCG, human chorionic gonadotropin; IgE, immunoglobulin E; RAST, radioallergosorbent test; UTI, urinary tract infection.

- *Skin biopsy* is useful to rule out urticarial vasculitis.
- *Skin stroking.* A gentle stroking of the skin can produce a wheal in dermatographism.
- *Application of heat.* In heat-induced urticaria, immersion of an extremity in warm water (42°C) for 15 minutes causes a wheal to appear in 2 to 20 minutes.
- *Application of ice.* In cold-induced urticaria, application of an ice pack for 10 minutes causes a wheal within 5 to 10 minutes after its removal.
- *Irradiation.* Exposure to 290- to 690-mm wavelength of light for 30 to 120 seconds can cause a wheal within 30 minutes after exposure. This test is useful in solar-induced urticaria.
- *C4 level* is decreased in hereditary angioedema.
- *C1 esterase inhibitor level* is decreased in hereditary angioedema.
- *Intradermal or skin patch test.* Usually of little diagnostic value. Can be helpful in atopic patients with chronic urticaria to establish sensitivity to certain provocative agents.
- *Radioallergosorbent testing (RAST)* offers no distinct advantages over skin patch or intradermal testing in detecting environmental, food, or inhalant causes.

Referral

Referral to a dermatologist or an allergist may be indicated for unresponsive or chronic cases of urticaria. In addition, some physicians prefer to consult a specialist as soon as the diagnosis of urticaria is made.

Management

Management consists primarily of discontinuation of precipitating factors. If history suggests a food or drug origin, begin an elimination diet of common agents [nonsteroidal antiinflammatory drugs (NSAIDs), antibiotics, strawberries, nuts, and eggs are common etiologic triggers]. Have the patient keep a log of food types ingested, times of ingestion, and occurrences of urticaria.

Medications

See Table 12.6.

In first occurrences, improvement is usually noted within 24 hours of treatment, with the hives disappearing completely within 2 weeks. Attacks of chronic urticaria can persist for 30 to 45 days before resolving on their own.

Other Treatment Modalities

- Avoidance of the offending agent, if identified, is most important.
- Patients with chronic urticaria can become increasingly frustrated when a cause is not found. Appropriate tests and referrals can alleviate anxiety.
- Patients who have bronchospasm during an episode of acute urticaria may be at risk for serious anaphylactic reactions in future episodes. These patients should be instructed to carry an emergency epinephrine autoinjector (EpiPen) or EpiPen Jr. (for children) at all times in case of unexpected exposure to the offending agent and subsequent anaphylaxis.

Follow-up

Patients with acute urticaria who do not respond to treatment in 7 to 10 days should be followed to determine whether referral is necessary or the diagnosis is correct.

Patient Education

Compliance

Patients should be urged to comply with the necessary lifestyle changes, including avoidance of offending agents.

T ABLE 12.6. Medical Treatment of Urticaria

Antihistamines (H₁ BLOCKERS)

Cetirizine (Zyrtec)
Availability:	Prescription only.
Dosage:	*Adults:* 10 mg daily orally.
	Children (over age 6 years): 5 to 10 mg daily (5 mg/5 mL) orally.
Duration:	Until symptoms resolve.
Side effects:	Some sedation.
Comments:	Useful for both acute and chronic urticaria.

Loratadine (Claritin)
Availability:	Prescription only.
Dosage:	*Adults:* 10 mg daily orally.
	Children (over age 6 years): 10 mg daily (5 mg/5 mL) orally.
Duration:	Until symptoms resolve.
Side effects:	Nonsedating; can cause headache.
Comments:	Useful for both acute and chronic urticaria.

Hydroxyzine (Atarax)
Availability:	Prescription only.
Dosage:	*Adults:* 25 to 100 mg daily orally every 6 hours.
	Children (under age 6 years): 2 to 5 mg/kg per day in 4 divided doses
	(25 mg/5 mL) orally; *(over age 6 years):* 25–50 mg every 6 hours orally.
Duration:	Until symptoms resolve.
Side effects:	May cause sedation.
Comments:	Useful for acute urticaria. Sedation is helpful if pruritus is causing insomnia.

Diphenhydramine (Benadryl)
Availability:	Over the counter.
Dosage:	*Adults:* 25 to 50 mg, 4 times daily orally.
	Children: 5 mg/kg per day in divided doses every 6 hours (12.5 mg/5 mL).
Duration:	Until symptoms resolve.
Side effects:	Sedation.
Comments:	Useful in acute urticaria.

Epinephrine (aqueous 1:1000)
Availability:	Prescription only.
Dosage:	*Adults:* 0.5 mL subcutaneously; may repeat 15 to 20 minutes for 3 to 4 doses.
	Children: 0.01 mL/kg subcutaneously; maximum single dose is 0.5 mL;
	may repeat 15 to 20 minutes for 3 to 4 doses.
Duration:	Until systemic symptoms resolve.
Side effects:	May cause arrhythmias, hypertension, headache, nausea, vomiting.
Comments:	Caution should be used when using epinephrine in older adults or
	in patients with coronary artery disease. Use in acute urticaria with
	symptoms of wheezing, chest tightness, shortness of breath, or dyspnea.

continued

T ABLE 12.6. *continued.* **Medical Treatment of Urticaria**

Prednisone (a corticosteroid)

Availability:	Prescription only.
Dosage:	*Adults:* 40 to 60 mg orally initially.
	Children: 1 mg/kg per day initially orally.
Duration:	Taper over 10 to 14 days.
Side effects:	Long-standing use of corticosteroids inhibits the pituitary-adrenal axis causing serious complications.
Comments:	Useful in acute urticaria.

Doxepin (a tricyclic antidepressant with potent H_1-blocking capabilities) (Sinequan)

Availability:	Prescription only.
Dosage:	10 to 25 mg orally 3 times daily.
Duration:	Should be used long-term.
Side effects:	Anticholinergic side effects of dry mouth, constipation, and lethargy, which frequently resolve over time.
Comments:	Useful in chronic urticaria.

Adjunctive therapy for chronic urticaria
H_2-Receptor blockers

Cimetidine (Tagamet)

Availability:	Prescription and over the counter.
Dosage:	*Adults:* 300 mg orally 3 times daily.
	Children: 20 mg/kg per day divided every 6 hours (300 mg/5 mL) orally.
Duration:	Until chronic symptoms have resolved.
Side effects:	Headache, mental confusion, diarrhea.
Comments:	For chronic urticaria; use in conjunction with H_1 antihistamines.

or

Rantidine (Zantac)

Availability:	Prescription and over the counter.
Dosage:	*Adults:* 150 mg orally twice daily.
	Children: 2.5 to 3.8 mg/kg per day divided every 12 hours (15 mg/5 mL) orally.
Duration:	Until chronic symptoms have resolved.
Side effects:	Headache, diarrhea, nausea, vomiting.
Comments:	For chronic urticaria; use in conjunction with H_1 antihistamines.

β-Adrenergic agents

Terbutaline (Bricanyl)

Availability:	Prescription only.
Dosage:	*Adults:* 2.5 to 5 mg orally 3 times daily.
	Children: Not for use in children under 12 years of age.
Duration:	Until chronic symptoms have resolved.
Side effects:	Nervousness, tremor, headache, nausea.
Comments:	For chronic urticaria; use in conjunction with H_1 antihistamines.

Family and Community Support

Patients should receive reassurance and emotional support, since urticaria and anaphylaxis can be frightening. Patients should also be made aware that urticaria can be
familial.

ANGIOEDEMA

The tissue reactions to histamine that occur in angioedema are similar to those that
occur in urticaria. In angioedema, however, reactions occur deeper within tissues and
on mucous membranes. This deep-tissue reaction often results in life-threatening
swelling of confined spaces, as occurs when the airway is compromised.

Chief Complaint

When angioedema is an acute, life-threatening reaction, the patient may not be able
to voice a complaint. Lip swelling, hoarse voice, and respiratory and gastrointestinal
tract symptoms may all be observed.

Clinical Manifestations

- Angioedema can cause shock, hypotension, and death.
- There may be marked facial swelling.
- Respiratory distress (wheezing, laryngeal edema, stridor) may also be present.

Epidemiology

Family History

Angioedema is acquired or hereditary; C1 esterase inhibitor deficiency is hereditary.

Age

Angioedema can occur at any age, although it is more common after 30 years of age.

Sex

It is equally prevalent in male and female patients.

Risk Factors

A history of food allergy, insect bites (venom), medication use [e.g., angiotensin-converting enzyme (ACE) inhibitors], or recent exposure to contrast dye may be elicited.

PATHOPHYSIOLOGY

There is dermal edema, dilation of blood vessels, dilated lymphatics, and a perivascular infiltrate
of mononuclear cells in the dermis and subcutaneous tissues.

Diagnosis

Clinical Presentation

The patient presents with marked facial swelling and respiratory distress, including
wheezing, laryngeal edema, or stridor. The patient may also have gastrointestinal tract
symptoms.

Diagnostic Tests

C4 level and C1 esterase inhibitor level may be low in angioedema. Also see Table 12.5.

Differential Diagnosis

Urticaria is a superficial allergic reaction that is rarely life threatening.

Referral

Referral to an allergist may be indicated following stabilization of the patient's airway.

Management

- Stabilizing the airway is vital, since angioedema can cause shock, hypotension, and death.
- Emergency care, with special attention to the Airway, Breathing, and Circulation (ABCs), should be rendered immediately in life-threatening situations.
- If an intravenous line can be started, patients can be given diphenhydramine (50 to 100 mg intravenously for adults; 1 to 2 mg/kg per dose intravenously, slowly, for children).
- Subcutaneous aqueous epinephrine 1:1000 is administered (0.5 mL for adults, repeated every 15 to 20 minutes as needed; 0.01 cc/kg per dose to a maximum dose of 0.5 cc for children, repeated every 15 to 20 minutes as needed); *And*
- Methylprednisolone is administered (125 mg initially for adults, repeated every 8 hours as needed; 10 to 30 mg/kg per dose over 1 hour for children, repeated every 8 hours as needed).

Follow-up

Patients should be admitted to the hospital for close observation following stabilization of the airway.

Patient Education

Compliance

- Patients should be advised that angioedema can recur and should be instructed in the appropriate management techniques.
- An EpiPen (EpiPen Jr. for children) should be issued to the patient, with full instructions regarding its use. Patients should be informed that the EpiPen must be carried at all times. Patients must understand the need for immediate medical care even if they have had some relief from the use of their EpiPen.
- Medical alert tags are also appropriate.
- Patients should be advised to avoid the offending agent.
- In severe cases involving the airway, strict compliance with a regimen of oral steroids, including tapering the medication according to the prescribed method, is necessary.

Family and Community Support

The patient's family should be educated on use of the EpiPen and other appropriate emergency medical care measures.

DERMATITIS HERPETIFORMIS

Dermatitis herpetiformis is an autoimmune disease, which may be chronic, characterized by grouped vesicles over the extensor surfaces of the body with marked pruritus. This disease may also be associated with gluten enteropathy. Dermatitis herpetiformis is not associated with herpes simplex.

Chief Complaint

Patients complain of a blistering rash preceded by intense burning and pruritus. The rash increases in severity over time.

Clinical Manifestations

- Dermatitis herpetiformis consists of multiple vesicular lesions distributed symmetrically and frequently seen on the buttocks, elbows, knees, scalp, shoulder, and neck (Figure 12.2, see color insert following page 170).
- New lesions appear as erythematous papules, becoming vesicular and eventually excoriated and forming a crust.
- The duration of these lesions varies from days to weeks, and areas of hypopigmentation may remain after lesions have healed.
- Dermatitis herpetiformis may be associated with steatorrhea, anemia, small bowel lymphoma, systemic lupus erythematosus (SLE), and thyroid disease. A variant of this disease, IgA bullous dermatitis, has different skin biopsy findings and spares the small bowel.
- Although there are usually no systemic symptoms, approximately 80% of patients have direct tissue damage to the small bowel, causing enteropathy and malabsorption.

Epidemiology

There is a human lymphocyte antigen (HLA) association (HLA-B8, HLA-DR3).

Age

The disease typically occurs in patients over the age of 20 years.

Sex

Dermatitis herpetiformis is more common in men than in women in a ratio of 2:1.

Risk Factors

- Allergy to gluten, the most common offending antigen, which is present in all grains except rice and corn.
- Male sex.

PATHOPHYSIOLOGY

Granular deposits of IgA along with neutrophils are present in the upper dermis (basement membrane).

Diagnosis

Skin biopsy of early lesions is always indicated to diagnose. Immunofluorescence studies help confirm the diagnosis.

Differential Diagnosis

See Table 12.7.

T ABLE 12.7.   Dermatitis Herpetiformis: Differential Diagnosis

Contact and atopic dermatitis	Adult distribution is usually on the flexor surfaces.
Scabies	Skin distribution is mainly on the wrists, finger webs, and groin.
	Skin scraping is positive.
	Other family members may also have symptoms.
Insect bite reactions	The rash fades in several days.
	Lesions are asymmetric on exposed skin.

Diagnostic Tests

Skin biopsy with immunofluorescence studies of a vesicle help differentiate the following conditions:

Dermatitis herpetiformis. Biopsy specimen reveals granular IgA deposition at the basement membrane.

Linear IgA bullous dermatitis. Biopsy specimen reveals granular IgA deposits at the dermal-epidermal junction.

Bullous pemphigoid. Biopsy specimen reveals immunoglobulin G (IgG) deposits at the basement membrane.

Small bowel biopsy during upper endoscopy is indicated if enteropathy is suspected; biopsy specimen reveals blunting and flattening of small bowel villi similar to those seen in celiac sprue.

Upper endoscopy for biopsy may be needed for diagnosis when the patient has gastrointestinal tract symptoms.

There is an association with HLA-B8 and HLA-DR3.

Referral

- Consultation with a dermatologist or an allergist is recommended to evaluate and treat the patient, as well as to monitor the systemic treatment.
- Referral may be necessary in patients requiring upper endoscopy for biopsy if the family physician does not perform this procedure.

Management
Medications
See Table 12.8.

Other Treatment Modalities
When strictly followed, a gluten-free diet that eliminates all wheat and grain can reduce the need for medications. Gluten-free foods are available through ENER-G Foods, Inc., 6901 Fox Avenue South, P.O. Box 24723, Seattle, WA 98124-0723.

Follow-up
Patients should be followed closely to monitor adherence to the treatment regimen.

Patient Education
Compliance
- Patients should be warned that compliance with a gluten-free diet is essential because symptoms will recur if the diet is abandoned.
- One-third of patients have spontaneous remission. Unless this spontaneous remission occurs, however, the diet or medications remain necessary.

T ABLE 12.8. **Medical Treatment of Dermatitis Herpetiformis**

Dapsone

Availability:	Prescription only.
Dosage:	100 to 200 mg orally, decreasing to the lowest effective dose (25 to 50 mg/day).
Duration:	May be required long-term.
Side effects:	There are numerous side effects. Before treatment, individuals at risk for G6PD deficiency (blacks, Asians, those of Mediterranean descent) require that glucose-6-phosphate levels be determined because of the risk of hemolytic anemia. Peripheral motor neuropathy, methemoglobinemia, hemolysis, and anemia are dose-related effects and occur to some degree in all patients. Therefore the CBC should be taken weekly for the first month, monthly thereafter for 6 months, then every 6 months. Coadministration of cimetidine can decrease the methemoglobinemia.
Comments:	Mechanism of action is not known.

Sulfapyridine

Availability:	Prescription only.
Dosage:	1 to 5 g/day orally.
Duration:	May be required long-term.
Side effects:	There is a rare complication of fever, malaise, lymphadenopathy, and hemolytic anemia.
Comments:	Can be used if dapsone is not tolerated.

G6PD, glucose-6-phosphate dehydrogenase; CBC, complete blood cell count.

Lifestyle Changes

Patients should be placed on a gluten-free diet and cautioned that it may be several months following the initiation of the diet before any gastrointestinal tract improvement is evident.

ERYTHEMA MULTIFORME

Erythema multiforme (EM) is a type III immune complex disease triggered by exposure to certain antigens or drugs. Stevens-Johnson syndrome and toxic epidermal necrolysis have been considered advanced, severe cases of EM. Much debate centers around whether they constitute a spectrum of disease versus independent diseases or variants of one another. Discussion about the intricacies and management of these diseases are beyond the scope of this textbook.

Chief Complaint

Patients report a pruritic, raised rash, which may be blistering and painful.

Clinical Manifestations

- EM begins as a central papule with concentric rings; it is a classic target lesion, which blanches on compression. The initial lesion can be followed by more severe disease with vesicle or bullae formation in multiple forms, sizes, and shapes (multiforme) (Figure 12.3, see color insert following page 170).
- The initial rash is asymmetrically arranged, nonbullous, and may last from 2 to 6 weeks.
- Blisters rupture easily and are followed by erosions or crustules.

- Postinflammatory hyperpigmentation may be seen at healed lesion sites.
- Lesions are usually confined to extensor surfaces, palms, genitals, and soles and, depending on the severity of the disease, may involve the mucous membranes. The milder forms of EM are associated with little mucous membrane involvement; however, 25% to 70% of patients have severe forms, affecting the mucous membranes.
- Corneal ulcers, anterior uveitis, and hematologic, cardiac, and renal involvement may occur but are very rare.
- Patients may have had a previous herpes simplex infection or *Mycoplasma* infection with a prodrome of itching before appearance of the rash.
- Approximately 33% of patients have a prodrome of upper respiratory tract symptoms.
- The most severe and life-threatening variant of EM is Stevens-Johnson syndrome. This is a type III immunologic reaction with immune complexes deposited in the cutaneous microvasculature. Physical signs include mucosal erosions, target lesions, and blisters covering 10% of the body surface. There is some speculation that Stevens-Johnson syndrome is a separate disease. When over 10% of the skin is involved, the condition is called toxic epidermal necrolysis, which has a 20% to 30% mortality rate.

Epidemiology

Disease can be recurrent in up to 33% of cases.

Age

EM occurs in patients from 20 to 40 years of age.

Sex

Men are affected more often than women.

Risk Factors

For risk factors see Table 12.9.

T ABLE 12.9.   Risk Factors for Erythema Multiforme

Medications	Bacterial infections
Allopurinol (Zyloprim)	Streptococcus
Oral corticosteroids	*Mycobacterium tuberculosis*
Tetracyclines	*Yersinia*
Carbamazepine (Tegretol)	**Viral infections**
Sulfonylureas	Herpes simplex
Sulfonamides	Hepatitis A and B
Penicillins	Infectious mononucleosis
NSAIDs	Herpes zoster
Barbiturates	**Fungal infections**
Phenytoin (Dilantin)	Coccidioidomycosis
Other origins	Histoplasmosis
Pregnancy (usually the latter half)	***Chlamydia* infections**
Cancer	Psittacosis
Radiation therapy	***Mycoplasma* infections**

NSAIDs, nonsteroidal antiinflammatory drugs.

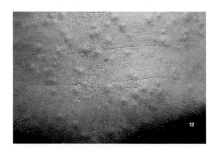

FIGURE 1.1. Closed comedones. [Courtesy of the Department of Dermatology, State University of New York–Health Science Center (SUNY–HSC) at Brooklyn, New York.]

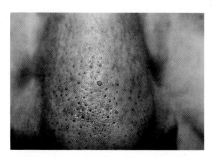

FIGURE 1.2. Open comedones. (Courtesy of the Department of Dermatology, SUNY–HSC at Brooklyn, New York.)

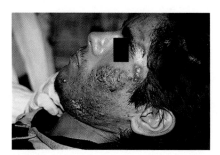

FIGURE 1.3. Nodular cystic acne vulgaris. (Courtesy of the Department of Dermatology, SUNY–HSC at Brooklyn, New York.)

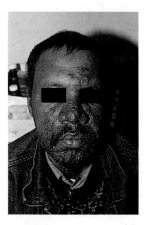

FIGURE 1.4. Rosacea. (Courtesy of the Department of Dermatology, SUNY–HSC at Brooklyn, New York.)

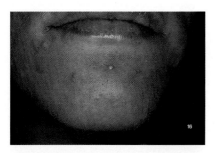

FIGURE 1.5. Perioral dermatitis. (Courtesy of the Department of Dermatology, SUNY–HSC at Brooklyn, New York.)

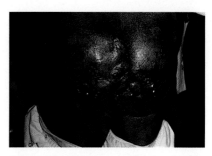

FIGURE 1.6. Hidradenitis suppurativa of the buttocks. (Courtesy of the Department of Dermatology, SUNY–HSC at Brooklyn, New York.)

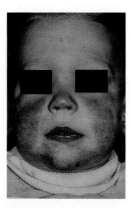

FIGURE 2.1. Atopic dermatitis in infancy. (Courtesy of the Department of Dermatology, SUNY–HSC at Brooklyn, New York.)

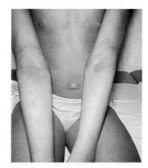

FIGURE 2.2. Atopic dermatitis on flexor surfaces. (Courtesy of the Department of Dermatology, SUNY–HSC at Brooklyn, New York.)

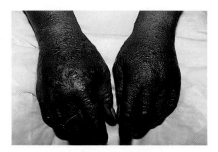

FIGURE 2.3. Contact dermatitis. (Courtesy of the Department of Dermatology, SUNY–HSC at Brooklyn, New York.)

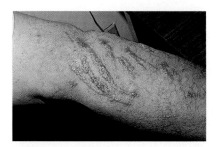

FIGURE 2.4. Poison ivy. (Courtesy of the Department of Dermatology, SUNY–HSC at Brooklyn, New York.)

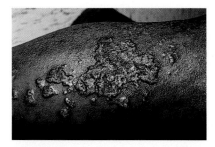

FIGURE 2.5. Lichen simplex chronicus. (Courtesy of the Department of Dermatology, SUNY–HSC at Brooklyn, New York.)

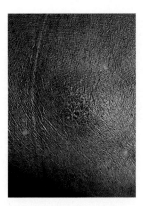

FIGURE 2.6. Nummular impetiginous eczema. (Courtesy of the Department of Dermatology, SUNY–HSC at Brooklyn, New York.)

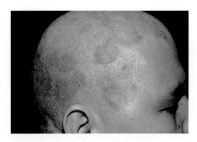

FIGURE 2.7. Seborrheic dermatitis. (Courtesy of the Department of Dermatology, SUNY–HSC at Brooklyn, New York.)

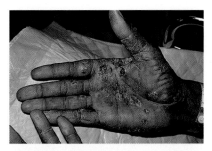

FIGURE 2.8. Dyshidrotic eczema. (Courtesy of the Department of Dermatology, SUNY–HSC at Brooklyn, New York.)

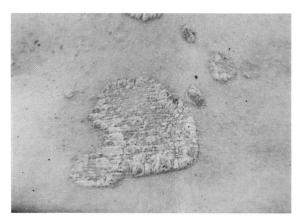

FIGURE 3.1. Erythematous plaques with thick white scales typical of psoriasis vulgaris. (From Roenigk HH. Psoriasis. In: Roenigk HH, ed. *Office dermatology.* Baltimore: Williams & Wilkins, 1981, Plate I, Fig. 8-1, with permission.)

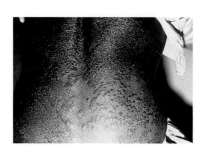

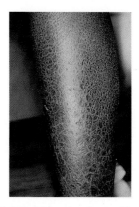

FIGURE 3.2. Diffuse psoriasis. (Courtesy of the Department of Dermatology, SUNY–HSC at Brooklyn, New York.)

FIGURE 3.3. Ichthyosis vulgaris. (Courtesy of the Department of Dermatology, SUNY–HSC at Brooklyn, New York.)

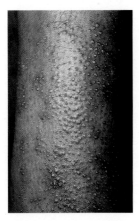

FIGURE 3.4. Keratosis pilaris. (Courtesy of the Department of Dermatology, SUNY–HSC at Brooklyn, New York.)

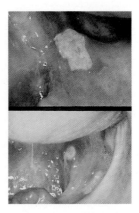

FIGURE 4.1. Aphthous ulcer. (Courtesy of the Department of Dermatology, SUNY–HSC at Brooklyn, New York.)

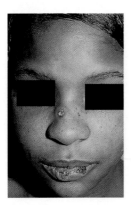

FIGURE 4.2. Herpes labialis. (Courtesy of the Department of Dermatology, SUNY–HSC at Brooklyn, New York.)

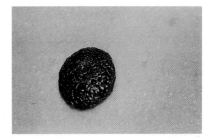

FIGURE 5.1. Junctional nevus. (Courtesy of the Department of Dermatology, SUNY–HSC at Brooklyn, New York.)

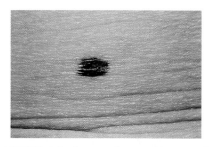

FIGURE 5.2. Compound nevus. (Courtesy of the Department of Dermatology, SUNY–HSC at Brooklyn, New York.)

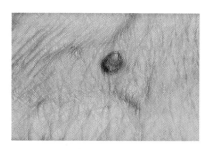

FIGURE 5.3. Blue nevus. (Courtesy of the Department of Dermatology, SUNY–HSC at Brooklyn, New York.)

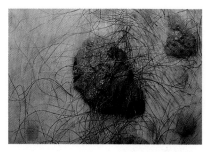

FIGURE 5.5. Seborrheic keratosis. (Courtesy of the Department of Dermatology, SUNY–HSC at Brooklyn, New York.)

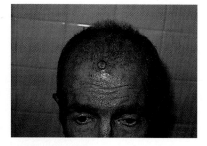

FIGURE 5.6. Keratoacanthoma. (Courtesy of the Department of Dermatology, SUNY–HSC at Brooklyn, New York.)

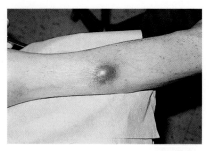

FIGURE 5.7. Dermatofibroma. (Courtesy of the Department of Dermatology, SUNY–HSC at Brooklyn, New York.)

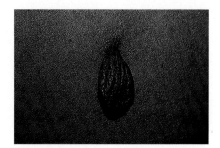

FIGURE 5.8. Skin tag. (Courtesy of the Department of Dermatology, SUNY–HSC at Brooklyn, New York.)

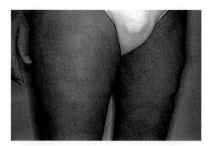

FIGURE 5.9. Lipoma. (Courtesy of Richard B. Odom, MD.)

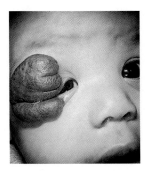

FIGURE 6.1. Hemangioma. (Courtesy of the Department of Dermatology, SUNY–HSC at Brooklyn, New York.)

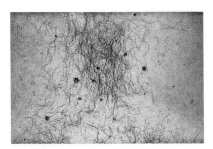

FIGURE 6.2. Multiple cherry angiomas. (Courtesy of the Department of Dermatology, SUNY–HSC at Brooklyn, New York.)

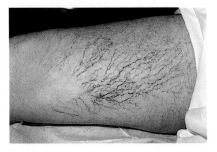

FIGURE 6.3. Spider angioma. (Courtesy of the Department of Dermatology, SUNY–HSC at Brooklyn, New York.)

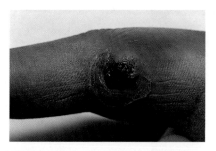

FIGURE 6.4. Pyogenic granuloma. (Courtesy of the Department of Dermatology, SUNY–HSC at Brooklyn, New York.)

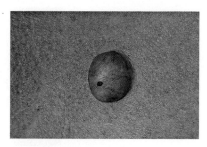

FIGURE 7.1. Epidermoid cyst. (Courtesy of the Department of Dermatology, SUNY–HSC at Brooklyn, New York.)

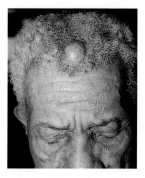

FIGURE 7.2. Trichilemmal cyst. (Courtesy of the Department of Dermatology, SUNY–HSC at Brooklyn, New York.)

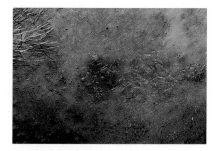

FIGURE 8.1. Actinic keratosis. (Courtesy of the Department of Dermatology, SUNY–HSC at Brooklyn, New York.)

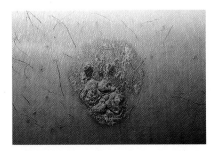

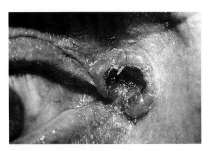

FIGURE 8.2. Squamous cell carcinoma. (Courtesy of the Department of Dermatology, SUNY–HSC at Brooklyn, New York.)

FIGURE 8.3. Basal cell carcinoma. (Courtesy of the Department of Dermatology, SUNY–HSC at Brooklyn, New York).

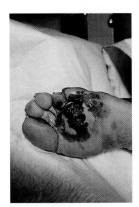

FIGURE 8.4. Nodular melanoma. (Courtesy of the Department of Dermatology, SUNY–HSC at Brooklyn, New York.)

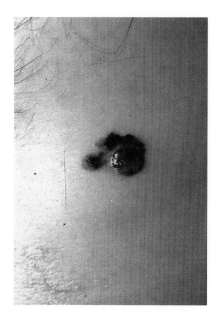

FIGURE 8.5. Malignant melanoma. (From Roenigk HH. Excision of common malignant tumors of the skin. In: Roenigk HH, ed. *Office dermatology*. Baltimore: Williams & Wilkins, 1981, Plate V, Fig. 28-8.)

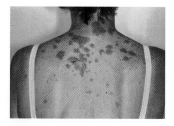

FIGURE 9.1. Photoallergic reaction. (Courtesy of Jeffrey D. Bernard, MD.)

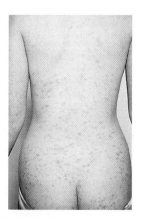

FIGURE 10.1. Pityriasis rosea. (Courtesy of the Department of Dermatology, SUNY–HSC at Brooklyn, New York.)

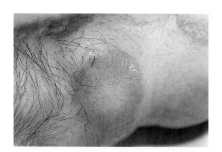

FIGURE 10.2. Granuloma annulare. (Courtesy of the Department of Dermatology, SUNY–HSC at Brooklyn, New York.)

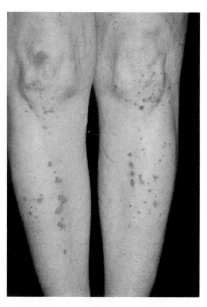

FIGURE 10.3. Lichen planus on both legs. (From Roenigk HH. Psoriasis. In: Roenigk HH, ed. *Office dermatology*. Baltimore: Williams & Wilkins, 1981, Plate II, Fig. 9-3, with permission.)

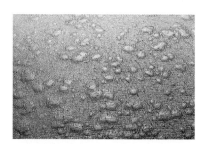

FIGURE 10.4. Eruptive lichen planus. (Courtesy of the Department of Dermatology, SUNY–HSC at Brooklyn, New York.)

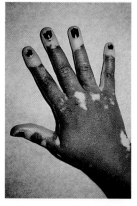

FIGURE 11.1. Vitiligo. (Courtesy of the Department of Dermatology, SUNY–HSC at Brooklyn, New York.)

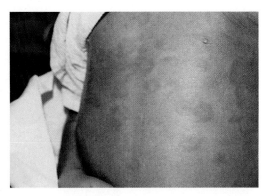

FIGURE 12.1. Urticaria. (Courtesy of the Department of Dermatology, SUNY–HSC at Brooklyn, New York.)

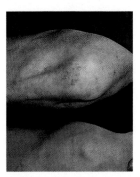

FIGURE 12.2. Dermatitis herpetiformis. (Courtesy of the Department of Dermatology, SUNY–HSC at Brooklyn, New York.)

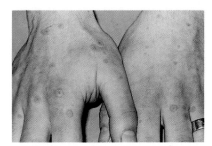

FIGURE 12.3. Erythema multiforme. (Courtesy of the Department of Dermatology, SUNY–HSC at Brooklyn, New York.)

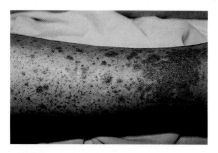

FIGURE 12.4. Vasculitis. (Courtesy of the Department of Dermatology, SUNY–HSC at Brooklyn, New York.)

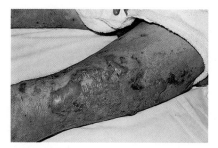

FIGURE 12.5. Bullous pemphigoid. (Courtesy of the Department of Dermatology, SUNY–HSC at Brooklyn, New York.)

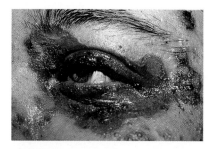

FIGURE 12.6. Pemphigus vulgaris. (Courtesy of the Department of Dermatology, SUNY–HSC at Brooklyn, New York.)

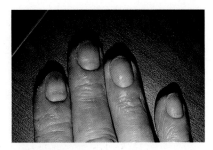

FIGURE 13.1. Beau lines. (Courtesy of the Department of Dermatology, SUNY–HSC at Brooklyn, New York.)

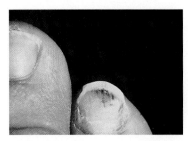

FIGURE 13.2. Splinter hemorrhages. (Courtesy of the Department of Dermatology, SUNY–HSC at Brooklyn, New York.)

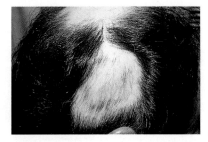

FIGURE 14.1. Alopecia areata. (Courtesy of the Department of Dermatology, SUNY–HSC at Brooklyn, New York.)

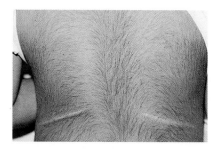

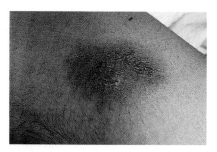

FIGURE 14.3. Hirsutism. (Courtesy of the Department of Dermatology, SUNY–HSC at Brooklyn, New York.)

FIGURE 15.1. Exanthematous drug eruption. (Courtesy of the Department of Dermatology, SUNY–HSC at Brooklyn, New York.]

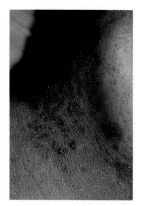

FIGURE 14.4. Pseudofolliculitis barbae. (Courtesy of the Department of Dermatology, SUNY–HSC at Brooklyn, New York.)

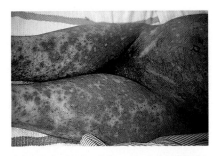

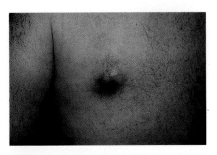

FIGURE 15.2. Fixed drug eruption. (Courtesy of the Department of Dermatology, SUNY–HSC at Brooklyn, New York.)

FIGURE 16.2. Abscess. (Courtesy of the Department of Dermatology, SUNY–HSC at Brooklyn, New York.)

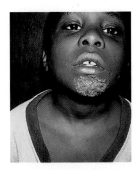

FIGURE 16.1. Impetigo. (Courtesy of the Department of Dermatology, SUNY–HSC at Brooklyn, New York.]

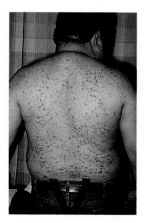

FIGURE 16.3. Infectious folliculitis. (Courtesy of the Department of Dermatology, SUNY–HSC at Brooklyn, New York.)

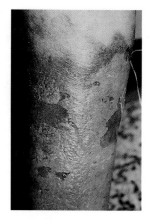

FIGURE 16.4. Erysipelas. (Courtesy of the Department of Dermatology, SUNY–HSC at Brooklyn, New York.)

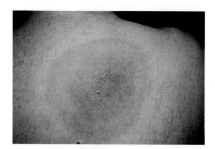

FIGURE 16.6. Erythema migrans. (Courtesy of the Department of Dermatology, SUNY–HSC at Brooklyn, New York.)

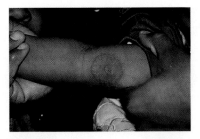

FIGURE 17.1. Tinea corporis. (Courtesy of the Department of Dermatology, SUNY–HSC at Brooklyn, New York.]

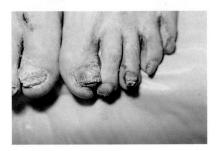

FIGURE 17.2. Tinea unguium and tinea pedis. (Courtesy of the Department of Dermatology, SUNY–HSC at Brooklyn, New York.)

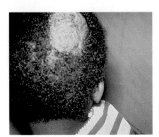

FIGURE 17.3. Kerion. (Courtesy of the Department of Dermatology, SUNY–HSC at Brooklyn, New York.)

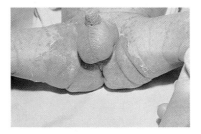

FIGURE 17.5. Diaper dermatitis secondary to *Candida* infection. (Courtesy of the Department of Dermatology, SUNY–HSC at Brooklyn, New York.)

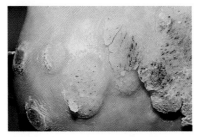

FIGURE 17.6. Pityriasis versicolor. (Courtesy of the Department of Dermatology, SUNY–HSC at Brooklyn, New York.)

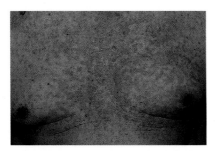

FIGURE 18.1. Plantar warts. (Courtesy of the Department of Dermatology, SUNY–HSC at Brooklyn, New York.]

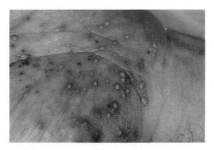

FIGURE 18.2. Hand-foot-and-mouth disease. (Courtesy of the Department of Dermatology, SUNY–HSC at Brooklyn, New York.)

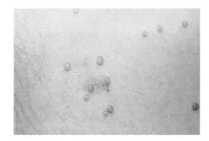

FIGURE 18.3. Molluscum contagiosum. (Courtesy of the Department of Dermatology, SUNY–HSC at Brooklyn, New York.)

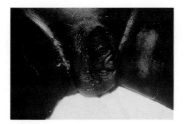

FIGURE 18.4. Kawasaki disease. (Courtesy of Neil S. Prose, MD.)

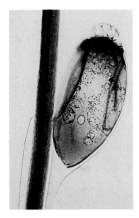

FIGURE 19.1. Nit from head or pubic louse. (Courtesy of Mervyn L. Elgart, MD.)

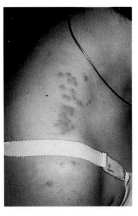

FIGURE 19.2. Cercarial dermatitis. (Courtesy of Mervyn L. Elgart, MD.)

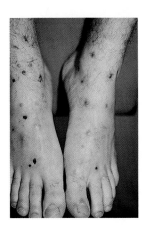

FIGURE 19.3. Flea bites. (Courtesy of Mervyn L. Elgart, MD.)

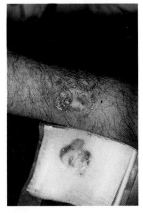

FIGURE 19.4. Spider bite. (Courtesy of the Department of Dermatology, SUNY–HSC at Brooklyn, New York.)

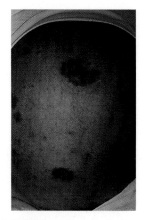

FIGURE C.1. Herpes gestationis.

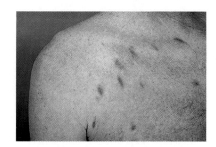

FIGURE E.1. Kaposi sarcoma.

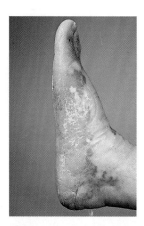

FIGURE E.2. Kaposi sarcoma.

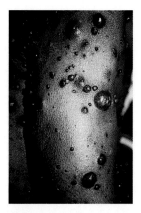

FIGURE E.3. Bacillary angiomatosis.

PATHOPHYSIOLOGY

EM is a type III inflammatory reaction. An infiltrate of lymphocytes is seen perivascularly in the upper dermis with focal damage to the epidermis.

Diagnosis

The diagnosis is mainly made from a thorough history (including a history of medications) and physical examination. The diagnostic criteria for EM include the following:

- An acute, self-limited course.
- Duration of skin lesions 2 to 6 weeks from onset to healing.
- Red, round rash symmetrically distributed and lasting at least 7 days.
- Presence of target lesions.
- Confirmation via positive skin biopsy.

Differential Diagnosis

See Table 12.10.

Diagnostic Tests

- A complete blood cell count (CBC), streptococcal throat culture, and antistreptolysin O (ASO) titer may be necessary if the patient gives a history of a recent infection, especially of the throat.
- A monospot test and CBC should be considered if the patient complains of malaise and has lymphadenopathy or hepatosplenomegaly.
- If the patient gives a history suggestive of hepatitis or the patient is jaundiced, a liver profile and hepatitis antibody profile may be necessary.

T ABLE 12.10.   Erythema Multiforme: Differential Diagnosis

Nonbullous disease	
Viral exanthems	Confluent erythematous rash with a different distribution than erythema multiforme.
Nummular eczema	No target lesions or mucosal involvement. Biopsy may be helpful to differentiate.
Urticaria	Rash lasts less than 24 hours; no target lesions. Biopsy may be helpful to differentiate.
Bullous disease	
Pemphigus vulgaris	No target lesions or intact bullae. Biopsy is necessary to differentiate.
Bullous pemphigoid	No target lesions; rash is usually flexural. Biopsy is necessary to differentiate.
Staphylococcal scalded skin syndrome	Rash includes diffuse erythema and blisters; limited mucosal involvement; no target lesions. Bacterial culture is often positive.

- Patients with chronic or recurrent EM should receive laboratory testing to determine the sources of chronic infection, carcinoma, or connective tissue disease. Suggested tests include CBC, erythrocyte sedimentation rate (ESR), Venereal Disease Research Laboratory (VDRL) test, radiologic studies, renal and liver profiles, antinuclear antibody (ANA) testing, and urinalysis, as dictated by history and physical examination.
- Allergy testing is usually not necessary unless it is indicated by the patient's history and physical examination.

Referral

- A rheumatology or dermatology referral may be indicated if the diagnosis is unclear or if the disease is unresponsive to treatment.
- EM can cause conjunctival scarring, especially in Stevens-Johnson syndrome. Early consultation with an ophthalmologist is recommended.

Management

- Identification and removal, if possible, of the etiologic agent is the primary goal of management.
- Consider hospitalization if vital signs are unstable and progression to Stevens-Johnson syndrome is suspected.

Medications

See Table 12.11.

Other Treatment Modalities

- If close monitoring indicates secondary bacterial infection, culture and treat the condition appropriately.
- Use viscous lidocaine for sore mouth caused by mucosal involvement.

Stevens-Johnson syndrome

- Rehydrate. If the patient is unable to take fluids by mouth, consider hospitalization for intravenous fluid therapy.
- Instruct patient to swish and expectorate viscous lidocaine 2% as needed for mouth pain from oral lesions or use 30 minutes before meals.
- Eye consultation is recommended to prevent conjunctival scarring.
- Treat secondary bacterial infection in adults for 10 days with:

  Cephalexin (Kelflex) 500 mg orally four times daily, or

  Erythromycin 500 mg orally, four times daily, or

  Dicloxacillin (Pathocil) 250 mg orally, four times daily.

  Instruct the patient to use Burow solution for exudative or weeping lesions. Soak gauze with solution, and apply topically for 20 minutes and then remove. Use two to three times daily. Avoid excessive drying with the solution.

Toxic epidermal necrolysis

- Hospitalize the patient immediately in a burn unit.
- Seek consultation with appropriate specialists.

Follow-up

- In severe disease it may be necessary to monitor the CBC, urinalysis, and renal and liver profiles for complications.

T ABLE 12.11. Medical Treatment of Erythema Multiforme

Acylovir (Zovirax)

Availability:	Prescription only.
Dosage:	400 mg orally twice daily or 200 mg orally 3 times daily.
Duration:	Ongoing.
Side effects:	Nausea, headache.
Comments:	Use suppressive dosing for prevention of EM by controlling recurrent herpes infection. Adjust dose in patients with renal disease (see PDR).

Famciclovir (Famvir)

Availability:	Prescription only.
Dosage:	250 mg orally twice daily.
Duration:	Ongoing.
Side effects:	Nausea, headache.
Comments:	Use suppressive dosing for prevention of EM by controlling recurrent herpes infection. Adjust dose in patients with renal disease (see PDR).

Valacyclovir (Valtrex)

Availability:	Prescription only.
Dosage:	500 mg orally once daily.
Duration:	Ongoing.
Side effects:	Nausea, headache.
Comments:	Use suppressive dosing for prevention of EM by controlling recurrent herpes infection. Adjust dose in patients with renal disease (see PDR). Use caution in immunosuppressed patients; can cause thrombotic thrombocytopenic purpura and hemolytic uremic syndrome in up to 3% of cases.

Topical corticosteroids (use potent topical agents; see Appendix A for details)

Availability:	Prescription.
Dosage:	Applied twice daily.
Duration:	Until rash resolves.
Side effects:	Long-term use can cause skin atrophy and telangiectasia.
Comments:	Useful in patients with limited skin involvement. Avoid use of potent corticosteroids on face and groin.

Oral steroids

Availability:	Prescription only.
Dosage:	60 to 80 mg orally daily, tapered over 3 weeks according to symptoms.
Duration:	3 weeks.
Side effects:	Long-term use can inhibit the pituitary-adrenal axis, causing severe systemic problems (see PDR).
Comments:	Helpful in adults with mild cases (limited skin involvement). Not recommended for children because the agents can increase the risk of bacterial infection.

EM, erythema multiforme; PDR, *Physicians' Desk Reference.*

- Close follow-up every 1 to 2 weeks is necessary to assess the severity of the illness and the hydration status of the patient and to ascertain whether the patient has developed a secondary bacterial infection.
- Severe disease can be worse in patients with diabetes because the disease can cause dehydration, fluctuations in serum glucose levels, and poor nutrition secondary to mucosal disease. Also, the use of corticosteroids can be problematic in patients with diabetes because it can raise the serum glucose level.

Patient Education

- Patients should be informed that the rash will last approximately 2 to 3 weeks, then regress spontaneously.
- Acetaminophen, taken accordingly to the manufacturer's dosing recommendations, may be used for relief.
- EM can be recurrent, but it is not contagious.
- To avoid recurrence, patients must avoid offending medications; if herpes simplex infections precipitate this rash, suppressive antiviral therapy is indicated.
- Patients should be cautioned that there may be postinflammatory hyperpigmentation.

ERYTHEMA NODOSUM

Erythema nodosum is an immunologically mediated hypersitity reaction with a variety of causes. Immune complexes have not been isolated, and it is believed to be a type IV, or delayed, reaction.

Chief Complaint

Patients complain of painful nodules (nodosum) of the lower legs or arms, arthralgias, fever, and malaise.

Clinical Manifestations

- Prodromal symptoms of erythema nodosum include malaise, fatigue, and arthralgias, which most commonly occur in the ankle joints.
- The rash begins to appear 1 to 3 weeks after the prodrome.
- The initial lesions are erythematous, tense, painful, hard nodules, bilaterally distributed but not symmetric.
- As the lesions progress, they become fluctuant and yellow in appearance, similar to an old bruise.
- Lesions range from 2 to 20 cm in diameter and are located in the subcutaneous fat.
- The extensor surfaces of the upper and, more commonly, lower extremities are affected, but lesions may also occur on the thighs and forearms.
- Joint symptoms include erythema, swelling, pain, and effusion.
- Lesions completely resolve in 3 to 8 weeks without sequelae.

Epidemiology

Age

Age of onset is variable, depending on underlying cause, but the condition generally occurs in patients ranging from 20 to 30 years of age.

Sex

Female patients are affected more than male patients in a 3:1 ratio.

Risk Factors

Erythema nodosum has a varied etiology, and a specific cause is found in only approximately 50% of cases (Table 12.12). Risk factors are listed in Table 12.12.

- Heredity.
- Female sex.
- Recent travel.
- Recent history of bacterial, viral, or fungal infection.

T ABLE 12.12.   Etiology of Erythema Nodosum

Medications	Behçet syndrome
Oral contraceptives	Infections
Sulfonamides	Streptococcal disease
Bromides	Psittacosis
Inflammatory bowel disease	Lymphogranuloma venereum
Ulcerative colitis	Histoplasmosis
Chron disease	Coccidioidomycosis
Lymphoma	Blastomycosis
Leukemia	Tuberculosis
Pregnancy	Infectious mononucleosis
Radiation therapy	*Yersinia* infection (enteritis)
Sarcoidosis	Idiopathic (40% of cases)

PATHOLOGY

Erythema nodosum is believed to be a type IV delayed-hypersensitity reaction. Early lesions show edema and neutrophilic infiltration with a fibrous septa in the subcutaneous fat.

Diagnosis

Diagnosis is based on clinical appearance and history. Skin biopsy is rarely needed.

Differential Diagnosis

See Table 12.13.

Diagnostic Tests

- Initial laboratory tests center on finding an underlying treatable cause.
- Recommended initial tests include the following:

T ABLE 12.13.   Etiology of Erythema Nodosum: Differential Diagnosis

Superficial and deep thrombophlebitis	Hard, tender veins, rather than nodules, can cause leg swelling.
Cellulitis/erysipelas	There are unilateral indurated areas that can rapidly expand. Bacterial culture may be positive for streptococci.
Insect bites	Lesions are usually pruritic nodules that regress in several days.
Vasculitis	The lesions are usually chronic, but may be indistinguishable from erythema nodosum. Biopsy may be necessary to differentiate.

A throat culture to rule out streptococci.

An ASO titer.

Chemistry profile.

Chest radiograph to rule out tuberculosis, fungal infections, and sarcoid.

A purified protein derivative (PPD) skin test.

An ESR.

Gastrointestinal tract symptoms warrant a stool culture (for *Yersinia* species).

- Further radiologic studies, such as a computed tomography (CT) scan of the chest or a gastrointestinal tract series, may be needed, especially if the initial chest radiograph is abnormal or the patient has gastrointestinal tract symptoms.
- Lymph node biopsy is warranted to rule out lymphoma if lymphadenopathy is present.

Referral

If the diagnosis is unclear or the lesions are unresponsive to treatment, referral is recommended.

Management

Management is focused on eliminating any inciting medication and treating any underlying disease.

Medications

See Table 12.14.

Other Treatment Modalities

- Bed rest with elevation of the involved area.
- Dressings for compression, such as support hose, elastic bandages, or Unna boots, may help.

Follow-up

Monitoring Patient Course

Patients should be followed up in 2 to 3 weeks to check on the progress of treatment. Further follow-up is warranted if the symptoms are unresponsive to treatment or if the nodules are persistent.

Potential Problems and Complications

There are problems of recurrence when the underlying cause is not treated. However, the nodules usually regress without sequelae.

Patient Education

- Patients should be advised that erythema nodosum is self-limited and resolves spontaneously, usually within weeks. Prolonged leg tenderness and ankle swelling may persist, however, for weeks thereafter.
- Erythema nodosum can recur, especially if the inciting agent or illness has not been treated.

T ABLE 12.14. Medical Treatment of Erythema Nodosum

NSAIDs or salicylates

Availability:	Over the counter.
Dosage:	Follow manufacturer's directions.
Duration:	Until pain resolves.
Side effects:	Gastrointestinal tract distress.
Comments:	For pain relief.

Prednisone

Availability:	Prescription only.
Dosage:	Initially, 40 to 60 mg daily, orally, tapered over 7 to 10 days.
Duration:	Tapered over 7 to 10 days.
Side effects:	Long-term use can inhibit pituitary-adrenal axis, causing severe systemic problems (see PDR).
Comments:	Effective, but rarely needed. Should only be used after the underlying infection has been treated or if the origin is unknown.

Potassium iodide (SSKI)

Availability:	Prescription only.
Dosage:	300 mg orally 3 times daily.
Duration:	3 to 4 weeks.
Side effects:	Stomachaches, nausea, vomiting, diarrhea, skin rash, and salivary gland swelling or pain.
Comments:	For resistant cases. Monitor thyroid function, since prolonged use can cause hypothyroidism.

NSAIDs, nonsteroidal antiinflammatory drugs; PDR, *Physicians' Desk Reference*; SSKI, saturated solution of potassium iodide.

HYPERSENSITITY VASCULITIS

- Vasculitis literally means inflammation of vessels, and vessels of any size may be affected. It encompasses many types, and has various mechanisms of pathogenesis. Hypersensitity vasculitis (HV) is the type most physicians see in practice and is discussed in detail in this chapter.
- The majority of vasculitides are associated with an immune complex deposition in the small vessels near the surface of the skin (Table 12.15). This deposition is recognized as a type III inflammation in which complement is activated and tissue damage results. Because blood vessels are involved, hemorrhages occur, which account for the typical small petechiae on the skin. As larger vessels become involved, the areas involved with the hemorrhage become confluent, resulting in scattered skin ulcers, infarction, and necrosis.
- The other mechanisms of vasculitis are less common and in some cases not known. Antineutrophil cytoplasmic autoantibody (ANCA) is present in Wegener granulomatosis and Churg-Strauss syndrome. Different autoantibodies play a role in Goodpasture and Kawasaki diseases. The direct tissue destruction within vessels of increasing size cause more physical damage on the skin along with increased severity.

Chief Complaint

Patients complain of erythematous papules, nodules, or hemorrhagic papules, which may become confluent into a larger, patchy, and painful rash that may be severe enough to cause vesicles, bullae, necrosis, and skin ulceration.

TABLE 12.15.   Types of Vasculitis

Small vessel disease	Large vessel disease

Leukocytoclastic (allergic reaction)
   Hypersensitivity vasculitis
   Henoch–Schönlein purpura (in children)
   Behçet syndrome
	Granulomatous vasculitis
	   Allergic granulomatous angiitis
	      (Churg–Strauss syndrome)
	   Wegener granulomatosis

Hypocomplementemic
   Urticarial vasculitis
	Lymphomatoid granulomatosis
	   Nodular vasculitis (erythema induratum)

Erythema elevatum diutinum (a rare, chronic vasculitis seen in HIV disease)	**Giant cell arteritis** (temporal arteritis) Takayasu arteritis
Malignant atrophic papulosis (Degos disease)	
Livedo vasculitis Polyarteritis nodosa	

Rheumatic vasculitis
   SLE
   Rheumatoid arthritis
   Scleroderma
   Polymyositis
   Dermatomyositis
   Sjögren syndrome
   Necrotizing vasculitis	

HIV, human immunodeficiency virus; SLE, systemic lupus erythematosus.

Clinical Manifestations

- HV begins with a prodromal period with fever, malaise, myalgias, and joint pain.
- Edema, nodules, erythema, and tenderness are present. The rash can range from small petechiae through coalesced (palpable) purpura to necrotic ulcers. The lesions may be painful and pruritic, or there may be no associated symptoms at all (Figure 12.4, see color insert following page 170).
- Distribution involves the lower extremities (legs and ankles), buttocks, and arms.
- In some cases, such as those involving reaction to medication, the lesions can last several days to several weeks; chronic vasculitis may last for years.
- Patients with HV may demonstrate a variety of systemic manifestations, including gastrointestinal tract bleeding or pain, glomerulitis, arthralgia or arthritis of joints, peripheral neuropathy, hemoptysis or dyspnea, and cardiac arrythmia.
- Henoch-Schönlein purpura is a type of hypersensitity vasculitis seen in individuals under 20 years of age. It is associated with diffuse abdominal pain (usually worse after meals), bloody diarrhea, arthralgia, and palpable purpura, usually seen below the waist. Kidney involvement includes hematuria and proteinuria. It usually follows an upper respiratory tract infection.

Epidemiology

Approximately 50% of the cases are idiopathic.

Age

Although HV usually occurs in patients from 20 to 30 years of age, it can occur in patients of any age.

Sex

HV occurs equally among male and female patients.

Risk Factors

- See Table 12.16.
- There is a hereditary factor in the development of HV.
- Recent infection, such as upper respiratory tract infection caused by group A streptococcus, is a risk factor for HV.
- Use of certain medications may be a precipitating factor.

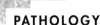

PATHOLOGY

Granulocytes are seen perivascularly and extravascularly in the upper dermis in both adult and childhood forms of vasculitis. Immunofluorescent studies show IgG and immunoglobulin M (IgM) deposits in the vascular wall in adults. IgA deposits predominate in Henoch-Schönlein disease.

Diagnosis

- Diagnosis consists of correctly identifying the rash as a vasculitis, then determining the underlying cause.
- One technique to distinguish vasculitis from other types of rashes is to place a glass slide over an area and press firmly; a lack of blanching when pressure is applied indicates a vasculitis.
- It is important to question the patient to determine whether a family history of autoimmune disease exists.

TABLE 12.16. Risk Factors for Hypersensitivity Vasculitis

Infectious

Viral: Hepatitis B and C, influenza, mononucleosis, and cytomegalovirus

Bacterial: Staphylococcus aureus and group A streptococcus, leprosy, tuberculosis, and *Escherichia coli*

Drugs/chemicals

Penicillin, sulfonamides, aspirin, quinidine, propylthiouracil, phenothiazines, allopurinol (Zyloprim), iodides, thiazides, insecticides, herbicides, petroleum products, and serum

Malignancy

Chronic lymphocytic leukemia, non-Hodgkin lymphoma, multiple myeloma, Hodgkin lymphoma, renal carcinoma, and hairy cell leukemia

Systemic diseases

SLE, rheumatoid arthritis, biliary cirrhosis, ulcerative colitis, hemolytic anemia, cryoglobulinemia, chronic active hepatitis, and Sjögren syndrome

Idiopathic (50% of cases)

SLE, systemic lupus erythematosus.

Differential Diagnosis

See Table 12.17.

Diagnostic Tests

Patients with HV may demonstrate a variety of systemic manifestations, including gastrointestinal tract bleeding or pain, glomerulitis, arthralgia or arthritis of joints, peripheral neuropathy, hemoptysis or dyspnea, and cardiac arrhythmia. A complete review of systems, with appropriate testing, is indicated to detect these extracutaneous manifestations.

- Initial laboratory tests should include ASO titer, ESR, platelet count, CBC, renal and liver profiles, chest radiograph, tests for human immunodeficiency virus (HIV), urinalysis, ANA, serum protein electrophoresis, throat culture, tests for hepatitis B and C, cryoglobulin determination, and test for rheumatoid factor.
- Skin biopsies should be performed with immunofluorescent studies if the diagnosis is uncertain (Table 12.18).

Referral

- Referral to a rheumatologist may be helpful for diagnostic testing if the origin is unclear.
- Other specialists, such as renal or pulmonary specialists, should be consulted, depending on the involved organ system.
- Referral to a dermatologist is recommended for patients who demonstrate deep ulcerations.

T ABLE 12.17. Hypersensitivity Vasculitis: Differential Diagnosis

Thrombocytopenic purpura	Can occur on extremities, chest, neck, and face. Platelet count is low, and bleeding time prolonged.
	Biopsy is useful to differentiate.
Disseminated intravascular coagulation	Disseminated purpura with hemorrhage. Bleeding studies prolonged; fibrinogen level low. Nonpalpable purpura.
Sepsis (meningococcal)	Severe systemic problems such as vascular collapse, fever, shock. Nonpalpable purpura.
	Biopsy may be useful early in the course.
Rocky Mountain spotted fever	Can cause septic vasculitis.
	Rash can occur anywhere, including the palms and soles.
	Nonpalpable purpura.
Exanthematous drug eruption	Blanching, red maculopapular rash is symmetric on upper trunk, neck, face, and extremities. History of recent drug ingestion.
	Nonpalpable purpura.
	Biopsy is useful to differentiate.
Senile purpura	Occurs as a response to minor trauma or secondary to medication (e.g., NSAIDs, warfarin) in older patients.
Nonpalpable purpura.	

NSAIDs, nonsteroidal antiinflammatory drugs.

T ABLE 12.18.   Diagnostic Criteria: Hypersensitivity Vasculitis

Hypersensitivity vasculitis (must have 3 out of 5 to confirm diagnosis)
Age greater than 16 years when the symptoms develop
Medication taken near or at onset of symptoms
Palpable purpura that does not blanche under pressure; no thrombocytopenia
Maculopapular rash
Biopsy findings showing granulocytes perivascularly and extravascularly; immunofluorescent studies showing
    IgM and IgG in vessel wall

Henoch–Schönlein purpura (must have 2 out of 4 to confirm diagnosis)
Age under 20 years
Palpable purpura; no thrombocytopenia
Abdominal pain worse after meals, probably related to bowel angina (ischemia), and bloody diarrhea
Biopsy findings showing granulocytes perivascularly and extravascularly; immunofluorescent studies show
    IgA in vessel wall

IgM, immunoglobulin M; IgG, immunoglobulin G; IgA, immunoglobulin A.
From Calabrese LH, Michel BA, Bloch DA, et al. The American College of Rheumatology 1990 criteria for the
classification of hypersensitivity vasculitis. *Arthritis Rheum* 1990;33(8):1108–1113; Mills JA, Michel BA, Bloch
DA, et al. The American College of Rheumatology 1990 criteria for the classification of Henoch-Schönlein purpura. *Arthritis Rheum* 1990;33(8):1114–1121, with permission.

Management

- Identifying and treating the underlying cause is the mainstay of treatment. Elimination of precipitating medication or chemical agents is essential. Lesions may resolve
  spontaneously when the underlying cause is treated or eliminated.
- Appropriate antibiotics should be used for primary or secondary bacterial infections.

Medications
See Table 12.19.

Other Treatment Modalities
Plasma exchange has been shown to be effective and should be performed by a physician who is trained and experienced in this treatment modality.

Henoch-Schönlein Purpura
- Children should be hospitalized, hydrated, and monitored closely for systemic
  organ involvement, especially renal disease.
- Oral prednisone 1 mg/kg daily may be administered initially, then tapered over 2 to
  3 weeks.

  Or

- Methylprednisolone may be administered intravenously, 10 to 30 mg/kg per dose,
  repeated every 8 hours. Switch to oral prednisone when vasculitis and systemic
  symptoms subside.

Follow-up

Patients should be followed up weekly until the vasculitis regresses, especially in
cases in which an underlying cause has not been identified. Purpura may progress to
necrotic ulcerations that could lead to gangrene, making close follow-up essential.

T ABLE 12.19.   Medical Treatment of Hypersensitivity Vasculitis

Colchicine

Availability:	Prescription only.
Dosage:	0.6 mg orally 2 to 3 times daily for 7 to 10 days, then taper off.
Duration:	Until lesions resolve.
Side effects:	Diarrhea (see PDR).
Comments:	For recurrent or persistent purpura. Contraindicated in children and pregnant women.

Azathioprine (Imuran)

Availability:	Prescription only.
Dosage:	100 to 250 mg orally once daily.
Duration:	4 to 8 weeks or until improvement is noted.
Side effects:	Leukopenia, thrombocytopenia, nausea, vomiting, or hepatitis.
Comments:	Monitor CBC, platelet count, and liver function tests weekly. Contraindicated in pregnant women.

Dapsone

Availability:	Prescription only.
Dosage:	25 to 75 mg orally twice daily.
Duration:	4 to 8 weeks or until improvement is noted.
Side effects:	Nausea, vomiting, abdominal pain, fever, tinnitus, vertigo, headache, phototoxity, and blurred vision (see PDR).
Comments:	Can cause hemolytic anemia in G6PD deficiency; determine G6PD level before use.

Prednisone

Availability:	Prescription only.
Dosage:	60 mg orally daily initially; taper slowly.
Duration:	Until improvement is noted.
Side effects:	Long-term use can cause inhibition of the pituitary-adrenal axis, causing severe systemic problems (see PDR).
Comments:	For severe disease with multiple ulcerations and/or multiple organ involvement. Can be used concomitantly with azathioprine to alleviate steroid use.

PDR, *Physicians' Desk Reference;* CBC, complete blood cell count; G6PD, glucose-6-phosphate dehydrogenase.

Patient Education

- Patients should be reassured that the prognosis of HV secondary to infection is very good. However, the possibility of systemic involvement is more problematic, since HV can affect major organ systems, including the cardiovascular system. For this reason, patients should be counseled to adhere closely to the prescribed regimen of steroid treatment, including the recommended tapering of dosage. Patients should also be counseled as to the side effects of steroids.
- Rest and elevation of the affected area provide temporary relief until treatment begins to take effect.
- In certain instances, allergic vasculitis can be caused by certain malignancies.
- HV is not contagious, but if an underlying infection has caused the disease, that infection may be contagious.

BULLOUS PEMPHIGOID

Bullous pemphigoid is a chronic autoimmune disease causing bullae in older patients.

Chief Complaint

Patients report a blistering, pruritic, and painful rash at many sites on the body.

Clinical Manifestations

- The prodrome of bullous pemphigoid is a spontaneous urticarial rash, which in some cases is preceded by pruritis (Figure 12.5, see color insert following page 170).
- The initial lesion evolves into a bullous rash after several weeks to months. These bullae may arise from an erythematous base or from normal skin.
- Bullae are round or oval, and tense. When bullae rupture, erosions and crusts appear.
- Lesions are found scattered randomly about the skin, or grouped in a specific area. Sites of predilection include lower legs, flexor surfaces of the forearms, medial aspects of the thighs, groin, and abdomen. Mucous membranes may be involved in 33% of cases.
- The rash may be asymptomatic or may be pruritic and painful.
- Bullous pemphigoid may persist for months, or as long as 5 to 7 years in chronic cases.
- Nikolsky sign (the shearing or sloughing off of normal skin after applying lateral pressure) is not present.
- Healing occurs in 90% of patients without scarring; however, the incidence of post-inflammatory hyperpigmentation is low.
- Secondary bacterial infection can occur in the erosions.
- Remissions and recurrences are common.

Epidemiology

- There is no association with an increased risk of occult malignancy.
- The mortality rate is low.

Age

Age of onset is 60 to 80 years of age.

Sex

The incidence is equal in men and women.

Risk Factors

- A familial predisposition for bullous pemphigoid is likely.
- Use of multiple medications may be a risk factor.
- Skin trauma from ultraviolet radiation may increase the risk of developing bullous pemphigoid.

PATHOLOGY

This is an autoimmune disease with circulating autoantibodies to the basement membrane of the skin. Antibodies (IgG) attach to the basement membrane in a linear fashion that activates complement and inflammatory mediators. These collect beneath the top layer of the skin and cause the bullae formation.

Diagnosis

Differential Diagnosis

See Table 12.20.

Diagnostic Tests

- Antibasement antibody (IgG) titer should be ordered when the diagnosis is suspected; antibodies are present in 70% of patients. Severity of the disease does not correlate with the titer.
- Skin biopsy is helpful, but not mandatory.
- A CBC shows eosinophilia, but is nonspecific.

Referral

It is recommended that patients with extensive disease be referred to a dermatologist, who can then manage the disease in concert with the primary care physician.

Management

Aggressive therapy is indicated because of the disfiguring nature of bullous pemphigoid.
- High-dose prednisone with or without the concomitant use of azathioprine (Imuran) is the initial choice of treatment for severe diseases. Patients in whom steroids (azathioprine) are contraindicated may be treated with azathioprine alone.
- Other agents, such as dapsone or tetracycline, can be tried if the initial therapy is not helpful.

Medications

See Table 12.21.

Other Treatment Modalities

Plasmapheresis has also been reported to be helpful in severe bullous disease. It should be left to physicians experienced in this treatment modality.

Follow-up

- Long-term use of corticosteroids is a real possibility in bullous disease, making close follow-up a necessity. Severe systemic side effects such as diabetes, hypertension, osteoporosis, decreased host response to infection, and poor wound heal-

---

T ABLE 12.20. Bullous Pemphigoid: Differential Diagnosis

Pemphigoid vulgaris	Tense, intact bullae are rare; there is more mucosal involvement.
	It is much more severe than bullous pemphigoid and is potentially fatal.
	Biopsy is necessary to differentiate the two.
Bullous drug eruption	Rash develops from use of a new medication or chronic use of medications (e.g., furosemide, sulfonamides).
	Biopsy is useful to differentiate.
Bullous erythema multiforme	There are targetlike lesions and a history of infection or medication use.
	Immunofluorescence test is negative for linear IgG antibodies.
Dermatitis herpetiformis	Grouped vesicles occur on extensor surfaces; occasionally lesions are excoriated.
	Biopsy is useful to differentiate.

IgG, immunoglobulin G.

T ABLE 12.21. Medical Treatment of Bullous Pemphigoid

High-potency topical corticosteroids

Availability:	Prescription only.
Dosage:	Apply twice daily.
Duration:	Taper to less potent creams over 4 to 5 weeks until the lesions are well healed.
Side effects:	Long-term use can cause skin atrophy and telangiectasia.
Comments:	For mild disease (localized bullae, urticarial rash, or pruritus).

Prednisone

Availability:	Prescription only.
Dosage:	50 to 100 mg orally daily or 1 mg/kg orally daily.
Duration:	Use high dosage until symptoms regress, then taper.
Side effects:	Long-term use can cause serious systemic side effects (see *Physician's Desk Reference*).
Comments:	Use to control symptoms initially. Lower dose should be used when remission has occurred.

Tetracycline

Availability:	Prescription only.
Dosage:	1 to 2.5 g orally daily.
Duration:	7 to 10 days.
Side effects:	Nausea, sun sensitivity, gastrointestinal tract upset.
Comments:	Helpful in reducing bullae formation in mild cases, although the mechanism is not understood. Useful in combination with nicotinamide in patients in whom steroids are contraindicated.

Azathioprine (Imuran)

Availability:	Prescription only.
Dosage:	Initially, 100 mg (1 to 1.5 mg/kg) orally daily; decrease to 50 to 100 mg per day for maintenance.
Duration:	Use until disease is suppressed (2 to 6 months after initiation), then continue for an additional 2 months. Can be reinstituted during flare-ups.
Side effects:	Leukopenia, thrombocytopenia, nausea, vomiting, and hepatitis. Long-term use requires weekly monitoring of CBC and liver function tests.
Comments:	For moderate to severe bullous disease. Can be used in conjunction with prednisone as a steroid-sparing agent. Recent studies suggest that this agent is not effective when used alone.

Dapsone

Availability:	Prescription only.
Dosage:	100 to 150 mg orally daily.
Duration:	Until remissions occur.
Side effects:	Nausea, vomiting, abdominal pain, fever, tinnitus, vertigo, headache, phototoxicity, and blurred vision.
Comments:	For mild cases, but not first-line choice in severe bullous disease. Can cause hemolytic anemia in G6PD-deficient patients; determine G6PD level before use.

Hydroxyzine

Availability:	Prescription only.
Dosage:	25 to 50 mg orally daily.
Duration:	As needed for pruritus.
Side effects:	Drowsiness.
Comments:	Helpful for severe pruritus.

CBC, complete blood cell count; G6PD, glucose-6-phosphate dehydrogenase.

ing can occur. Blood pressure and serum glucose levels should be monitored every 1 to 2 weeks initially. As the dosage of prednisone is tapered, the frequency of the follow-up visits can be decreased.

- Secondary bacterial infection can occur in the skin erosions. Patients should be monitored closely to identify the infections quickly and treat them with antibiotics.
- Medication side effects, especially those associated with azathioprine, should also be monitored periodically.

Patient Education

Patient should be reassured that remission and cure, without any residual scarring, occurs in 90% of cases. Lesions typically heal without scarring unless secondary bacterial infection occurs in the erosions. However, bullous pemphigoid may last from a few months to 5 to 7 years.

Compliance

Compliance with systemic corticosteroids is mandatory.

Lifestyle Changes

- Patients should be counseled to avoid scratching and to use oral antihistamines if necessary to help control the pruritis.
- Sunlight exposure should be avoided, since it frequently worsens bullae.

Family and Community Support

The cosmetically disfiguring nature of this disease makes supportive counseling from the physician advisable.

PEMPHIGUS VULGARIS

Pemphigus vulgaris (PV) is a serious, chronic autoimmune disease causing bullae on the skin and mucous membranes. PV can be fatal if not treated aggressively with immunosuppressants.

Chief Complaint

Patients may initially complain of sores in the mouth or a painful throat, which precedes the skin involvement by several months, or they may present with a blistering, painful rash that is *not pruritic.*

Clinical Manifestations

- PV usually begins in the mouth, with painful erythematous lesions on the soft palate. On the skin, vesicular lesions are seen predominately on the axilla, groin, umbilicus, face, scalp, and chest (Figure 12.6, see color insert following page 170).
- Burning or itching is minimal with new lesions. However, the lesions are very painful when they rupture, and they rupture easily, leaving behind erythematous erosions with surrounding crusting and scaling skin. The lesions also bleed easily. Secondary bacterial infections can occur in erosions.
- Blisters or bullae are flaccid, skin-colored, and round and may be localized or generalized in distribution.
- Oral mucosal pain secondary to denuded mucous membranes can lead to dehydration and nutritional difficulties. Weakness, malaise, and even weight loss may result from the patient's inability to eat.
- Nikolsky sign is pathognomonic for this disease. It is demonstrated by pressing on a bulla and observing the extravasation of fluid laterally, thus extending the bulla into normal skin. This occurs because of the loss of cohesion between the cells.

- Lesions heal without scarring in 90% of cases, although some scarring may occur in areas of eroded lesions with secondary infection.

Epidemiology

- PV is relatively rare, with an incidence ratio of 1:100,000.
- PV occurs in higher incidence in Ashkenazi Jewish people of Mediterranean extraction.
- The disease usually occurs in patients ranging from 40 to 60 years of age and occurs equally among men and women.
- The mortality rate is 5% to 10%, with death usually occurring secondary to sepsis or complications resulting from corticosteroid use.

Risk Factors

- Minor burns, sunburn, and skin injury may be risk factors.
- Use of certain medications, including penicillamine, captopril (Capoten), rifampin (Rifadin), and phenylbutazone (Butazolidin), may precipitate development of PV.
- Heredity may be a risk factor.
- Myasthenia gravis, thymoma, and non-Hodgkin lymphoma have all been associated with PV and occur more frequently in patients with PV.

PATHOLOGY

IgG antibodies are involved. The tissue destruction is different in pemphigus vulgaris than in bullous pemphigoid because the antibodies do not attack the basement membrane but attack the keratinocyte surface glycoproteins, which in turn forces cells to lose their cohesiveness and causes the top layer of skin to separate just above the basal cell layer (acantholysis).

This disease is associated with the HLA-DR4/HLA-DR6 phenotype.

Diagnosis

Diagnosis of this disease and its variants can be difficult, and correct diagnosis is necessary. It is recommended that cases of suspected PV be referred to a dermatologist.

Differential Diagnosis

See Table 12.22.

Diagnostic Tests

- A serum pemphigus antibody titer (IgG autoantibodies targeting desmoglein III) should be drawn initially. The amount of antibody correlates well with the disease severity, which is useful during treatment.
- Routine skin biopsy should be performed to reveal the characteristic acantholysis. Direct and indirect immunofluorescence biopsy should be obtained to reveal the presence of IgG antibodies.

Referral

Referral to a dermatologist is recommended for diagnosis and treatment of this potentially fatal disease. The treatments are immunosuppressive and require close follow-up.

T ABLE 12.22. Pemphigus Vulgaris: Differential Diagnosis

Bullous pemphigoid	Tense bullae occur on extensor surfaces. There is less oral mucosal involvement than in pemphigus vulgaris.
	Biopsy is necessary to differentiate the two; linear IgG antibodies are noted in the biopsy.
Bullous drug eruption	Rash occurs from use of a new medication or with chronic use of medication.
	Biopsy is useful to differentiate from pemphigus vulgaris.
Bullous erythema multiforme	Targetlike lesions occur on the skin and oral mucosa. There is a history of infection or medication use.
	Immunofluorescence test is negative for IgG antibodies.
	Biopsy does not show acantholysis; therefore it helps to differentiate the two.
Dermatitis herpetiformis	Grouped vesicles occur on extensor skin surfaces.
	Biopsy is helpful to differentiate the two.

IgG, immunoglobulin G.

Management

The extensiveness and potential lethality of PV requires referral to a dermatologist.

Medications

See Table 12.23.

Other Treatment Modalities

- Antibiotics, cleansing baths, and loose dressings can help treat and prevent infection.
- Fluids for electrolyte disturbances may be needed.
- To reduce antibody levels with poorly controlled disease, plasmapheresis may be helpful. A physician experienced in this treatment modality should be consulted.

Follow-up

- The physician should monitor patients weekly until treatment reduces the oral involvement. Patients with severe oral involvement may require hospitalization for parenteral hydration and nutritional support.
- Patients should also be monitored weekly for secondary bacterial infection. The erosions usually become infected, necessitating use of oral or parenteral antibiotics, depending on the severity of the infection.
- Infections in patients taking high-dose corticosteroids and immunosuppressants can be problematic and may lead to sepsis, which is one of the leading causes of mortality in this disease.
- Long-term corticosteroid use can cause diabetes, hypertension, osteoporosis, decreased host immune response, and poor wound healing. Patients should be monitored weekly with blood glucose determinations and blood pressure readings.
- Occult neoplasia has been associated with PV. The physician should perform diagnostic tests, including CBC, chest radiograph, and CT scan of the chest and abdomen to diagnose these associated tumors.

Patient Education

Patients should be advised that the disease and bullae will resolve in about 6 to 12 months. They may be reassured that blisters usually heal without scarring unless a secondary bacterial infection occurs.

T ABLE 12.23. Medical Treatment of Pemphigus Vulgaris

Prednisone

Availability:	Prescription only.
Dosage and duration:	2 to 3 mg/kg orally daily. Use high dosage initially until new blister formation ceases, then taper rapidly by 10 mg over 7 to 10 days (until the rash is almost cleared), then taper slowly to an effective maintenance dose.
Side effects:	Long-term use can lead to serious systemic side effects (see *Physician's Desk Reference*).

Azathioprine (Imuran)

Availability:	Prescription only.
Dosage and duration:	2 to 3 mg/kg daily orally. Use high dose initially until the rash is completely cleared, then taper to 1 mg/kg and continue for several months.
Side effects:	Leukopenia, thrombocytopenia, nausea, vomiting, and hepatitis.
Comments:	Use concomitantly with prednisone for sparing effect. Monitor CBC and liver profile weekly.

Methotrexate (Rheumatrex)

Availability:	Prescription only.
Dosage:	25 to 35 mg/kg daily, orally or parenterally. Use high dose until lesions have cleared, then taper to lowest dose to maintain clearing.
Duration:	Discontinue when pemphigus antibody titer is negative for 3 months.
Side effects:	Stomatitis, leukopenia, nausea, abdominal distress, and hepatotoxicity.
Comments:	Not as effective as cyclophosphamide or azathioprine. Monitor CBC and liver profile weekly. Contraindicated in pregnant women.

Cyclophosphamide (Cytoxan)

Availability:	Prescription only.
Dosage:	Bolus of 1000 mg intravenously each week for 2 weeks followed by maintenance dose of 50 to 100 mg orally every day; or 100 to 200 mg orally daily for 2 weeks, then reduced to 50 to 100 mg daily for maintenance.
Duration:	Reduce high-dose therapy when the lesions clear, maintain lower dose until the pemphigus antibody titer is negative for 3 months.
Side effects:	Bone marrow suppression, hemorrhagic cystitis, bladder fibrosis, sterility, alopecia, and increased risk of malignancy.
Comments:	Monitor CBC and urinalysis weekly for side effects. Can be used concomitantly with oral prednisone for its sparing effect. Probably more effective than azathioprine for adjunctive therapy, but has more serious side effects.

CBC, complete blood cell count.

BIBLIOGRAPHY

Calabrese LH, Michel BA, Bloch DA, et al. The American College of Rheumatology 1990 criteria for the classification of hypersensitivity vasculitis. *Arthritis Rheum* 1990;33(8):1108-1113.

Korman N. Pemphigus. *J Am Acad Dermatol* 1988;18:1219-1238.

Mahmood T. Urticaria. *Am Fam Physician* 1995;51(4):811-816.

Mertz GJ, Loveless MO, Levin MJ, et al. Oral famciclovir for suppression of recurrent genital herpes simplex virus infection in women: a multicenter, double-blind, placebo-controlled trial. *Arch Intern Med* 1997;157(3):343-349.

Mills JA, Michel BA, Bloch DA, et al. The American College of Rheumatology 1990 criteria for the classification of Henoch-Schönlein purpura. *Arthritis Rheum* 1990;33(8):1114-1121.

Stevens GL, Adelman HM, Wallach PM. Palpable purpura: an algorithmic approach. *Am Fam Physician* 1995;52:1355-1362.

CHAPTER 13

Nail Disorders

CHIEF COMPLAINT

The patient reports a change in texture, color, or both, of some or all nails, including both the fingernails and toenails. Likewise, the patient may report a distortion of any or all of the nails, including abnormal color, shape, and thickness of the nail plate.

CLINICAL MANIFESTATIONS

Nail Matrix Abnormalities

The nail matrix is composed of modified epithelium, which produces the keratin that forms the nail plate. The proximal nail fold overlies the nail matrix. The distal aspect of the matrix that can be seen through the translucent nail plate is called the lunula (the white half-moon noted in the proximal nail bed). The cuticle is formed from a keratin layer of the proximal nail fold and overlies the proximal nail plate. The cuticle serves as a functional barrier to the nail matrix from infection.

Nail matrix abnormalities are generally caused by inflammatory conditions, which affect the modified epithelium of the matrix, thereby affecting normal keratin production. These abnormalities in normal keratin production result in nail pitting and ridging.

Pitting

Pitting can be a normal variant of the nail, with isolated pitting, or may be indicative of the following:

Psoriasis

Nails may be asymptomatic (i.e., there are no symptoms of pain, burning, pruritus, etc.).

There are a few to multiple pitted disruptions of the nail plate involving some or all nails (usually fingernails).

There may be more subtle depressions to deeper, more sharply defined, punched-out lesions.

Subungual hyperkeratosis heralds the onset of onycholysis (separation of the nail plate from the underlying nail bed).

Eczema and atopic dermatitis

Nails may be asymptomatic.

Larger, irregular pitting of the nails is noted.

Eczema is seen around the nail.

Alopecia areata

Alopecia areata is associated with patches of hair loss in the scalp. Alopecia is a cause of nail pitting which is a poor prognostic sign for hair regrowth. Alopecia involves the nail in 7% to 66% of cases.

Nail pitting is usually irregular, diffuse, and small.

Scotch-plaid pitting or transverse rippling, which is characteristic of alopecia areata, is seen.

There may also be opacification of the nail.

Transverse Ridging

Transverse ridging may be a normal variant of the nail, or it may indicate the following:

Eczema

As with pitting, any form of eczema surrounding the nail may disrupt the nail matrix and manifest as transverse ridging. Nail is asymptomatic.

Paronychia

Paronychia is an acute or chronic infection of the nail fold that can be caused by *Staphylococcus aureus, Candida* species, dermatophytes, or herpes. It is painful and throbbing.

There is red, tender swelling of the paronychia.

Ridging of the nail is caused by persistent pressure to the nail matrix.

Beau lines

Beau lines can be caused by a systemic disease (e.g., high fever, shock, myocardial infarction, pulmonary embolism) that results in a period of low cell division, causing a thin nail plate. For example, in scarlet fever, a transverse ridge (Beau line) secondary to an arrest of nail growth occurs in all of the nails at the same place. Following resolution of the systemic illness, the nail matrix returns to normal function and nail growth returns to normal (Figure 13.1, see color insert following page 170).

Transverse linear depression in several or all nails usually is distributed symmetrically.
  The thumbs and toenails are most commonly affected.

There may also be white discoloration of the nail.

Beau lines can be seen in infants as young as 4 to 5 weeks of age.

Longitudinal Ridging

Longitudinal ridging may be a normal finding, especially in children, or it may be indicative of the following:

Lichen planus

Approximately 10% of cases of lichen planus involve the nail. Longitudinal ridging is the most common nail change associated with lichen planus, which is associated with other cutaneous findings, including the four Ps: purple, pruritic, planar, and polyangular findings.

There is fine longitudinal ridging of the nails parallel to the long axis of the digit.

Thinning and brittleness of the nail may also be seen.

Median nail dystrophy

Median nail dystrophy is idiopathic or in some cases is caused by chronic picking or biting of the proximal nail fold (habit-tic deformity of the nail). The injured matrix then gives rise to a dystrophic nail plate.

The nails themselves may be asymptomatic.

Median nail dystrophy is usually seen in a single nail, most often affecting the thumb.

The longitudinal ridging has an "upside-down Christmas tree" appearance.

A broad nail groove made up of numerous concave longitudinal ridges can be seen in the habit-tic variant.

Warts

Warts are common in nail biters on the skin bordering the nail plate, at the base of the nail or the tip of the finger. They cause longitudinal ridging by persistent pressure to the proximal nail fold.

Myxoid cyst

Myxoid cyst is a focal collection of mucin and commonly occurs at the base of the nail. It occurs more commonly in women.

It is associated with some nail pain.

It usually occurs on the dorsal aspect of the distal interphalangeal joint of the finger; it is less common on the toe.

It causes persistent pressure to the proximal nail fold, disrupting the nail matrix and causing ridging.

Darier disease

Darier disease (keratosis follicularis) has diagnostic nail signs in 92% of cases.

The disease is autosomal dominant.

All nails are affected.

Regular, fine, longitudinal ridges are seen, with notching at the end of the nail.

Red or white subungual streaks may also be noted.

Nail Bed Abnormalities

The nail bed is the epithelium that lies beneath the nail plate. It is a highly vascular area with parallel longitudinal grooves to facilitate nail plate growth. The nail bed extends from the lunula to the areas known as the *hyponychium* (a small segment of the epidermis at the distal end of the digit, which lacks adherence to the nail plate). It begins at the distal end of the nail bed and ends at the anatomic structure known as the *distal groove.*

Discoloration

Nail bed abnormalities are manifested by color changes beneath the translucent nail plate and include the following:

Psoriasis

In addition to the other cutaneous and nail findings associated with psoriasis, the disease may cause a yellow-orange to brown discoloration of the nail bed, known as a salmon patch.

Malignant melanoma

Melanoma in the nail bed presents as a brown or black discoloration, with progressive widening of the discoloration over time. Usually only one nail is involved.

The discoloration can spread to the proximal nail fold.

The condition is usually ignored by the patient.

Junctional nevus

The nail may be asymptomatic.

There is a round or oval area of brown discoloration of the nail bed.

Malignant melanoma should be suspected if the color becomes variegated or the lesion changes in any way.

Glomus tumor

Glomus tumor is a benign tumor, which may present as a tender area under the nail plate. Seventy-five percent of these tumors are found in the hand (fingertips), particularly subungually.

Pain under the nail is associated with pressure or the cold.

There may be a pink discoloration to the nail.

Glomus tumor occurs in adults between the ages of 30 and 50 years, with women affected more frequently than men.

Half-and-half nail

Half-and-half nail is a sharp demarcation between the proximal white and distal pink or brown half of the nail bed. It is associated with chronic renal failure.

Half-and-half nail is seen in 9% to 50% of patients with chronic renal failure.

The nail bed may also appear white or pale.

Pruritus, eccymosis, and yellow hyperpigmentation of the skin may also occur in association with chronic renal failure.

Splinter hemorrhages

Splinter hemorrhages are red or brown streaks localized to an individual nail usually at the midportion of the nail bed and seen more frequently in male patients (Figure 13.2, see color insert following page 170); the first three fingers of both hands are those commonly involved. They are associated with the following:

Subacute bacterial endocarditis, which also demonstrates systemic signs and symptoms, such as weakness, fatigue, fever, chills, and night sweats. Splinter hemorrhages associated with subacute bacterial endocarditis are rare and are located proximally.

Minor trauma. Brown or red streaks typically occur at the distal portion of the nail bed.

Subungual hematoma

Subungual hematoma is associated with a history of significant trauma to the nail.

A brown or black hematoma is noted below the nail plate.

There is often throbbing pain.

The hematoma may stain the nail plate, and it advances with nail growth.

Terry nail

Terry nail is a condition in which the color of the proximal two-thirds of the nail bed is white and the distal third is red. Terry nail is associated with hypoalbuminemia, hepatic cirrhosis, and congestive heart failure, as follows:

Hypoalbuminemia

The nail bed is usually pale or white, although it may demonstrate the distinct coloration of Terry nail.

When hypoalbuminemia is associated with nephrotic syndrome, a nail condition known as *Muehrcke nail* may demonstrate transverse white bands separated by a normal bed color; this bed color remains stationary as the nail grows. Muehrcke nail is rarely seen on the thumb and occurs more commonly on the second, third, or fourth finger.

Hypoalbuminemia can cause generalized body edema.

Hepatic cirrhosis

The characteristic Terry nail is associated with hepatic cirrhosis.

Other signs include palmar erythema, spider telangiectasia, and clubbing.

Systemic symptoms include anorexia, nausea, vomiting, fatigue, weakness, and jaundice.

Congestive heart failure

Symptoms include shortness of breath, peripheral edema, paroxysmal nocturnal dyspnea, or orthopnea.

Terry nail may also occur.

Nail Plate Abnormalities

The nail plate is a hard, translucent plate of dead keratin formed from the nail matrix. Nail plate abnormalities are often the most visible feature of skin disorders such as alopecia areata or psoriasis; changes are also seen as a result of trauma and underlying systemic disease.

Discoloration

Blue nails

Blue nail plate discoloration (blue or blue-gray) may be the result of a variety of medications, dyes, chemicals, occupational exposures, as well as systemic diseases such as hemochromatosis, ochronosis, and Wilson disease.
Hemochromatosis is caused by increased iron absorption and excessive iron stores.

The nail plate may have a blue or blue-gray discoloration.

Weakness, abdominal pain, and/or arthralgia may be associated findings.

Wilson disease is a chronic, inherited (autosomal recessive) metabolic disorder characterized by neurologic symptoms caused by toxic accumulation of copper in the brain, liver, and other organs.

The nail plate has a blue or blue-gray discoloration.

Kayser-Fleischer rings (deposits of copper in the cornea) are found on physical examination.

Associated findings include tremor, chorea, and spasticity.

Brown nails

Brown nails are a normal variation in African Americans. They may also be indicative of the following:

Hemochromatosis.

Gold therapy and *arsenic intoxication.*

Addison disease.

> Addison disease is due to autoimmune-induced or tuberculosis-induced hypofunction of the adrenal glands.

> Patients may present with hyperpigmentation of the mucous membranes, palm folds, and the areola, as well as brown nail discoloration.

> Adrenal hypofunction, with aldosterone and cortisol deficiency, may cause weakness, fatigue, and weight loss.

Malignant melanoma.

> Malignant melanoma may present with a brown-black nail streak.

> Pigmentation may spill over into the proximal nail fold (Hutchinson sign).

Yellow nails

Yellow nail syndrome is a systemic (usually pulmonary) familial illness, probably due to a congenital abnormality of the lymphatics, and associated with cancer, pleural effusion, bronchiectasis, Hodgkin lymphoma, endometrial cancer, or malignant melanoma.

It is characterized by yellow-green nails, lymphatic abnormalities (i.e., lymphangitis and lymphedema of the face and extremities), absent cuticles, and onycholysis. There is no nail growth. Both fingernails and toenails are affected.

Pulmonary symptoms such as shortness of breath and cough may be present. There may be abnormal vaginal or uterine bleeding.

It is more commonly seen in adults; males and females are equally affected.

White nails

Leukonychia is a white discoloration of the nails, although the nail plate rarely is totally white. Leukonychia is a normal finding in some individuals and can be inherited as an autosomal dominant trait.

White spots on individual nails are probably due to minor trauma or manipulation of the cuticle (as can occur with an overly aggressive manicure).

White lines do not extend the entire width of the nail.

Leukonychia usually regresses spontaneously as the nail grows out.

Thickening

Onychomycosis causes a gradual onset of nail plate thickening of one or more digits caused by dermatophyte infection (90% are caused by *Trichophyton rubrum*).

The nail plates of toes are most often affected (by the dermatophyte infection) because of their slow rate of growth compared with fingernails.

Nail plates are chalk white or yellow and thickened.

Change in Shape

Clubbing

Clubbing is the chronic, gradual onset of overcurvature of the nail. The angle between the normally curved nail plate and the proximal nail fold (Lovibond angle) is greater than 160 degrees.

Clubbing can be a normal variant. The normal variant can be distinguished from acquired clubbing by the Schamroth window test, which demonstrates a small diamond-shaped space formed by the angles of two opposed fingernails. There is no diamond-shaped window formed by opposing two truly clubbed fingernails.

Clubbing can be congenital, inherited as an autosomal dominant trait.

Approximately 80% of clubbing cases involve the pulmonary system [e.g., chronic obstructive pulmonary disease (COPD), bronchiectasis, cystic fibrosis, neoplasm, tuberculosis] or the cardiovascular system (e.g., cyanotic congenital heart disease, endocarditis, secondary polycythemia).

Acquired clubbing can also be due to gastrointestinal tract disease, such as cirrhosis, chronic obstructive jaundice, ulcerative colitis, as well as thyrotoxicosis.

Koilonychia

Koilonychia (spoon-shaped nails) can be a normal finding in children, especially newborns.

Spoon-shaped nails are often brittle.

The concavity is caused by softening and thinning of the nail plate, usually of the thumb, index, and middle fingernails.

Koilonychia is an associated finding in iron deficiency anemia, Plummer-Vinson syndrome (dysphagia and glossitis), Raynaud disease, hemochromatosis, and trauma.

EPIDEMIOLOGY

Ten percent to 50% of patients with systemic disease have nail involvement, as in the following examples:
* Forty percent to 60% of patients with melanoma are affected on the hand or foot; 3% of melanomas in whites have subungual lesions, and 15% to 20% of melanomas in African Americans have subungual lesions.
* Approximately 50% of adults with psoriasis have nail involvement.
* Half-and-half nail is present in 9% to 50% of patients with chronic renal disease.

RISK FACTORS

* *Underlying disease,* such as chronic renal disease, pulmonary disease, congestive heart failure, endocarditis, hepatic cirrhosis, Wilson disease, diabetes, thyroid disease, hypoalbuminemia, hemochromatosis, anemia, Raynaud disease, and ulcerative colitis.
* *Dermatologic conditions,* such as psoriasis, atopic dermatitis, lichen planus, eczema, junctional nevus, and melanoma.
* *Occupational exposure;* for example, excessive contact with water as experienced by dishwashers, sewer workers, and domestic workers; arsenic, solvent, and x-ray exposure.
* *Trauma to the nails* or manipulation to the nails, such as nail biting or an aggressive manicure.
* *Irritants,* such as nail polish, nail-polish remover, nail wraps, false nails.
* *Drug exposure;* for example, antimalarials, quinolones, thiazides, minocycline (Minocin), allopurinol (Zyloprim), silver nitrate, and gold therapy, as well as alcohol and cigarettes.
* *Infections,* such as viruses (warts), *S. aureus, Candida* species, dermatophytes, and tuberculosis.

PATHOLOGY

The pathology of the various nail abnormalities varies widely according to the underlying cause. Pitting and ridging of the nail matrix are generally caused by inflammatory conditions affecting the modified epithelium of the matrix, thereby altering normal keratin production. Nail matrix disorders commonly are associated with a spongiosis in the epithelium of the matrix on biopsy. Color changes in the nail bed may be caused by a number of different conditions, including localized lesions to individualized nail beds or manifestations of more systemic disorders. Gradual and chronic development of nail changes is typically associated with concomitant systemic disease or skin disorder, while sudden changes are generally the result of trauma.

DIAGNOSIS

Diagnosis of changes in the nail matrix, bed, or plate is usually based on history and physical examination followed by appropriate testing for nail infections and for the diagnosis of suspected underlying disease associated with nail symptoms.

Differential Diagnosis
See Tables 13.1-13.3.

Diagnostic Tests
Most of the nail abnormalities can be diagnosed by history and physical examination. When the diagnosis of the nail disorder is in doubt, biopsy of the skin lesion may help differentiate the nail disorder.

Nail Matrix Abnormalities

Paronychia

Candidal or dermatophytic causes can be confirmed by potassium hydroxide (KOH) preparation or fungal culture, if necessary. Bacterial culture often grows *S. aureus*.

T ABLE 13.1.   Differential Diagnosis: Nail Matrix Disorders

Pitting	Transverse ridging	Longitudinal ridging
Alopecia areata	Beau lines	*Normal finding*
Pityriasis rosea	Severe dysmenorrhea	Lichen planus
Psoriasis	Raynaud disease	Rheumatoid arthritis
Eczema	Carpal tunnel syndrome	Darier disease
Reiter syndrome	Chronic eczema	Myxoid cysts
	Overzealous manicures	Warts
	Habit-tic deformity	Median nail dystrophy
	Psoriasis	Habit-tic deformity
	Chronic paronychia	Mechanical injury
		Raynaud disease

T ABLE 13.2. Differential Diagnosis: Splinter Hemorrhage

High-altitude sickness	Thyroid disease
Arterial emboli	Leukemia
Severe anemia	Trauma
Thrombocytopenia	Septicemia
Cirrhosis	Vitamin C deficiency
Cystic fibrosis	Sarcoidosis
Darier disease	Amyloidosis
Diabetes	Chronic renal disease
Drug exposure (tetracylines)	Chronic pulmonary disease
Eczema	Psoriasis
Heart disease (endocarditis)	Psittacosis
Hemochromatosis	Raynaud disease
Hepatitis	Onychomycosis
HIV infection	Occupational hazards
Hypertension	

HIV, human immunodeficiency virus.

Nail Bed Abnormalities

- When the diagnosis is in doubt, biopsy of the lesion can differentiate *malignant melanoma* from *junctional nevus* and *glomus tumor.*
- *Half-and-half nail.* Chronic renal failure is confirmed by an abnormal renal profile.
- *Splinter hemorrhages.* If endocarditis is suspected, blood cultures can be performed.
- *Terry nail.* Serum albumin measurements can determine the diagnosis of *hypoalbuminemia.* A chest x-ray can confirm *congestive heart failure.* Liver function tests and liver biopsy can confirm *hepatic cirrhosis.*
- *Muehrcke nail.* An abnormal renal profile and serum albumin measurements can determine the diagnosis of hypoalbuminemia associated with nephrotic syndrome.

Nail Plate Abnormalities

Blue nails

Elevated levels of serum ferritin and transferrin saturation can help diagnose *hemochromatosis.*

Elevated serum ceruloplasmin levels and the presence of Kayser-Fleischer rings in the eyes confirm *Wilson disease.*

Brown nails

Elevated levels of serum ferritin and transferrin saturation can help diagnose *hemochromatosis.*

T ABLE 13.3. Differential Diagnosis: Nail Plate Disorders

Leukonychia	Red nails	Clubbing	Koilonychia
Hereditary condition	Heart disease	Hereditary condition	Hereditary, congenital condition; normal variant in children
Onychomycosis	Alopecia areata	Chronic pulmonary disease	Anemia (iron-deficiency)
Anemia	Psoriasis	Thoracic tumor	Polycythemia
Drug exposure (chemotherapeutic agents)	Vitiligo	Heart disease (cyanotic heart disease, congestive heart failure)	Coronary artery disease
Cirrhosis	Chronic urticaria	Raynaud disease	Syphilis
Renal disease	Thyroid disease	Gastrointestinal tract cancer	Fungal infections
Kawasaki disease	Irritable bowel syndrome	Ulcerative colitis	Hemochromatosis
Ulcerative colitis	Chronic anemia	Familial polyposis	Diabetes
Leprosy	Cirrhosis	Chronic active hepatitis	Thyroid disorders
Hypoalbuminemia	Tuberculosis	Grave disease	Trauma
Alopecia areata	Pneumonia	Polycythemia	Occupational exposure (oils, solvents, acids)
Erythema multiforme	Alcohol and tobacco abuse	Hypervitaminosis A	Avitaminosis (B_2, C)
Hodgkin disease	Malnutrition	Malnutrition	Raynaud disease
Heart disease	Carbon monoxide poisoning	SLE	Lichen planus
Occupational exposure	SLE	Occupational exposure	Psoriasis
Pneumonia	Drug exposure (procainamide)	Congenital (transient)	Alopecia areata
Arsenic, lead toxicity	Arthritis	Trauma	Darier disease
Renal failure	Trauma		Carpal tunnel syndrome
Sickle cell disease	Hodgkin disease		Kidney transplant
Trauma			Connective tissue disorders
Zinc, nicotinic acid deficiency			Plummer-Vinson syndrome
Trichinosis			

SLE, systemic lupus erythematosus.

High serum potassium, blood urea nitrogen (BUN), and renin levels and low serum sodium and cortisol levels, along with abdominal computed tomography (CT) (to assess the adrenal glands) can confirm suspected *Addison disease.*

Nail bed biopsy will confirm *malignant melanoma.*

Yellow nail syndrome

Chest radiograph and/or chest or abdominal CT support the history and physical findings associated with systemic illness or cancer.

Onychomycosis

Dermatophyte infection as the cause of abnormal nail plate thickening can be confirmed by KOH preparation of nail scrapings or culture to demonstrate branching hyphae.

Referral

Because many nail abnormalities are symptoms of underlying disease, the physician may wish to refer the patient to the appropriate specialist. In cases of nail abnormalities caused by skin disorders, if the physician does not feel comfortable with the extensiveness of the disorder and its systemic treatment, referral is indicated.

Management

Treatment of the underlying disorder or elimination of the offending agent or medication is often the only way to improve the nail disorder. Specific treatments that improve the nail are listed in Tables 13.4–13.6.

T ABLE 13.4.   Treatment of Nail Matrix Disorders

Disorder	Treatment
Psoriasis	Treatment of the underlying condition with photochemotherapy can help the pitting. Cosmetic cover-up with nail polish is useful.
Eczema and atopic dermatitis	There is no specific treatment for nail matrix changes. Treat the underlying disorder. Pitting usually clears when eczema is controlled.
Alopecia areata	There is no specific treatment for nail matrix changes. Treat the underlying disorder. Hair regrowth can accompany an improvement in the nail matrix changes.
Paronychia	Incise and drain if a pustule is present. Empiric treatment with cephalexin (Keflex), dicloxacillin (Pathocil), or erythromycin (see Chapter 17 for details). If fungal or candidal infection is suspected, use oral antifungal agents such as ketoconazole (Nizoral) or terbinafine (Lamisil).
Beau lines	No specific treatment. Following resolution of the systemic illness, the nail matrix returns to normal and nail growth resumes.
Lichen planus	There is no specific treatment for the nail disorder. Treat the underlying skin disease, and the nail matrix problem usually disappears.
Habit-tic deformity/ Median nail dystrophy	It is very difficult to help the patient break the habit-tic that caused the deformity. The median nail dystrophy usually resolves spontaneously in a few months.
Warts	Treatment includes salicylic acid, cantharidin, or cryotherapy (see Chapter 18 for details).
Myxoid cyst	Lesion is benign and may be ignored. Lesions have reportedly resolved after several weeks of daily firm compression. Incision and drainage, cryosurgery with liquid nitrogen, and intralesional steroid injections have all been employed with varying results. Surgical excision can be used for the painful or bothersome lesion if necessary.
Darier disease	Treatment is not helpful for the nail disorder. Nails should be kept short, and nail trauma avoided.

T ABLE 13.5. Treatment of Nail Bed Disorders

Disorder	Treatment
Malignant melanoma	Nail bed tumor should be removed by a surgeon or dermatologist.
Glomus tumor	Perform biopsy of lesion if diagnosis is in doubt.
	Treatment consists of complete surgical excision and ablation of the base by an experienced surgeon.
Junctional nevus	Perform biopsy of lesion if diagnosis is in doubt. If the lesion is benign, there is no need to treat, as long as it is asymptomatic.
Subungual hematoma	Incise the nail plate by boring a hole with a 27-gauge needle or the use of hot cautery and evacuate the blood through the hole.
Psoriasis	Treat the underlying skin condition. There is no specific treatment of the nail bed disorder.
Half-and-half nail	There is no specific treatment of nail bed changes. Standard treatment of the underlying disorder is warranted. Renal transplantation has been shown to clear the nail disorder completely.
Splinter hemorrhages	If caused by trauma, lesions usually regress spontaneously as the nail grows out. Otherwise, treatment of the underlying disease is warranted.
Terry nail/Muehrcke nail	There is no specific treatment of nail bed changes. Standard treatment of the underlying disorder is warranted.

T ABLE 13.6. Treatment of Nail Plate Disorders

Disorder	Treatment
Blue nail plate discoloration	Withdrawal of offending agent, medication, or exposure when appropriate.
	There is no specific treatment of nail plate changes. Standard treatment of the underlying disorder is warranted.
Brown nail plate discoloration	Withdrawal of offending agent or exposure when appropriate.
	There is no specific treatment of nail plate changes. Standard treatment of the underlying disorder is warranted.
Yellow nail syndrome	No specific treatment is necessary, since spontaneous resolution of the nail discoloration can be seen. However, intradermal triamcinolone or oral vitamin E (600 to 1200 U daily) have been reported to clear the nail discoloration.
	Treatment of the underlying disorder is warranted to help clear the nail discoloration.
Leukonychia	Lesions usually regress spontaneously as the nail grows out.
Onychomycosis	Oral antifungal agents are helpful to treat fungal infections of the nails (see Chapter 17 for complete treatment details).
Clubbing	There is no specific treatment of nail plate changes. Standard treatment of the underlying disorder is warranted.
Koilonychia	There is no specific treatment of nail plate changes. Standard treatment of the underlying disorder is warranted.

Follow-up

Follow-up is primarily dictated by the treatment of the underlying condition or elimination of the offending agent or medication. When the nail will not improve, no specific follow-up is necessary.

Patient Education

- To improve the health of the nail, it is important for the patient to understand that a routine regimen of nail care must be followed, including trimming, filing, and cuticle care.
- Nail biting and picking at the cuticle should be discouraged to reduce chances for infection and dystrophic nails.
- The patient should avoid vigorous nail manicures, since extensive manipulation can lead to infections and ridging.
- Artificial or sculptured nails can lead to onycholysis.

BIBLIOGRAPHY

Baran R, Dawber RPR, eds. *Diseases of the nails and their management.* Oxford: Blackwell Science, 1994.

Noronha PA, Zubkov B. Nails and nail disorders in children and adults. *Am Fam Physician* 1997;55(6):2129–2140.

CHAPTER 14

....

Hair Disorders

BASICS

Hair growth occurs in cycles. Periods of growth are followed by periods without growth. The growth cycle is called the anagen phase. The nongrowth cycle is called the telogen, or resting, phase. A longer telogen phase, resulting in slower growth, occurs in the eyebrows, eyelashes, and axillary and pubic hair; a short telogen phase occurs in the hair of the scalp and beard, which grows faster. A brief transition phase between the growing and resting phases is called the catagen phase.

ALOPECIA

Loss of hair is termed effluvium; baldness is termed alopecia. Alopecia is divided into nonscarring conditions, which occur without skin inflammation and scarring, and scarring conditions, which lead to fibrosis and formation of scar tissue, permanently destroying the hair follicle.

Scarring Alopecia

Scarring alopecia is the destruction or damage of hair follicles by infectious or non-infectious inflammatory processes. The inflammation heals with scarring, which leads to patches of hair loss. Table 14.1 lists the causes of scarring alopecia, some of which

T ABLE 14.1. Etiology of Scarring Alopecia

Infections	Caustic agents (acid and alkali)
Syphilis (tertiary)	Freezing (cryotherapy)
Staphylococcus aureus	
Tinea capitis	**Inflammatory diseases**
Herpes zoster	Systemic lupus erythematosus
Severe folliculitis	Scleroderma
Leprosy	Dermatomyositis
Tuberculosis	Pemphigoid
	Amyloidosis
Neoplasms	Sarcoidosis
Basal cell carcinoma	Pseudopelade
Melanoma	Dissecting perifolliculitis of the scalp
Lymphomas	Acne keloid (dermatitis papillaris capillitii)
Metastatic carcinoma	Lichen planus
	Necrobiosis lipoidica
Physical/chemical agents	
Trichotillomania	**Congenital defects**
Burns	Aplasia cutis congenita
Radiation exposure	Darier disease (keratosis follicularis)

are discussed in other chapters of this book. A dermatologic text should be consulted for more details.

Nonscarring Alopecia

ALOPECIA AREATA

Alopecia areata is hair loss without visible inflammation in the scalp, eyebrows, or eyelashes. Alopecia totalis involves the loss of all scalp hair and eyebrows; alopecia universalis involves hair loss over the entire body.

Chief Complaint

Patients report a sharply outlined area without hair, or bald spot, on the scalp and express consternation about their appearance.

Clinical Manifestations

- Alopecia areata is a scattered, discrete loss of hair occurring over weeks to months (Figure 14.1, see color insert following page 170). The hair loss is usually asymptomatic, without pain or pruritis of the affected area. Also, there is no attendant scarring or skin atrophy.
- Occasionally, broken-off, stubby hairs called "exclamation point" hairs can be seen in the area of alopecia.
- Hair follicles are present at the periphery and can be pulled out easily.
- The area of hair loss is usually sharply defined.
- Hair growth disturbance is commonly seen in the scalp, eyebrows, eyelashes, pubic hair, or beard. The fingernails can also show dystrophic changes, with hundreds of tiny depressions, or pits.
- The initial regrowth of hair may be fine and white-yellow in appearance.

Epidemiology

Alopecia areata is a relatively common hair growth disturbance, with a prevalence of about 0.1% and an incidence of 1.7% of the United States population.

Family History

About 20% to 30% of patients have a positive family history; the disease is autosomal dominant with variable penetrance.

Age

- Adults under 25 years of age are the most commonly affected, but the disease can be seen in all ages.
- When the alopecia areata occurs after puberty, 80% of patients have regrowth of the lost hair.

Sex

The disease occurs in equal proportions among men and women in the United States.

Risk Factors

Alopecia areata can be associated with Hashimoto thyroiditis, vitiligo, myasthenia gravis, pernicious anemia, and stress.

PATHOLOGY

Alopecia areata is a disturbance of the anagen (growth) phase in which the hair follicles are reduced in size. There is a noticeable increase of telogen (resting phase) hair. Biopsy findings often show T-cell infiltrates around the hair follicles.

Diagnosis

Diagnosis of alopecia areata is based on clinical findings, laboratory tests, and patient history.

Differential Diagnosis

See Table 14.2.

Diagnostic Tests

- A 4-mm punch biopsy of the hair follicle can be performed if the diagnosis is uncertain.
- Antinuclear antibody and Venereal Disease Research Laboratory (VDRL) testing should be performed on patients with alopecia areata to rule out systemic lupus erythematosus and secondary syphilis.
- A potassium hydroxide (KOH) preparation or fungal culture should be obtained to rule out tinea capitis.
- Because 20% of children with alopecia areata have subclinical hyperthyroidism, a thyroid profile is warranted.
- Alopecia in adults is also associated with thyroid disease and pernicious anemia; therefore a thyroid profile and complete blood cell count (CBC) are also warranted in these patients.

T ABLE 14.2. Alopecia Areata: Differential Diagnosis

Secondary syphilis	Areas of hair loss with "moth-eaten" margins. VDRL test, punch biopsy are useful to differentiate.
Cutaneous (discoid) lupus erythematosus	Inflammatory type of alopecia with prominent hair follicles and scale; permanent hair loss. Punch biopsy, ANA test are useful to differentiate.
Tinea capitis	Hair loss with scaling and inflammation. KOH preparation, fungal culture are useful to differentiate.
Trichotillomania	Broken hairs of variable length; no "exclamation point" hairs are evident. Punch biopsy is useful to differentiate.
Androgenetic alopecia	Gradual onset of hair loss; typical male or female loss pattern. Punch biopsy is useful to differentiate.
Traction alopecia	Use of brush rollers, hot combs, vigorous brushing, scalp massages, and certain hairstyles causing hair loss. Punch biopsy is useful to differentiate.

VDRL, Venereal Disease Research Laboratory; ANA, antinuclear antibody; KOH, potassium hydroxide.

Referral

Referral to a dermatologist may be appropriate in cases with poor prognostic signs or for patients who are not responsive to initial therapy.

Management

- The treatment goal for alopecia areata is to achieve hair regrowth that is cosmetically appealing. No evidence is available to suggest that treatment causes remission or alters the course of the disease. Curative therapy is not always available for alopecia areata. Alopecia areata occurring before puberty, positive patient history of asthma or atopic dermatitis, positive circulating antinuclear or thyroid autoantibodies, the development of alopecia totalis or alopecia universalis, and alopecia areata lasting for more than 5 years, are all poor prognostic signs for hair regrowth.
- Most of the problems and complications in the treatment of alopecia areata revolve around the use of systemic corticosteroids, cyclosporine (Sandimmune), or photochemotherapy. The physician should alert the patient to the systemic problems with each of these three modalities.
- Chronic medication use is often necessary to maintain hair regrowth. Sometimes this is necessary for life or until a spontaneous remission occurs.

Medications

See Table 14.3.

Other Treatment Modalities

Systemic cyclosporine induces regrowth of hair loss but, as with systemic corticosteroids, alopecia returns when the drug is discontinued. Therefore it is not a recommended first-line treatment and should be administered only by physicians who are experienced in its use, because of the potential for serious side effects.

- *Oral psoralen ultraviolet A-range (PUVA) photochemotherapy* may be administered; however, it is only effective in about 30% of cases. Therefore it is not a recommended first-line treatment and should be administered only by physicians who are experienced in its use, because of the potential for serious side effects.
- *Patients should be informed* that, while claims have been made that treatments such as hypnosis, hair massage, or acupuncture will help treat alopecia areata, these claims are unsubstantiated by any controlled studies.

Follow-up

Patients should be monitored periodically, with the first follow-up 3 months after start of treatment and follow-up every 3 to 4 months thereafter, to assess regrowth of hair and to continue to provide psychological support.

Patient Education

Patients should be reassured that alopecia areata is temporary. In more than 80% of patients, the hair regrows spontaneously; regrowth may begin immediately or occur from several months to years after the hair loss began. In about 90% of patients with alopecia areata, hair regrows within 2 years.

Compliance

Compliance with drug treatment and follow-up should be emphasized because alopecia areata is a recurrent disease. New patches can occur after other patches have gone into remission.

Lifestyle Changes

Patients who wish to wear a wig, hairpiece, hat, or head wrap should be reassured that wearing any of these items will not affect hair regrowth.

T ABLE 14.3. Medical Treatment of Alopecia Areata

Topical corticosteroid:
betamethasone dipropionate 0.05% (cream, lotion, or ointment) (Diprosone)
Availability: Prescription.
Dosage: Applied to area of hair loss and at least 1 cm beyond, twice daily.
Duration: Use for 3 months and evaluate results; longer use is permissible if improvement is seen
without evidence of cutaneous side effects.
Side effects: Long-term use can cause skin atrophy and telangiectasia; can also inhibit the adrenal-pituitary axis.
Comments: More useful for large patches of hair loss or in alopecia totalis.

Intralesional triamcinolone acetonide
Availability: Prescription.
Dosage: Inject 1 to 3 mL (depending on size of lesion) directly into the hair-loss area with the wheals of
medication touching each other to cover the entire area. Use 2.5 to 5 mg/mL concentration for
eyebrows, beard; 10 to 15 mg/mL for scalp.
Duration: Single injection, repeated every 6 to 8 weeks if needed.
Side effects: May produce skin atrophy and scalp pain.
Comments: Treatment of choice for small, discrete patches of hair loss.

Anthralin (Drithocreme 0.5% or 1%), to induce hair growth
Availability: Prescription.
Dosage: Begin with 0.5% cream; leave on affected area 10 to 20 minutes, rinse with lukewarm
water, shampoo. Increase to 1% cream if unresponsive and there is no irritant reaction.
Duration: Applied every 2 days initially for 2 weeks; if tolerated, use daily. Reevaluate
treatment in 3 months; may take up to 1 year before response is noted.
Side effects: Erythema and scaling occur; some irritation is desired.
Comments: Stains hands and clothes brown; wash hands immediately.

Minoxidil 2% or 5% solution, to induce hair growth
Availability: Over the counter.
Dosage: Applied twice daily to the affected areas.
Duration: Ongoing; hair growth will stop if treatment is halted. Reevaluate treatment in 3 months;
may take up to 1 year before response is noted.
Side effects: Dryness, skin irritation, pruritus, contact dermatitis; 23% of patients develop low blood pressure. Can also
cause tachycardia and edema; use caution in prescribing for patients with cardiovascular disease.
Comments: 2% solution is indicated for mild, smaller areas of loss. May be used in conjunction with betamethasone
dipropionate 0.05%, twice daily in adults and children, or with anthralin in adults.

Prednisone
Availability: Prescription.
Dosage: 60 to 80 mg orally per day, for 2 to 3 days, tapered by 10 to 20 mg
every 2 to 3 days until response is noted, then maintain.
Duration: May be needed for 2 to 3 months.
Side effects: Long-term use of systemic steroids can inhibit the adrenal-pituitary axis,
causing serious systemic side effects; see *Physician's Desk Reference*.
Comments: Risk associated with long-term use contraindicates continued use in alopecia areata.
Can induce regrowth, but when treatment is discontinued, alopecia frequently returns.

Family and Community Support

- Both patients and family members should be counseled that, unlike some hair loss caused by fungus, alopecia areata is not contagious and it will not spread to other parts of the body, but new hair-loss patches can develop on the scalp, eyebrows, beard, or groin, in addition to the original site.
- For many patients, the most important factor in managing alopecia areata is psychosocial support. The physician must elicit the aid of family members to help the patient cope with this disease. The National Alopecia Areata Foundation (714 C Street, San Raphael, CA 94901; telephone: 415-456-4644) can also be useful in identifying local resources.

ANDROGENETIC ALOPECIA

Androgenetic alopecia, or male pattern baldness, is a common progressive balding that occurs in either sex because of a genetic predisposition to the action of androgens on hair follicles in the scalp (Figure 14.2).

Chief Complaint

Patients report gradual thinning of the hair or balding. Some female patients report hair loss after pregnancy.

Clinical Manifestations

- Men often have a receding anterior hairline with a resultant bald spot on the crown or occiput of the head.
- Alopecia in women typically begins mildly, with a decrease in hair density in the crown, while the frontal hairline is retained. In some instances of female androgenetic alopecia, younger women show other physical signs of excess androgens, such as acne, hirsutism, irregular menses, or virilization signs.
- The hair shaft becomes very fine, shorter, and smaller in diameter than normal.
- Androgenetic alopecia has been associated with seborrheic dermatitis, creating an excess oil in the scalp.
- No other skin lesions are noted.

Epidemiology

Age

Androgenetic alopecia occurs in about 30% to 40% of adults.

Race

This type of hair loss occurs in all races.

Sex

- Androgenetic alopecia is more common in men.
- Men may begin to demonstrate hair loss anytime after the onset of puberty, but the loss is usually fully apparent in the fifth decade of life.
- Women have androgenetic alopecia later in life, with about 40% of cases occurring in the sixth decade of life.

Risk Factors

Androgenetic alopecia tends to be autosomal dominant in men and autosomal recessive in women.

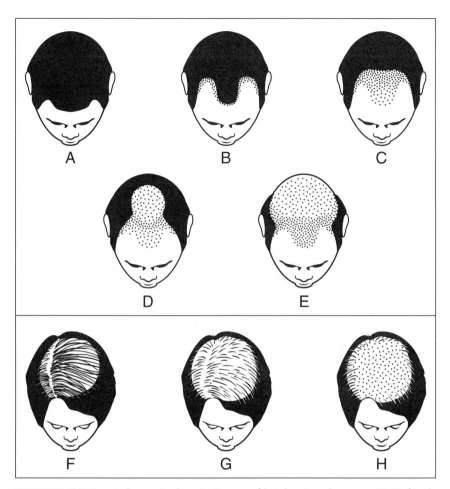

FIGURE 14.2. Androgenetic alopecia: Patterns of hair loss in male patients **(A–E)**; female patients **(F–H)**. Taken from Fitzpatrick TB, Johnson RA, Wolff K, et al. Color atlas and synopsis of clinical dermatology, 3rd ed. New York: McGraw-Hill, 1997:section 2, 23.

PATHOLOGY

Androgenetic alopecia is a result of the combined effects of androgens on the hair follicles in the scalp and a genetic predisposition to balding. This results in thinning and shortening of the hair.

Diagnosis

Diagnosis of androgenetic alopecia is based on a strong family history and physical examination. The diagnosis can be made by determining the number of anagen and telogen hairs in the patient's scalp, by plucking at least 50 hairs or more and counting the number of growing (or anagen) hairs and the number of telogen hairs (with a clublike or bulbous base). Patients normally have 80% to 90% of hairs in the anagen phase. In androgenetic alopecia there is an increase in the percentage of telogen hairs.

Differential Diagnosis
See Table 14.4.

Diagnostic Tests
- Laboratory studies should include thyroid hormone, serum iron, VDRL, antinuclear antibody testing and CBC.
- Female patients with virilizing signs and symptoms require total testosterone, free testosterone, prolactin, and dehydroepiandrosterone (DHEA) studies.

Referral
In patients whose hair loss is unresponsive to topical minoxidil (Rogaine), referral to a cosmetic surgeon or a dermatologist who is experienced in hair transplantation may be helpful. Patients may also be referred for other types of hair enhancements, such as wigs or hair weaves.

Management
There is no one effective treatment to prevent the progression of androgenetic alopecia.

Medications
See Table 14.5.

Other Treatment Modalities
- Spironolactone (Aldactone) and cimetidine (Tagamet) bind to androgen receptors, blocking the action of hydrotestosterone on the scalp. These medications can be effective in treating female patients with elevated adrenal androgen levels (total testosterone and DHEA values); however, these agents *should not* be used to treat androgenetic alopecia in male patients.

T ABLE 14.4.   Androgenetic Alopecia: Differential Diagnosis

Alopecia areata	More acute onset; different distribution.
	Punch biopsy or hair pull test is needed to differentiate.
Telogen effluvium	Can be clinically indistinguishable from androgenetic alopecia in women.
	Punch biopsy and/or hair pull test useful to differentiate.
Secondary syphilis	Can cause diffuse hair loss, but distribution is different.
	VDRL is useful to differentiate.
Systemic lupus erythematosus	Can cause diffuse hair loss, but distribution is different.
	ANA test is useful to differentiate.
Iron deficiency anemia	Can cause diffuse hair loss, but distribution is different.
	CBC is useful to differentiate.
Hypothyroidism	Can cause diffuse hair loss, but distribution is different.
	Thyroid profile is useful to differentiate.
Hyperthyroidism	Can cause diffuse hair loss, but distribution is different.
	Thyroid profile is useful to differentiate.

VDRL, Venereal Disease Research Laboratory; ANA, antinuclear antibody. CBC, complete blood cell count.

T ABLE 14.5.   Medical Treatment of Androgenetic Alopecia

Topical minoxidil (2% and 5% solution) (Rogaine)

Availability:	Over the counter and prescription.
Dosage:	Apply 1 mL to scalp twice daily.
Duration of use:	Ongoing; hair growth will stop if treatment is halted.
Side effects:	Can cause irritant and contact dermatitis as well as pruritus of the scalp. Should be used with caution in patients with cardiovascular disease, as treatment can cause tachycardia and edema.
Comments:	May reduce rate of loss or partially restore lost hair. Approximately 20% to 40% of men respond with reduced hair loss or partial regrowth of hair between 4 and 12 months; the effect on women is not yet known. Recent reports show promise using a combination of topical minoxidil 2% and topical retinoic acid (0.05%). The 5% solution shows 45% more hair regrowth than the 2% solution, with results occuring on average within 2 months rather than 4 months. 5% solution not recommended for women since it has now been shown to be more effective.

Finasteride (Propecia)

Availability:	Prescription.
Dosage:	Male patients only; 1 mg per day.
Duration:	Ongoing; improvement should be noted within 3 months.
Side effects:	In 2% of cases, there was a loss of libido, impotence, and a decrease in the amount of semen. This is reversible with the cessation of medication.
Comments:	**For male patients only.** Inhibits the conversion of testosterone to DHT. About 83% of patients have regrowth of hair after 2 years; decrease in hair loss has also been noted. Not for use in female patients of child-bearing years; may cause abnormalities in the sex organs of the male fetus.

DHT, dihydrotestosterone.

- In female patients (20 to 40 years of age), who present evidence of androgen excess and where virilizing tumors have been excluded, a birth control pill with low androgen potential (Demulen 1/35) is useful to restore hair loss.
- Because some patients express a great deal of emotional disturbance about hair loss, psychological support and counseling about hair loss and the various treatments available may be useful.

Follow-up

Close follow-up is not necessary in androgenetic alopecia.

Patient Education

- Patients should be reminded that treatment with topical minoxidil or oral finasteride (in men) is a continuing process, since hair growth will regress if this treatment is stopped.
- Patients should also be cautioned about various commercial preparations (including hair tonics, vitamins, shampoos, and other treatments) that make claims about regrowing hair. To date, there is no guaranteed method of regrowing hair.

TELOGEN EFFLUVIUM

Telogen effluvium is a transient shedding of resting, or telogen phase, hair follicles secondary to a shift from the growth, or anagen, phase resulting in an increased daily hair loss, which in turn produces a visible generalized thinning of hair.

Chief Complaint

Patients report an increased hair loss on the scalp.

Clinical Manifestations

- Hair loss is usually diffuse, with the degree of hair thinning varying across the scalp.
- Usually 50% of hair must be lost before it is cosmetically apparent.
- Peak hair loss occurs approximately 3 to 4 months after the inciting event.
- Patients with telogen effluvium demonstrate no abnormalities of the scalp.
- During hair examination several hair shafts may have clubbed or telogen phase hairs.
- In the hair-pull test, a count of greater than five telogen hairs out of two to three dozen is a positive sign for telogen effluvium.

Epidemiology

Age

Telogen effluvium can occur at any age.

Sex

This disease is more common in female patients.

Risk Factors

- *Health and nutrition.* Risk factors include trauma or systemic disease, such as prolonged fever, poor nutritional states, accident, surgical shock, stress, hemorrhage, childbirth, excessive dieting, collagen vascular disease, syphilis, human immunodeficiency virus (HIV), or thyroid disease.
- *Drugs.* Use of certain medications, including warfarin (Coumadin), heparin, beta-blockers, allopurinol (Zyloprim), doxepin (Sinequan), haloperidol (Haldol), lovastatin (Mevacor), levodopa (Larodopa), indomethacin (Indocin), amitriptyline (Elavil), lithium, and nitrofurantoin (Furadantin) may also be the precipitating factor.

PATHOLOGY

Microscopic examination of hair shafts reveals clubbed hairs with straight hair shafts and depigmented bases.

Telogen effluvium is the second most common cause of alopecia after androgenetic alopecia.

Diagnosis

Diagnostic Tests

Diagnosis of telogen effluvium is based on history and close examination of the hair shafts. Examination consists of removing approximately 50 hairs and examining the hair shafts. In a normal growth pattern, 80% to 90% of the hair shafts are in the anagen phase. More than 10% to 20% of hair shafts in the telogen phase indicates the presence of telogen effluvium.

Differential Diagnosis
See Table 14.6.

Diagnostic Tests
Laboratory tests, including CBC, serum iron, thyroid-stimulating hormone, antinuclear antibody, and VDRL testing, should be performed to rule out other causes of alopecia.

Referral
If the diagnosis is uncertain, referral is indicated.

Management
Medications
No specific medication is recommended for telogen effluvium.

Other Treatment Modalities
- Shampoos such as Progaine or Vivagen help the hair look fuller.
- Hair styling can also make the hair appear fuller.

Follow-up
The physician can monitor the hair shafts every 1 to 2 months to determine whether there is a restoration of the anagen hairs, signaling a resolution of the problem.

Patient Education
- Patients should be reassured that telogen effluvium is a normal reaction following any of the predisposing problems mentioned previously, and that this hair loss will not be total and is usually reversible.

T ABLE 14.6. Telogen Effluvium: Differential Diagnosis

Androgenetic alopecia	Patient has gradual hair loss over many years. Punch biopsy is useful to differentiate the two.
Anagen effluvium	Acute, almost total hair loss; rapid onset, usually following use of certain medications. Punch biopsy is useful to differentiate, but diagnosis is usually made by the history and physical examination.
Hyperthyroidism	Can cause diffuse hair loss. Thyroid profile or punch biopsy is useful to differentiate.
Hypothyroidism	Can cause diffuse hair loss. Thyroid profile or punch biopsy is useful to differentiate.
Systemic lupus erythematosus	Can cause diffuse hair loss. Antinuclear antibody test or punch biopsy is useful to differentiate the two.
Secondary syphilis	Can cause diffuse hair loss. VDRL test or punch biopsy is useful to differentiate the two.
Drug-induced alopecia	Can cause diffuse hair loss. Usually a history of medication use.

VDRL, Venereal Disease Research Laboratory.

- It can take up to a year for telogen effluvium to dissipate and normal hair growth to return, after which it may take approximately 6 months for full regrowth of hair to occur.
- Patients should be cautioned that in some cases of severe or recurrent hair loss, such as hair loss that recurs following successive pregnancies, complete regrowth may not occur.

ANAGEN EFFLUVIUM

Anagen effluvium is a diffuse hair loss involving the entire scalp. Its rapid onset of 10 to 14 days distinguishes this disease from telogen effluvium, which has an onset of 3 to 4 months.

Chief Complaint

Patients report complete hair loss, occurring approximately 2 weeks after their first chemotherapy session.

Clinical Manifestations

- Anagen effluvium demonstrates diffuse hair loss involving the entire scalp.
- This disease has a rapid onset (10 to 14 days) and is far more pronounced than telogen effluvium.
- Patients usually present no other skin symptoms.
- About 80% to 90% of hair is observed to be in the anagen phase.
- The hair is thin and fragile, and breaks off as soon as it reaches the skin surface.
- Total scalp alopecia may also be observed.

Epidemiology

Anagen effluvium occurs equally among male and female patients.

Risk Factors

- *Drugs.* Anagen effluvium is often associated with medications such as warfarin (Coumadin), heparin, beta-blockers, allopurinol (Zyloprim), chemotherapeutic agents, doxepin (Sinequan), haloperidol (Haldol), lovastatin (Meracor), levodopa (Larodopa), indomethacin (Indocin), amitriptyline (Elavil), lithium, and nitrofurantoin (Furadantin).
- *Environmental and occupational.* Intoxication and heavy metal poisoning such as thallium, mercury, or lead poisoning may also be precipitating factors.

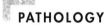

PATHOLOGY

Arrest or damage to the anagen hairs causes these hairs to be dystrophic, with narrowed or broken proximal shafts and pigmented bases.

Diagnosis

Diagnosis of anagen effluvium is based on history and physical examination. The hair pull test demonstrates most hairs to be in the anagen phase.

Differential Diagnosis

See Table 14.7.

T ABLE 14.7.   Anagen Effluvium: Differential Diagnosis[a]

Telogen effluvium	Diffuse, gradual hair loss.
	Punch biopsy is useful to differentiate.
Alopecia totalis	Can cause a total loss of hair on scalp.
	Punch biopsy is useful to differentiate.
Androgenetic alopecia	Gradual hair loss, characteristic pattern.
	Punch biopsy is useful to differentiate.

[a]See other causes of diffuse hair loss in Table 14.6.

Diagnostic Tests

- Punch biopsy demonstrates the characteristic disease of the hair shaft.
- Anagen effluvium in most cases is caused by medication, but other causes of diffuse hair loss should be eliminated by obtaining CBC, VDRL, thyroid profile, antinuclear antibody and serum iron studies.

Referral

Referral is usually not indicated for patients with anagen effluvium unless the hair loss is not related to medication.

Management

Medications

No specific medication is recommended for treatment of anagen effluvium.

Other Treatment Modalities

Patients should be reassured that regrowth usually occurs after the cessation of the medication or chemotherapeutic drug.

Patient Education

- Patient should be counseled about the use of head wraps, hats, or wigs to camouflage hair loss until regrowth occurs.
- It takes hair 1 year to grow about 6 inches, so it may take upwards of a year for full regrowth to occur.

Follow-up

The physician should follow these patients every 2 to 3 months after the cessation of the medication to identify hair regrowth.

HIRSUTISM AND HYPERTRICHOSIS

- Hirsutism is an excessive growth of androgen-dependent hair that occurs on the face, chest, areolae, linea alba, lower back, buttocks, inner thighs, and external genitalia of women. This is in distinction to the non–androgen-dependent hair that is usually found on the scalp.
- Hypertrichosis is excessive hair growth occurring in areas that are not androgen sensitive.

Chief Complaint

Female patients report excessive hair growth on the face, chest, or other areas.

Clinical Manifestations

- Hair overgrowth is usually noticed relatively abruptly and is not associated with the signs of puberty (Figure 14.3, see color insert following page 170).
- Common sites of hirsutism include the face, chest, abdomen, upper back, and shoulders.
- Virilization symptoms such as androgenetic alopecia, facial acne, deep voice, obesity, increased muscle mass, amenorrhea, or changes in menstruation may also be present.
- Clitoral hypertrophy may be present.
- These patients may also have elevated blood pressure.
- If violaceous striae, obesity, or muscle wasting signs, or a combination of these, are also noticed, Cushing syndrome may be present.

Epidemiology

About 15% of hirsute cases are idiopathic.

Family History

If there is a strong family history of excessive hair growth, it is probable that female offspring of hirsute patients may exhibit the same excessive hair growth pattern.

Race

Hirsutism is more commonly seen in lighter-skinned individuals than in those of African or Asian descent.

Risk Factors

- Use of androgens, anabolic steroids, phenothiazines, acetazolamide (Diamox), or oral contraceptives.
- Hyperprolactinemia.

PATHOLOGY

Androgens convert vellus hairs to coarse terminal hairs in androgen-sensitive hair follicles.
The common causes of hirsutism are categorized as idiopathic, familial, medication-induced, and androgen excess syndromes (ovarian, adrenal, and pituitary).

Diagnosis
Differential Diagnosis
See Table 14.8.

Diagnostic Tests

- A urinary 17-ketosteroid measurement is helpful in determining the amount of androgen secretion.
- If the patient has menstrual dysfunction, prolactin, follicle-stimulating hormone (FSH), and total testosterone levels should also be checked.
- If the patient has virilizing symptoms, DHEA should be checked.

T ABLE 14.8.   Hirsutism: Differential Diagnosis

Cushing syndrome	Patient presents with excessive hair growth, and abdominal striae predominate.
	If Cushing disease is suspected, refer patient to an endocrinologist.
Androgen-producing adrenal tumors	There are virilizing signs and symptoms and excessive hair growth.
	Cortisol level with dexamethasone suppression test is useful to differentiate the two.
Congenital adrenal hyperplasia	There are virilizing signs and symptoms and excessive hair growth.
	Urinary 17-ketosteroids, serum testosterone, and serum DHEA determinations are needed to differentiate the two.
Ovarian neoplasms	Patient presents with excessive hair growth, sometimes menstrual irregularities, and virilizing symptoms.
	Obtain CT scan of abdomen to rule out ovarian tumor.
	Obtain prolactin level, LH, FSH, 17-OH progesterone, serum testosterone, and cortisol levels if any menstrual abnormalities are present.
Polycystic ovarian syndrome	Patient has excessive hair growth and, occasionally, menstrual irregularities.
	Obtain CT scan of pelvis, perform pelvic examination, and obtain prolactin level, LH, FSH, 17-OH progesterone, serum testosterone, and cortisol levels if any menstrual irregularities are present.

DHEA, dehydroepiandrosterone; CT, computed tomography; LH, luteinizing hormone; FSH, follicle-stimulating hormone; 17-OH, 17-hydroxyprogesterone.

Referral

- If congenital adrenal hyperplasia or Cushing syndrome is suspected or the cause of hirsutism is unclear, referral to an endocrinologist is indicated.
- If ovarian neoplasm or polycystic ovarian syndrome is suspected, referral to a gynecologist is indicated.

Management

Hirsute patients with a normal menstrual history, a strong family history of hirsutism, and no physical findings indicative of an endocrine cause do not require treatment.

Medications

See Table 14.9.

Other Treatment Modalities

- *Physical and environmental*
- Cosmetic measures such as shaving, bleaching, waxing, depilatory creams, or electrolysis are useful to remove unwanted hair.
- In the hands of an experienced electrolysis practitioner, the excessive hair can be permanently removed. New laser treatments are being developed that will also permanently remove unwanted hair.
- *Psychological.* The physician should be cognizant of the emotional distress hirsute patients can experience. Patients should undergo a complete history and physical examination, including an evaluation of the common etiologic diseases. Patients should also be given options for treatment including both cosmetic and medical management.

TABLE 14.9. Medical Treatment of Hirsutism

Spironolactone (Aldactone)

Availability: Prescription.

Dosage: 50 mg twice per day, orally, from day 4 through day 22 of each menstrual cycle. The dose can be increased as high as 100 mg twice per day.

Duration: Continue use indefinitely to prevent hirsutism.

Side effects: Can cause hyperkalemia.

Comments: Antiandrogen medication helpful in decreasing androgen excess. Also helpful in idiopathic hirsutism. Will cause a significant reduction in hair shaft diameter within 6 months. Avoid use during pregnancy; can cross over to fetal circulation; counsel patients about contraception.

Cimetidine (Tagamet)

Availability: Over the counter.

Dosage: 300 mg orally, 5 times per day.

Duration: Use for at least 3 months, then reevaluate.

Side effects: Can cause diarrhea, skin rash, gynecomastia, headaches, and mental confusion.

Comments: Less effective than spironolactone. Can interact with warfarin (Coumadin), phenytoin, theophyline, and lidocaine.

Dexamethasone

Availability: Prescription.

Dosage: 1 mg per day, at bedtime.

Duration: Use continuously to suppress excessive hair growth.

Side effects: Long-term use inhibits the adrenal-pituitary axis; see *PDR*.

Comments: Useful for treatment of congenital adrenal hyperplasia.

Oral contraceptives with ethinyl estradiol (30 to 35 mcg), in combination with a low-dose progestin (1 mg of norethindrome, 0.25 mg norgestimate, 0.15 mg desogestrel, or 1 mg ethynodiol diacetate).

Availability: Prescription.

Dosage: One combination pill daily for 21 days, followed by no pill or placebo pills for the next 7 days.

Duration: Continue indefinitely to suppress excessive hair growth.

Side effects: Can cause many serious side effects; see PDR.

Comments: Suppresses adrenal androgen production by decreasing LH and FSH.

PDR, *Physicians' Desk Reference;* LH, luteinizing hormone; FSH, follicle-stimulating hormone.

Follow-up

Patients who have adrenal or ovarian causes should be closely followed by either the family physician or the endocrinologist managing treatment.

Patient Education

- Many patients are embarrassed to ask about unsightly or excessive hair growth. However, the possibility of a serious systemic cause suggests that the physician may wish to broach this matter if the patient does not mention it.
- Patients should be reminded that shaving does not increase hair growth.

- Patients should be advised that in some cases lacking an underlying cause, excessive hair growth will continue for a lifetime; however, if an underlying cause is found and can be successfully treated, the hirsutism will disappear.

PSEUDOFOLLICULITIS BARBAE

Pseudofolliculitis barbae (PFB) is a foreign-body inflammatory reaction in which tightly curled or coiled hair ends reenter the skin. These papules can become secondarily infected by *Staphylococcus aureus*.

Chief Complaint

Patients report lumps within the beard area that may be pruritic.

Clinical Manifestations

- Multiple papules may be present in the beard or other hair-bearing surfaces of the face, the back of the neck, the axilla, and the legs (Figure 14.4, see color insert following page 170).
- A portion of a hair often protrudes from the papules (this is a characteristic sign).
- Patients are usually asymptomatic; however, pruritus or pain can occur.
- Complications include scarring, keloid formation, secondary infection, and post-inflammatory hyperpigmentation.

Epidemiology

Pseudofolliculitis barbae occurs predominately among men of African descent; 50% of darker-skinned men develop this disease, as opposed to only 3% of lighter-skinned men.

Risk Factors

Frequent or extremely close shaving predisposes patients to these inflammatory lesions.

PATHOLOGY

Pseudofolliculitis barbae occurs when tightly curled or coiled hair ends reenter the skin and cause inflammation around the hair shafts resulting in the formation of papules.

Diagnosis

Diagnosis of pseudofolliculitis barbae is based on a clinical finding of hair protruding from one or more papules.

Differential Diagnosis

See Table 14.10.

Diagnostic Tests

If pustules are present, Gram stain and culture may reveal the presence of *S. aureus*.

Referral

When the diagnosis is unclear or treatment is not effective, referral may be indicated.

T ABLE 14.10. Pseudofolliculitis Barbae: Differential Diagnosis

Infectious folliculitis	Infectious folliculitis is caused by *Staphylococcus aureus* and tinea capitis. Culture and Gram stain, KOH preparation, or fungal culture is useful to differentiate the two.
Varicella zoster	Patient presents with inflammation and/or infection of the hair follicle itself. Viral culture and skin biopsy are useful to differentiate the two.

KOH, potassium hydroxide.

Management

- Although there is no curative treatment for PFB, avoidance of close shaving prevents its recurrence.
- Chronic PFB can lead to abscess formation from secondary bacterial infection, postinflammatory hyperpigmentation, and keloid formation.

Medications

See Table 14.11.

Other Treatment Modalities

- *Military personnel, food handlers, and other individuals* whose occupations necessitate daily shaving may require a waiver to present to their employer specifying that the patient should not shave for 2 to 3 days. This allows the beard to grow over ¼-inch long, thereby becoming less likely to embed into the skin.
- *Depilatories* such as Royal Crown and Magic Shave may be useful. These agents may cause inflammation if used daily; therefore use should be limited to once every 3 days. Depilatories can cause severe irritation resulting in postinflammatory hyperpigmentation and therefore should be used cautiously. A test of a small area should be conducted initially before application to the entire beard.
- *Hair releasing* is another method of treating PFB. The patient should be instructed to hydrate the facial skin by showering before shaving or by applying warm compresses for 10 minutes three to four times daily. Then the embedded hair shafts can be removed by tweezers, or a sterilized needle, or by use of a hair-releasing kit such as the Hair Bump Kit.
- Before shaving, apply a warm compress for 10 to 15 minutes. Then apply a generous amount of lubricating shave gel (e.g., Easy-Shave or PFB Bump Fighter shaving gel), and use a sharp, guarded razor (e.g., PFB Bump Fighter). These razors have a serrated foil guard covering 30% of the blade's cutting surface. Studies show a 25% greater reduction in the number of bumps using this razor. The Gillette standard adjustable razor with a setting from 0 to 4 is also useful to avoid a close shave. Always shave in the direction of hair growth. After shaving, rinse face and apply cold-water compresses for 5 minutes.
- Patients may also use an electric razor, such as the Norelco Triple Header. Allow the beard to grow for 2 to 3 days. Use preshaving lotion before shaving, and use the trimmer to cut down the hair to about ¹/₁₆ inch. Shave very lightly with rotary blades; then rinse face with cool water after shaving.
- Patients should be reminded that the idea is not to get a close shave, but to leave approximately 1 mm of hair protruding from the skin. This should prevent the hair

T ABLE 14.11.   Medical Treatment of Pseudofolliculitis Barbae

Hydrocortisone cream 1% to 2.5%

Availability:	Over the counter and prescription.
Dosage:	Applied to inflamed areas twice daily.
Duration:	Use until inflammation resolves.
Side effects:	Long-term use can cause skin atrophy or telangiectasia.
Comments:	For acutely inflamed or infected lesions. Do not use fluorinated corticosteroids on the face.

Topical erythromycin solution

Availability:	Prescription.
Duration:	Applied to inflamed area twice daily.
Duration of use:	Use until pustules resolve.
Comments:	Apply if pustules are seen.

Topical retinoin 0.5% cream or gel (Retin-A)

Availability:	Prescription.
Dosage:	Applied to inflamed area daily.
Duration of use:	Use daily.
Side effects:	Can cause burning, stinging, erythema.
Comments:	Especially helpful for moderate to severe pseudofolliculitis barbae. Regular use alleviates hyperkeratosis developed after daily shaving.

Cephalexin (Keflex), dicloxacillin (Pathocil), or erythromycin

Availability:	Prescription.
Dosage:	Cephalexin: 500 mg 2 to 4 times per day; dicloxacillin: 250 mg 4 times per day; or erythromycin: 500 mg 4 times per day.
Duration:	Use for 10 days.
Comments:	Systemic antibiotics for secondary infection with *Staphylococcus aureus*.

from embedding into the skin and is acceptable for most employers, including the military.

Patient Education

Compliance

Patients should be informed that the best preventive techniques are to grow a beard or avoid close shaves.

Family and Community Support

Patients and family members should be reassured that PFB is not transmissible and cannot be given to close contacts.

Follow-up

Close follow-up is not usually necessary; however, in cases of secondary infection or unsatisfactory results after the first course of treatment, close follow-up may be indicated.

BIBLIOGRAPHY

Barth JH. Alopecia and hirsuties: current concepts in pathogenesis and managment. *Drugs* 1988;35:83-91.

Brodin MB. Drug-related allopecia. *Dermatol Clin* 1987;5(3):571-579.

Burke KE. Hair loss: what causes it and what can be done about it? *Postgrad Med* 1989;85(6):52-77.

Coquilla BH, Lewis CW. Management of pseudofolliculitis barbae. *Military Med* 1995; 160:263-269.

Kaufman KD. Androgen metabolism as it affects hair growth in androgenetic alopecia. *Dermatol Clin* 1996;14(4):697-711.

Kvedar JC, Gibson M, Drusinski PA. Hirsutism: evaluation and treatment. *J Am Acad Dermatol* 1983;12(2, pt 1):215-225.

Modly CE, Wood CM, Burnett JW. Evaluation of alopecia: a new algorithm. *Cutis* 1989; 43:148-152.

Nielsen TA, Reichel M. Alopecia: diagnosis and management. *Am Fam Physician* 1995; 51(6):1513-1522.

Rubin MB. Androgenetic alopecia: battling a losing proposition. *Postgrad Med* 1997; 102(2):129-136.

Safavi KH, Muller SA, Suman VJ, Moshell AN, Melton III LJ. Incidence of alopecia areata in Olmsted County, Minnesota: 1975 through 1989. *Mayo Clin Proc* 1995;70: 628-633.

Sauder DN. Alopecia areata: an inherited autoimmune disease. In: Brown AC, Crounse RG, eds. *Hair, trace elements and human illness.* New York: Praeger, 1980: 343-347.

Sawaya ME. Clinical updates in hair. *Dermatol Clin* 1997;15(1):37-43.

Sawaya ME, Hordinsky MK. The antiandrogens: when and how they should be used. *Dermatol Clin* 1993;11(1):65-72.

Sawaya ME, Price VH. Different levels of 5a-reductase type I and II, aromatase, and androgen receptor in hair follicles of women and men with androgenetic alopecia. *J Invest Dermatol* 1997;109(3):296-300.

Spencer LV, Callen JP. Hair loss in systemic disease. *Dermatol Clin* 1987;5(3):565-570.

Steck WD. Clinical evaluation of pathologic hair loss. *Cutis* 1979;24:293-301.

CHAPTER 15

....

Skin Disorders Secondary to Medications

The two most common drug reactions seen by physicians are the exanthematous drug eruption and the fixed drug eruption, which occur in 1% of outpatients and in 1% to 3% of hospitalized patients. The keys to diagnosis and treatment of the common drug reaction are a good history and a physical examination that reveals a symmetric distribution of the rash and associated physical findings such as urticaria, arthralgia, mucosal involvement, facial edema, purpura, fever, or adenopathy.

EXANTHEMATOUS (MACULOPAPULAR) DRUG ERUPTION

Exanthematous (maculopapular) drug eruption, the most common type of dermatologic drug reaction (approximately 45% to 75% of drug eruptions are exanthematous reactions), may occur with a low-grade fever and is a source of annoyance to many patients taking medication. Penicillins are the most common offenders, but drug reactions have been reported with almost every class of pharmacologic agents that are either ingested or given parenterally. Topical drugs can cause photosensitivity reactions or contact dermatitis, which are addressed in Chapter 9.

Chief Complaint
Patients report a pruritic red rash, which may have developed as early as the same day the medication was started or may have developed as long as 2 weeks after the start of the medication.

Clinical Manifestations
Cutaneous manifestations
- The erythematous rash begins on the trunk and may spread symmetrically to the face and extremities (Figure 15.1, see color insert following page 170).
- The rash is usually symmetric, pink to red, and maculopapular.
- Lesions vary in size from 1 mm to 2 mm, but may be as large as 1 cm and may occasionally be confluent as well.
- These rashes may involve the palms and soles, but there is no involvement of the mucous membranes.
- In the thrombocytopenic patient the exanthematous rashes may appear like a vasculitis because they contain small hemorrhages.
- The lesions blanch under pressure.
- Patients may also have a low-grade fever.

Allergic manifestations.
- Allergic manifestations that can occur in addition to cutaneous reactions include rhinitis, conjunctivitis, and reactive airway disease.

Epidemiology
- Reactions can occur at any age and any time, and are not more prevalent among any race or gender.
- Reactions occur in 1% to 3% of hospitalized patients and 1% of outpatients.

Risk Factors
- Use of a new medication is a risk factor for the type of rash discussed in this section.
- Medication used for several treatment regimens over the previous months or years may sensitize the patient to its use, eventually causing a reaction on resumption of use.
- Approximately 50% to 100% of patients receiving ampicillin (Principen) for treatment of Epstein-Barr virus (infectious mononucleosis) develop an exanthematous drug eruption.
- Approximately 50% to 60% of patients with human immunodeficiency virus (HIV) develop an exanthematous drug eruption when given sulfonamides.

PATHOLOGY

Exanthematous drug eruptions are probably due to a type II or III hypersensitivity reaction, although the exact mechanism is not known (see Chapter 12). This reaction causes damage to small vessels, resulting in vasodilation and skin erythema.

Diagnosis
- Diagnosis is based on physical examination and patient history. It is important to note the date that use of the medication started, dose given, duration of use, and interruptions in use of the medication.
- Patients should also be asked about the use of herbal preparations and over-the-counter products. Any drugs consumed in the 2-week period before onset of the rash should be disclosed (Table 15.1).

Differential Diagnosis
See Table 15.2.

Diagnostic Tests
- In patients with systemic symptoms such as arthralgia, malaise, fever, or adenopathy, consider other organ systems that may be involved such as the vascular (vasculitis), renal, hematopoietic, and hepatic systems. Screening for systemic involvement includes complete blood cell count (CBC), platelet count, liver and renal profiles, and urinalysis.
- CBC with differential cell count may show eosinophilia.

Referral
Patients who have previously reacted to medications such as penicillin, which is known to cause type I mediated reactions, should be referred to an allergist for appropriate testing.

T ABLE 15.1.   Common Causes of Exanthematous Drug Eruptions

More likely to cause reactions	Less likely to cause reactions
Amoxicillin	Erythromycin
Ampicillin (Principen)	Tetracycline
Sulfonamides	Chloramphenicol (Chloromycetin)
Nitrofurantoin (Furadantin)	Gentamicin
Streptomycin	Phenytoin (Dilantin)
Allopurinol (Zyloprim)	Barbiturates
Carbamazepine (Tegretol)	Calcium channel blockers
Gold salts	Isoniazid
NSAIDs	Phenothiazines
	Benzodiazepines
	Quinidine
	Trazodone (Desyrel)

NSAIDs, nonsteroidal antiinflammatory drugs.

Management

Use of any medication that may be causing the drug eruption should be halted immediately.

Medications

See Table 15.3.

Other Treatment Modalities

• An understanding of immunology is important in managing these patients. The majority of drug reactions are not immunologically mediated, and the pathogenesis of the rash is not clearly understood. That is, some drug reactions directly trigger mast cell release of histamines. Therefore treatment with antihistamines is helpful.

T ABLE 15.2.   Exanthematous Drug Eruption: Differential Diagnosis

Viral exanthems	Lesions appear as a symmetric, red, macular rash; can be indistinguishable from exanthematous drug eruption.
	Punch biopsy is needed to differentiate the two.
Urticaria	Erythema and edema that can change location, size, and shape; are not always caused by medication; can involve mucous membranes.
	Punch biopsy is useful to differentiate the two.
Pityriasis rosea	Lesions usually appear as a herald patch; red, macular rash with centripetal scale.
	Punch biopsy is useful to differentiate the two.
Secondary syphilis	Rash is characterized by scaling papules and plaques on the trunk, palms, soles, and mucous membranes.
	Syphilis serologic test results will probably be positive.

T ABLE 15.3.   Medical Treatment of Exanthematous Drug Eruptions

Diphenhydramine (Benadryl)

Availability:	Over the counter.
Dosage:	*Adults:* 25 to 50 mg every 6 to 8 hours.
	Children under 12 years of age: 5 mg/kg divided every 6 hours (12.5/5 mL).
Duration:	Use until pruritis resolves.
Comments:	Sedation.

Hydroxyzine (Atarax)

Availability:	Prescription.
Dosage:	*Adults:* 25 to 50 mg every 6 to 8 hours.
	Children: 2 to 5 mg/kg per day, divided every 6 hours (25 mg/5mL).
Duration:	Use until pruritis resolves.
Comments:	Sedation.

Loratidine (Claritin)

Availability:	Prescription.
Dosage:	*Adults:* 10 mg daily.
	Children from 6 to 12 years of age: 10 mg daily (5 mg/5mL).
Duration:	Use until symptoms resolve.
Comments:	Preferred because less sedating.

Cetirizine (Zyrtec)

Availability:	Prescription.
Dosage:	*Adults:* 10 mg daily.
	Children from 6 to 12 years of age: 5 to 10 mg daily (5 mg/5mL).
Duration:	Use until symptoms resolve.
Comments:	Preferred because less sedating.

Hydrocortisone cream 1%, nonprescription[a]
Hydrocortisone cream 2.5%, prescription[a]

Dosage:	Applied 2 to 3 times per day.
Duration:	Use until rash and pruritis resolve.
Side effects:	Long-term use can cause skin atrophy.
Comments:	May be used on children. May be used on face or groin.

Triamcinolone cream 0.1%

Availability:	Prescription.
Dosage:	Applied 3 times per day.
Duration:	Use until rash and pruritis resolve.
Side effects:	Long-term use can cause skin atrophy and telangiectasia.
Comments:	Do not prescribe for children. Avoid use on face and groin.

continued

T ABLE 15.3.   *continued.*   **Medical Treatment of Exanthematous Drug Eruptions**

Prednisone

Availability:	Prescription.
Dosage:	40 to 60 mg orally, daily.
Duration:	7 to 10 days. Taper by 10 increments every 2 days.
Side effects:	Long-term use can cause severe systemic effects; see *Physician's Desk Reference*.
Comments:	Use for extensive rash or edema.

Eucerin or Sarna

Availability:	Over the counter.
Dosage:	Applied to rash once daily.
Duration of use:	Use until pruritis resolves.
Side effects:	None.

Colloidal oatmeal (Aveeno)

Availability:	Over the counter.
Dosage:	Several times per day.
Duration:	Use until pruritis resolves.
Side effects:	None.

*See **Appendix A.**

- The remaining immunologically mediated rashes are types I to IV reactions. Certainly, immunoglobulin E (IgE)–mediated type I immediate reactions are the most frightening, since anaphylaxis and urticaria can occur in this type.
- Paying close attention to the medication history is important, especially if a patient has had a previous Type 1 reaction (anaphylaxis or urticaria), in deciding whether to rechallenge the patient with the medication.
- If no other drug can be used to treat the patient, skin patch testing may be necessary to make a determination about the presence of an allergy. Referral to an allergist who is familiar with skin testing and prepared to treat anaphylactic reactions is indicated for these patients.
- Be aware of cross-sensitivity when prescribing new medications to the patient who has had a drug eruption; for example, the use of cephalosporins in a patient who is sensitive to penicillin carries approximately a 6% risk for cross-reactivity.
- Some patients may require desensitizing to a drug such as trimethoprim/sulfa, which is needed to prevent or treat *Pneumocystis carinii* pneumonia in patients with acquired immunodeficiency syndrome (AIDS).

Follow-up

Patients should be followed up within 1 to 2 weeks; if the rash has not resolved, another cause—either infection or environmental exposure—may be indicated.

Patient Education

- Patients should be advised that a reaction may occur some time after initiation of offending medications, since some drugs require a sensitization period before causing a noticeable reaction.
- The allergic rash may take up to several weeks to clear, even when treated.
- Patients should also be informed that generic drugs, brand-name medications, and even herbal preparations are equally likely to cause drug eruptions.

FIXED DRUG ERUPTION

- Fixed drug eruption is a hypersensitivity reaction to medications that occurs asymmetrically. When patients are rechallenged with the medication, a similar rash forms at the same site. The fixed drug eruption is only caused by ingested or parenteral medications or foods and not caused by topical agents.
- Certain foods, such as peas and beans, may also cause a reaction.

Common Causes of Fixed Drug Eruptions
See Table 15.4.

Chief Complaint
Patients report a localized, occasionally blistering, macular rash that may have been preceded by itching.

Clinical Manifestations
- Fixed drug eruptions are usually preceded by a local area of pruritus, followed by single or multiple red, round, edematous plaques with sharp borders (Figure 15.2, see color insert following page 170).
- The rash is asymmetric, in contrast to the symmetric rash of exanthematous drug eruptions.
- The plaques can form bullae, crust, and desquamate.
- Erosions can occur if bullae rupture.
- The rash may occur anywhere, but the genitals and oral mucosa are the most common sites.
- The reaction frequently occurs within hours of ingesting the offending agent.
- The lesions can be pruritic and cause a burning sensation.
- Fixed drug reactions resolve slowly, and postinflammatory hyperpigmentation (macules) may remain for several weeks after the lesions resolve.
- Patients who are reexposed to the offending agent develop a rash at the previous site, as well as additional lesions at other sites.

Epidemiology
Age
The reaction may occur at any age, although it is rare in children.

T ABLE 15.4.   Common Causes of Fixed Drug Eruptions

Sulfonamides	Fiorinal
Tetracycline	Barbiturates
Metronidazole (Flagyl)	Gold salts
Fluoroquinolones	Quinine (tonic water)
Penicillins	Oral contraceptives
Erythromycin	Meprobamate (Miltown)
Nystatin (Mycostatin)	Chlordiazepoxide (Librium)
Salicylates	Foods (peas, beans, lentils, and food coloring)
Acetaminophen	Phenolphthalein (certain over-the-counter laxatives)
NSAIDs	

NSAIDs, nonsteroidal antiinflammatory drugs.

Sex
Fixed drug reaction occurs in the same frequency in both male and female patients.

Risk Factors
Genetic predisposition may be a risk factor for development of fixed drug reactions.

PATHOLOGY
The exact causative mechanism is unknown, but probably represents a localized form of a delayed hypersensitivity reaction.
It is unclear whether this reaction is immunologically mediated.

Diagnosis
Diagnosis is based on physical examination and patient history, including history of recurrent lesions, usually at the same site, and precedent medication use.

Differential Diagnosis
See Table 15.5.

Diagnostic Tests
Diagnostic tests are rarely necessary.

Referral
Medication rechallenge or patch testing may be necessary in patients whose reactions are suspected to result from a necessary medication. These patients should generally be referred to an allergist.

Management
Medications
See Table 15.6.
- The offending agent should be eliminated if possible.
- Because it is unknown whether this reaction is immunologically mediated, it is unclear whether antihistamines or systemic steroids will be useful for these patients.

T ABLE 15.5. Fixed Drug Eruption: Differential Diagnosis

Herpes simplex	Lesions are grouped vesicles with erythematous base, confined to one location. The patient has no history of medication use. Tzanck smear is positive.
Erythema multiforme	Characterized by a symmetric rash that does not recur at the same site.
Ecchymosis	The rash appears as multiple pigmented lesions with no bullae, and does not recur at the same site. There is no recent medication use. Biopsy is useful to differentiate the two.

T ABLE 15.6. Medical Treatment of Fixed Drug Eruption

Burrow solution

Dosage:	Soak gauze in cool solution and apply to erosions for 20 minutes 2 or 3 times per day.
Duration:	Use until erosions resolve.
Comments:	Skin dryness or fissuring.

Moderate-potency topical corticosteroids [a]

Availability:	Prescription.
Dosage:	Applied 2 times per day.
Duration:	Use until pruritus resolves.
Side effects:	Long-term use can cause skin atrophy.
Comments:	Do not use on face or groin.

[a] See **Appendix A.**

Other Treatment Modalities

- Topically applied antibiotics, such as triple antibiotic ointment or silver sulfadiazine (Silvadene), under a dressing for infected erosions may be useful.
- The physician should be aware of cross-reactivity with similar drugs that can produce the same reaction, such as cephalosporins, which are cross-reactive with penicillin.
- These eruptions may become significantly worse, forming bullae in some patients, if the drug is continued or used again. Avoidance of the drug is most beneficial, but in some cases identification of the offending agent is a time-consuming process.

Follow-up

Patients should be followed up in 2 to 3 weeks if the rash has not resolved in that time, but should be counseled to return sooner if secondary infection or erosions occur.

Patient Education

- Patients should be reassured that the lesion will resolve but may leave an area of hyperpigmentation that may persist for months.
- With reexposure, the rash will probably recur at the same site of the original rash, and new rash sites may develop as well.

BIBLIOGRAPHY

Bigby M, Jick S, Jick H, Arndt K. Drug-induced cutaneous reactions. *JAMA* 1986;256: 3358-3363.

Roujeau JC, Stern RS. Severe adverse cutaneous reactions to drugs. *N Engl J Med* 1994;331:1272-1285.

Shear NH. Diagnosing cutaneous adverse reactions to drugs. *Arch Dermatol* 1990; 126:94-97.

CHAPTER 16

....

Bacterial Infections Affecting the Skin

In this chapter we discuss skin diseases precipitated by bacterial infection, including impetigo and ecthyma; abscesses, furuncles, and carbuncles; infectious folliculitis; erysipelas and cellulitis; erysipeloid; erythrasma; scarlet fever; and Lyme borreliosis. Etiologic agents include streptococci, *Staphylococcus aureus*, *Escherichia coli*, *Pseudomonas aeruginosa*, *Bacteroides* species, *Haemophilus influenzae*, and *Borrelia burgdorferi*.

IMPETIGO AND ECTHYMA

Impetigo and ecthyma are acute, contagious skin infections caused by bacteria *S. aureus* or group A streptococci. Impetigo is defined as infection that occurs strictly within the epidermis, while infection that extends more deeply into the dermis is known as ecthyma (Figure 16.1, see color insert following page 170).

Chief Complaint

Patients report honey-colored or yellow crusts and a variable degree of pruritus. Ecthyma may present similarly, but is typically more painful and tender, with the lesions located mainly on the legs.

Clinical Manifestations

Impetigo (Bullous or Nonbullous Forms)

Bullous form

- Bullous impetigo demonstrates the development of vesicles and bullae on otherwise normal skin, typically without surrounding erythema.
- Bullous impetigo generally appears on the trunk, face, hands, intertriginous areas, ankles or dorsa of the feet, and thighs and buttocks.

Nonbullous form

- Nonbullous impetigo generally begins with erythematous lesions, which develop transient vesicles or pustules and ultimately rupture, leaving erosions with the classic honey-colored crust typically associated with impetigo.
- Nonbullous impetigo generally appears on the face, arms, legs, and buttocks.
- *Lesions* are generally scattered and discrete, from 1 to 3 cm in diameter; however, the lesions may become confluent, forming larger-appearing lesions.
- *Satellite lesions* are typical and occur through autoinoculation, such as touching or scratching the infected areas, then touching unaffected skin.
- The duration of impetigo is days to weeks.
- If left untreated, these lesions may progress to involve the dermis, thereby forming ecthyma, which is a large ulceration with a hemorrhagic crust, particularly in individuals with poor hygiene or wound care.

Ecthyma

- Ecthyma occurs as ulcerations into the dermis rather than the simple erosions of the epidermis observed in impetigo.
- The lesions are generally larger and associated with more tenderness and induration on palpation.
- Ecthyma lesions are more common on lower extremities, generally appearing on the ankles, thighs, buttocks, or dorsa of the feet.
- The lesions give an impression of depth rather than breadth; the crust, which is thick and adherent to the ulceration, is generally hemorrhagic in appearance.
- Regional lymphadenopathy may be an associated finding of either impetigo or ecthyma.
- Ecthyma has a duration of weeks to months.

Epidemiology

Population

Superficial epidermal infection, or impetigo, is a common disorder that represents up to 10% of all skin disorders seen by dermatologists or family physicians.

Age

- Primary impetigo is most common in children, while secondary impetigo infections of preexisting dermatoses may occur at any age.
- Bullous impetigo is most often seen in children and young adults. Eighty percent of cases of bullous impetigo are caused by a strain of *Staphylococcus,* which is capable of producing an exotoxin and has been implicated as a cause of staphylococcal scalded skin syndrome.
- Colonization with *S. aureus* is common in these patients; the same individual may also be colonized by group A streptococci.

Risk Factors

- *Dermatologic.* Risk factors for secondary impetigo include any underlying dermatosis, such as atopic dermatitis, stasis dermatitis, psoriasis vulgaris, severe contact dermatitis, porphyria cutaneous tarda, acne vulgaris, stasis ulcers, dermatophytosis, or herpetic lesions.
- *Trauma.* Any compromise in the integrity of the epidermis, such as those caused by traumatic abrasions, lacerations, burns, or punctures, is also a risk factor for secondary impetigo.
- *Breaks in the stratum corneum* caused by excoriation (eczema), bug bites, scabies, or varicella zoster virus (either chickenpox or shingles), predispose patients to primary impetigo.
- *Health and environmental.* Warmth, high humidity, patient age, hygiene, diabetes, crowded living conditions, and the poor care of minor trauma are all factors that can aid in fostering the colonization of skin by *Staphylococcus* and *Streptococcus* organisms.

PATHOLOGY

Impetigo causes vesicle formation in the subcorneal region with a dermal perivascular infiltration of neutrophils and lymphocytes. Gram-positive cocci in chains or clusters can be seen in the bullous fluid or within the neutrophils.

Diagnosis

Diagnosis is based on history and clinical presentation.

Differential Diagnosis

See Table 16.1.

Diagnostic Tests

- Testing is generally needed only if the patient is unresponsive to the current empiric treatment. Confirmation of the etiologic pathogen can be supported by Gram stain and cultures with sensitivity testing.
- Gram stain of the lesions typically demonstrates streptococcal (gram-positive organisms in chains) or staphylococcal (gram-positive organisms in clusters) organisms.
- Cultures most commonly demonstrate *S. aureus*, group A streptococci, or a mixture of the two.

T ABLE 16.1.   Impetigo and Ecthyma: Differential Diagnosis

Nonbullous impetigo

Scabies	Lesions are distributed on hands, fingers, feet, groin, and wrists.
	Scabies preparation is usually positive, and bacterial cultures are usually negative.
Dermatophytosis	Rash usually has central clearing and responds to antifungal agents.
	A positive KOH preparation and bacterial culture may be useful to differentiate the two.
Herpes simplex	Lesions usually take the form of a grouped vesicular rash.
	Tzanck smears are often positive, and a bacterial culture may also be useful to differentiate the two.
Contact dermatitis	Lesions are sharply demarcated and pruritic with secondary bacterial infection.
Seborrheic dermatitis	Greasy scales appear on the face or scalp.
	A bacterial culture is usually negative.

Bullous impetigo

Bullous pemphigoid	Bullous pemphigoid occurs in an older population and responds slowly to antibiotics.
Dermatitis herpetiformis	Lesions take the form of a vesicular rash on the extensor surfaces and are intensely pruritic.
Thermal burns	Erythema and/or bullae appear at the site of the thermal injury.
Herpes zoster	Neuralgic pain precedes the onset of vesicular lesions, which can also be pruritic. Tzanck smear is often positive.
Herpes simplex	Lesions usually take the form of a grouped vesicular rash. Tzanck smear is often positive, and a bacterial culture may be useful to differentiate the two.
Porphyria cutanea tarda	Bullae and vesicles appear on sun-exposed areas of the skin.

Ecthyma

Venous stasis	Lesions occur as swollen, aching ulcerations of the medial aspect of the lower extremity. The patient usually has a history of chronic venous insufficiency. Biopsy may be useful to differentiate the two.
Hypersensitivity vasculitis with ulceration	Painful, pruritic ulcerations that are usually seen on the lower extremities. Biopsy may be useful to differentiate the two.

KOH, potassium hydroxide.

- Antibiotic sensitivity testing aids in the selection of the most efficacious antibiotic. If specific culture data with antibiotic sensitivity test results are not available and the lesion is not improving with conventional antibiotics, consider methicillin-resistant *Staphylococcus aureus* (MRSA).

Referral

Referral to a specialist may be warranted if diagnosis is uncertain or the patient is unresponsive to conventional treatment.

Management

The lesions respond quickly to antibiotic treatment.

Medications

See Table 16.2.

Other Treatment Modalities

- Crusts should be removed with warm compresses before applying topical antibiotics.
- Daily washes with benzoyl peroxide 2.5% cleansers (Benzac AC 2.5% wash) or antibacterial soap such as Dial are a good preventive measure.
- In cases of recurrent superficial skin infections, it is advocated that all family and household members be checked via nasal culture and treated if it is found that they are persistent carriers of causative organisms.

Follow-up

Monitoring Patient Course

Patients should be followed up 1 to 2 weeks after initiation of antibiotic treatment to monitor the disease course.

Potential Problems and Complications

- Impetigo and ecthyma can recur, usually resulting from failure to completely eradicate the offending organism with antibiotics, or reinfection from a family member.
- In severe cases of nonbullous or bullous impetigo and ecthyma, patients may be concerned with resultant scarring after resolution of the skin lesions. They should be reassured that, in general, impetigo does not leave a scar. However, ecthyma, because of its deeper involvement with the dermis, often heals with scarring.
- Impetigo can lead to poststreptococcal glomerulonephritis. While prompt treatment of impetigo is needed to prevent the spread of the infection to others, it does not diminish the risk of developing kidney disease.
- Other complications occurring from group A streptococci skin infections may include guttate psoriasis, scarlet fever, suppurative lymphadenitis, lymphangitis, cellulitis, erysipelas, and bacteremia.

Patient Education

Compliance

- Patients should be advised that proper handwashing technique (using an antibacterial soap) is a key preventive measure.
- Proper wound care also fosters the resolution of the superficial skin infections.

Lifestyle Changes

- Patients should be informed that lifestyle changes are directed toward reducing risk associated with the colonization of skin by *S. aureus* or group A streptococci. Such measures include strict control of glucose in diabetics; proper hygiene,

T ABLE 16.2.   Medical Treatment of Impetigo and Ecthyma[a]

Topical antibiotics
Mupirocin 2% (Bactroban)
Availability: Prescription only.
Dosage: Applied topically to affected area 3 times daily.
Duration: 7 to 10 days.
Comments: Effective against *Staphylococcus aureus,* methacillin-resistant *S. aureus* (MRSA), and
   group A streptococci. First-line treatment for mild cases.

Chronic colonization of the nares by *S. aureus*
Dosage: Apply mupirocin 2% ointment topically into nares twice daily.
Duration: 5 days.
Comments: Eliminates carrier state in 90% of patients for up to 6 months.

Oral antibiotics
Amoxicillin, clavulanate potassium (Augmentin)
Availability: Prescription only.
Dosage: *Adults:* 500 mg orally 2 times daily.
   Children: 25 to 45 mg/kg per day orally in 2 divided doses (200 or 400 mg/5 mL).
Duration: 10 days.
Comments: Treatment of staphylococcal and streptococcal disease.

Azithromycin (Zithromax)
Availability: Prescription only.
Dosage: *Adults:* 500 mg orally on day 1, then 250 mg daily for the next 4 days.
   Children: 10 mg/kg per day orally on day 1 (500 mg, maximum dose), then
   5 mg/kg per day orally daily on days 2 to 5 (100 and 200 mg/5 mL).
Duration: 5 days.
Comments: Treatment of staphylococcal and streptococcal disease.

Cephalexin (Keflex)
Availability: Prescription only.
Dosage: *Adults:* 1 to 2 g/day orally in 2 divided doses.
   Children: 30 to 40 mg/kg per day orally in 2 divided doses (250 mg/5 mL).
Duration: 10 days.
Comments: First-line treatment for multiple lesions and for group A streptococcal and *S. aureus* disease.

Ciprofloxacin (Cipro)
Availability: Prescription only.
Dosage: *Adults:* 500 mg orally 2 times daily.
   Children: N/A.
Duration: 7 days.
Comments: Treatment of MSRA; *not for use* in children under 18 years of age or in pregnant women,
   since it can cause problems with cartilage in children.

Clarithromycin (Biaxin)
Availability: Prescription only.
Dosage: *Adults:* 250 mg orally 2 times daily.
   Children: 7.5 mg/kg per day orally in 2 divided doses (125 or 250 mg/5 mL).
Duration: 7 to 10 days.
Comments: Treatment of staphylococcal and streptococcal disease in penicillin-allergic patients.

continued

TABLE 16.2.   *continued.*   **Medical Treatment of Impetigo and Ecthyma**[a]

Erythromycin

Availability: Prescription only.
Dosage: *Adults:* 250 mg orally 4 times daily.
 Children: 30 to 50 mg/kg per day orally in 4 divided doses.
Duration: 10 days.
Comments: Treatment of group A streptococcal disease in penicillin-allergic patients.
 Some resistance associated with *S. aureus.*

Minocycline (Minocin)

Availability: Prescription only.
Dosage: *Adults:* 100 mg orally 2 times daily.
 Children: N/A.
Duration: 10 days.
Comments: Treatment of MRSA; *not for use* in children under 12 years of age or in pregnant women,
 since treatment can cause staining of bone and teeth in children.

Oxacillin (Bactocill), Dicloxacillin (Pathocil)

Availability: Prescription only.
Dosage: *Adults:* 1 to 2 g/day orally in 4 divided doses.
 Children: 50 to 100 mg/kg per day in 4 divided doses (125 to 250 mg/5 mL).
Duration: 10 days.
Comments: Alternate treatment for penicillinase-resistant staphylococci.

Penicillin V

Availability: Prescription only.
Dosage: *Adults:* 250 mg orally 4 times daily.
 Children: 25,000 to 50,000 U/kg per day orally in 4 divided doses.[b]
Duration: 10 days.
Comments: Used in confirmed group A streptococcal disease *only,* since there are many resistant strains of *S. aureus.*

Trimethoprim-sulfamethoxazole (TMP-SMX) (Bactrim)

Availability: Prescription only.
Dosage: *Adults:* 1 double strength tablet (160 mg TMP/800 mg SMX) twice daily.
 Children: 8 to 10 mg/kg per day of TMP orally (40 mg TMP/200 mg SMX/5 mL) in 2 divided doses.
Duration: 10 days.
Comments: Treatment of MRSA.

Parenteral antibiotics
Benzathine penicillin

Availability: Prescription only.
Dosage: *Adults:* 1.2 million U intramuscularly.
 Children: >6 years of age, 600,000 U intramuscularly; <6 years of age, 300,000 U intramuscularly.
Duration: Once.
Comments: Used in confirmed group A streptococcal disease *only,* since there are many resistant strains of *S. aureus.*

[a] For side effects see Table 16.21.
[b] 250 mg = 400,000 U; 500 mg = 800,000 U.

particularly in individuals who live in a warm and highly humid environment; and proper care of minor skin trauma.
• Impetigo is highly infectious; children being treated for this disease should be removed from school or daycare for at least 24 to 48 hours after initiation of treatment.

ABSCESS, FURUNCLE, AND CARBUNCLE

• An abscess is a large, deep, walled-off collection of pus that may develop from folliculitis, a deeper source of infection, or from penetrating foreign bodies.
• A furuncle, or boil, is usually caused by *S. aureus* and typically arises from an extensive infection of a hair follicle.
• A carbuncle is an extensive infection comprising several adjoining hair follicles or furuncles that drain to the surface of the skin through multiple openings.

Chief Complaint
Patients report acute, deep-seated, red-hot, tender nodules, which may demonstrate fluctuance and, in the case of furuncles and carbuncles, purulent drainage.

Clinical Manifestations
• Abscesses, furuncles, and carbuncles begin as tender nodules under the skin surface that progress to exquisitely tender lesions.
• The lesions typically present for only a few days.

Abscesses
• Abcesses may be present anywhere on the skin (Figure 16.2, see color insert following page 170).
• They are often deep within the dermis, subcutaneous fat, muscle, or deeper structures.
• Lesions begin as small, tender nodules that may be firm on palpation.
• They progress in tenderness and size, becoming indurated and ultimately fluctuant with exquisite tenderness to palpation as pus begins to fill the central portion of the lesion. Sometimes the epidermis moves freely over the abscess.
• Surrounding cellulitis may be evident.
• Regional lymphadenopathy may develop.

Furuncles and carbuncles
• Furuncles evolve from a single infected hair follicle.
• Carbuncles comprise interconnecting, infected hair follicles.
• Lesions initially begin as firm, tender nodules approximately 1 to 2 cm in diameter with a central necrotic plug.
• The lesions may be accompanied by surrounding cellulitis.
• Tenderness and erythema become increasingly severe, and superficial pustules may occur.
• Ultimately, purulent drainage is evident on the skin surface, with multiple openings for drainage noted in carbuncles.
• Furuncles and carbuncles appear in the hair-bearing areas of the skin, including the axilla, buttocks, posterior area of the neck, occipital scalp, and beard area.
• Individuals with large abscesses or carbuncles may report accompanying fever and malaise.

Epidemiology

Furunculosis is most commonly seen without predisposing factors in healthy individuals and can recur.

Age

Abscesses, furuncles, and carbuncles occur primarily in children, adolescents, and young adults, with furuncles being uncommon in children but occurring with increased frequency after puberty.

Sex

Lesions most commonly affect men.

Risk Factors

- *Health and hygiene.* Risk factors for abscesses, furuncles, and carbuncles include a chronic *Staphylococcus* carrier state (usually in the nares, perineum, or axillae), diabetes, poor hygiene, obesity, and decreased immunity.
- *Endocrine.* Recurrent furuncles often are associated with diabetes mellitus.
- *Trauma, friction, moisture, or bruises* may all precipitate the development of these lesions.
- *Family history.* May occur in multiple family members at about the same time.

PATHOLOGY

Purulent infection arises from the hair follicle and extends into the dermal layer (abscess) and the subcutaneous tissue (furuncle), and can be lobulated (carbuncle). Gram stain usually shows gram-positive organisms in clusters with many polymorphonuclear neutrophils. The bacterial culture usually reveals *S. aureus,* but can reveal both anaerobes and aerobes in some sites.

Diagnosis

Diagnosis of furuncles, carbuncles, and abscesses is generally made by the history and clinical presentation.

Differential Diagnosis

See Table 16.3.

Diagnostic Tests

- *Gram stain and culture* of the purulent drainage may be used to support and confirm the diagnosis; *S. aureus* is typically the bacterial pathogen involved.
- *Sensitivity testing* of the bacteria may help to guide the antibiotic treatment.
- Although *S. aureus* is, as mentioned above, by far the most common origin of these lesions, other organisms have also been implicated, including *E. coli, P. aeruginosa,* and *Streptococcus fecalis* and anaerobic bacteria including *Bacteroides* species, *Lactobacillus* and *Peptococcus* species, and *Peptostreptococcus* species.
- Approximately 5% of all abscesses are sterile.

Referral

Referral may be indicated if the diagnosis is uncertain or the lesion is unresponsive to conventional treatment.

T ABLE 16.3.   Abscesses, Furuncles, and Carbuncles: Differential Diagnosis

Ruptured epidermal cyst	Usually a long-standing cyst accompanied by recent pain and enlargement.
Ruptured pilar cyst	Usually a long-standing cyst accompanied by recent pain and enlargement.
Hidradenitis, suppurative	Lesions take the form of tender red abscesses that eventually break through the skin. They are limited to the axilla or groin area and have a tendency to scar.

- Referral for the infections is recommended when they have connections to deeper structures, such as those around the perineal area, or for infections on the face which are located at a site that drains into the cavernous sinus.
- Dental abscesses should be referred to a dentist for treatment.

Management
- Furuncles, carbuncles, and abscesses generally respond well to incision and drainage. Using sterile technique, anesthetize the area with a local infiltration of 1% lidocaine (Xylocaine). A sharp incision is made in the epidermis. Bacterial cultures should be taken from the purulent drainage, followed by blunt dissection to break down any septa (carbuncle) that may have formed. Sterile (Iodoform) gauze should be used to pack large abscess cavities; this may be removed in 24 to 48 hours.
- Incision and drainage should be performed only on lesions that demonstrate fluctuance (looseness of the epidermis over abscess) on physical examination.

Medications
See Table 16.4.

Other Treatment Modalities
- *Benzoyl peroxide soap, povidone-iodine soap,* or *4% chlorhexidine solution* may be used daily while bathing and are also recommended to prevent skin colonization.
- *Prophylactic treatment* can be considered in individuals with recurrent furunculosis, beginning with a full dose of antibiotics until all lesions resolve, followed by a single daily dose given for a period of 2 to 3 months. Controlling or eradicating the carrier state of the causative organism is the goal of this regimen.
- *Adjuvant therapy* includes the application of dry heat, such as a heating pad or hot-water bottle. This therapy is useful in nondraining lesions. The application of heat often "draws" the infection toward the surface of the skin and may promote spontaneous drainage of the lesion.

Follow-up
Monitoring Patient Course
Patients with recurrent furunculosis should be followed up every 3 months for a culture of the anterior nares to monitor the effectiveness of treatment. If cultures are positive, a full course of antibiotics should be repeated and a repeat culture performed in 3 months.

Potential Problems and Complications
- Possible complications of the lesions include bacteremia with resultant bacterial seeding of heart valves, joints, bones, spine, and viscera, particularly in the kidneys.
- Deeper infections, such as carbuncles, may cause sepsis, especially in diabetics or immunocompromised patients.

T ABLE 16.4. **Medical Treatment of Abscesses, Furuncles, and Carbuncles**[a]

Topical antibiotics
Mupirocin 2% (Bactroban)

Availability:	Prescription only.
Dosage:	Apply ointment topically into nares twice daily.
Duration:	5 days.
Comments:	Treatment of recurrent infection by chronic *Staphylococcus aureus* colonization of the nares. Eliminates carrier state in 90% of patients for up to 6 months.

Oral antibiotics
Amoxicillin, clavulanate potassium (Augmentin)

Availability:	Prescription only.
Dosage:	*Adults:* 500 to 875 mg orally twice daily.
	Children: 25 to 45 mg/kg per day orally in 2 divided doses (200 or 400 mg/5 mL).
Duration:	10 days or until the swelling and redness resolves.
Comments:	Expensive alternate treatment.

Azithromycin (Zithromax)

Availability:	Prescription only.
Dosage:	*Adults:* 500 mg orally on day 1, then 250 mg daily for the next 4 days.
	Children: 10 mg/kg per day orally on day 1 (500 mg, maximum dose), then 5 mg/kg per day orally daily on days 2 to 5 (100 and 200 mg/5 mL).
Duration:	5 days.
Comments:	Expensive alternative for penicillin-allergic patients.

Cephalexin (Keflex)

Availability:	Prescription only.
Dosage:	*Adults:* 1 to 2 g/day orally in 4 divided doses.
	Children: 30 to 40 mg/kg per day orally in 4 divided doses (250 mg/5 mL).
Duration:	10 days or until redness and swelling resolve.
Comments:	Alternate first-line treatment.

Ciprofloxacin (Cipro)

Availability:	Prescription only.
Dosage:	*Adults:* 500 mg orally twice daily.
	Children: N/A.
Duration:	7 days.
Comments:	Treatment of methacillin-resistant *S. aureus* (MRSA); *not for use* in children under 18 years of age or in pregnant women.

Clarithromycin (Biaxin)

Availability:	Prescription only.
Dosage:	*Adults:* 250 to 500 mg orally twice daily.
	Children: 7.5 mg/kg per day orally in 2 divided doses (125 or 250 mg/5 mL).
Duration:	10 days or until redness and swelling resolve.
Comments:	A more expensive treatment of staphylococcal and streptococcal disease in penicillin-allergic patients.

continued

T ABLE 16.4.   *continued.*   **Medical Treatment of Abscesses, Furuncles, and Carbuncles**[a]

Erythromycin

Availability:	Prescription only.
Dosage:	*Adults:* 250 to 500 mg orally 4 times daily.
	Children: 30 to 50 mg/kg per day orally in 4 divided doses.
Duration:	10 days or until swelling and redness resolve.
Comments:	Treatment of group A streptococcal disease in penicillin-allergic patients.
	Some resistance associated with *S. aureus.*

Minocycline (Minocin)

Availability:	Prescription only.
Dosage:	*Adults:* 100 mg orally twice daily.
	Children: N/A.
Duration:	10 days.
Comments:	Treatment of MRSA; *not for use* in children under 12 years of age or in pregnant women.

Oxacillin (Bactocill), Dicloxacillin (Pathocil)

Availability:	Prescription only.
Dosage:	*Adults:* 1 to 2 g/day orally in 4 divided doses.
	Children: 50 to 100 mg/kg per day in 4 divided doses (125 to 250 mg/5 mL).
Duration:	10 days or until redness and swelling resolve.
Comments:	First-line treatment of abscesses, furuncles, and carbuncles.

Rifampin (Rifadin)

Availability:	Prescription only.
Dosage:	*Adults:* 300 mg orally twice daily.
	Children: 10 mg/kg per day orally twice daily (maximum, 600 mg/day).
Duration:	14 days.
Comments:	Use for recurrent infection caused by chronic colonization of *S. aureus* of the nares in conjunction with oxacillin or dicloxacillin, since rifampin resistance develops when given alone. Eliminates carrier state for 3 months.

Trimethoprim-sulfamethoxazole (TMP-SMX) (Bactrim)

Availability:	Prescription only.
Dosage:	*Adults:* 1 double strength tablet (160 mg TMP/800 mg SMX) twice daily.
	Children: 8 to 10 mg/kg per day of TMP orally (40 mg TMP/200 mg SMX/5 mL) in 2 divided doses.
Duration:	10 days.
Comments:	Treatment of MRSA.

Parenteral antibiotics
Vancomycin (Vancocin)

Availability:	Prescription only.
Dosage:	*Adults:* 1 g intravenously every 12 hours.
	Children: 20 mg/kg per day intravenously in 4 or 6 divided doses.
Duration:	Until patient is less toxic, fever is decreasing, and infection is subsiding; then switch to oral antibiotics for 10 days.
Comments:	Treatment of hospitalized MRSA patients with high fever and possible sepsis.

N/A, nonapplicable.

[a]For side effects see Table 16.21.

Patient Education

Compliance

- Patients should be counseled on the importance of taking the entire course of prescribed antibiotic to ensure healing of the infection. Since the infections are contagious, patients should be treated for 1 to 2 days before returning to work or
school to prevent the spread of infection.
- They should also be advised that showering is permissible only if the lesion has not
been surgically drained.
- In patients with diabetes, strict control of blood sugars is mandatory to aid in
reducing the incidence of recurrence.

Lifestyle Changes

- Patients with recurrent furunculosis should be told to change towels, sheets, and
washcloths on a daily basis. They should be instructed to clean shaving instruments
on a daily basis and avoid such behaviors as nose picking, which can cause bacteria such as *S. aureus* to spread to other skin sites.
- When washing, the patient should be advised to use an antibacterial soap to help
prevent skin colonization.

INFECTIOUS FOLLICULITIS

Infectious folliculitis is an infection of the upper portion of the hair follicle, or hair
shaft, usually resulting in a follicular pustule. The infection can be superficial or deep;
the deep infections may progress to a carbuncle or furuncle.

Chief Complaint

Patients report numerous small red pustules that are confined to hair shafts.

Clinical Manifestations

- Infectious folliculitis appears as a papule or pustule, usually surrounded by ery-
thema, at the upper portion of the hair follicle (Figure 16.3, see color insert following page 170).
- The pustule may rupture, leading to a crustule.
- The affected area may be pruritic and slightly tender to palpation.
- Regional lymph nodes may also be tender to palpation, and lymphangitis, inflam-
mation, or infection of the draining lymphatics causing a red streak to emanate
from the point of infection may also be seen.
- The lesions may be scattered, individual, or grouped.
- The distribution normally seen for infectious folliculitis includes the beard, scalp,
neck, legs, trunk, and, sometimes, buttocks.
- The lesions usually have a duration that may be as short as a few days, but may also
become chronic.
- Infectious folliculitis may progress to become abscesses or furuncles.
- In some darkly pigmented patients, postinflammatory hypopigmentation or hyper-
pigmentation can occur.

Epidemiology

- Superficial folliculitis is more common in children, whereas deep folliculitis can
occur at any age.
- Folliculitis often is seen in patients living in climates with high temperatures and
high humidity.
- The etiology of infectious folliculitis is varied; common etiologic factors include
bacteria, fungi, yeast, viruses, syphilis, and insects (Table 16.5).

T ABLE 16.5.   Etiology of Infectious Folliculitis

Bacterial
Staphylococcus aureus

Location	*Superficial:* face, beard area, scalp, neck, legs (shaving), trunk, axillae (shaving), and buttocks.
	Deep (sycosis): beard area.
Clinical manifestations	Grouped or clustered follicular papules and pustules.
	Ruptured pustules leading to erosions and crustules.
	Possible keloidal scarring.
	Carbuncles and furuncles.
Diagnosis	Gram stain showing gram-positive cocci in clusters with polymorphonuclear leukocytes.
	Bacterial culture.
	Can be predisposed by diabetes.

Pseudomonas aeruginosa

Location	Trunk
Clinical manifestations	"Hot tub" folliculitis; manifests several days after using a hot tub.
	Multiple follicular pustules.
	Usually resolves spontaneously in 7 days.
Diagnosis	Gram stain showing gram-negative rods.
	Bacterial culture.

Gram-negative folliculitis
   (*Proteus and Klebsiella
   species, Escherichia coli*)

Location	Face, trunk.
Clinical manifestations	Patients with worsening acne treated by oral antibiotics.
	Small follicular pustules.
	Sometimes, abscess formation.
Diagnosis	Gram stain showing gram-negative rods.
	Bacterial culture.

Fungal
Dermatophytic folliculitis

Location	Head, beard, groin, and trunk.
Clinical manifestations	*Tinea barbae:* Papulopustules coalescing to form kerion in beard area.
	Tinea capitis: Occurring in "gray patch" or "black dot" dermatophytic infection (see Chapter 17 for more details); also seen in kerion of the scalp.
	Tinea cruris or tinea corporis: Granuloma formation and scattered papules and nodules.
Diagnosis	KOH positive with hyphae.
	Fungal culture.

continued

T ABLE 16.5. *continued.* **Etiology of Infectious Folliculitis**

Pityrosporum folliculitis
Location | Trunk, upper arms, back; face and neck less commonly.
Clinical manifestations | Multiple small follicular papulopustules.
Intensely pruritic.
Mimics acne vulgaris (absence of comedones).
Patient usually from a tropical climate.
Diagnosis | Causative agent: *Pityrosporum ovale.*
Appears as "spaghetti and meatballs" in KOH preparation.
Fungal culture.

Yeast
Candida folliculitis
Location | *Occluded skin:* backs of hospitalized patients, under plastic dressings,
and in intertriginous areas of overweight patients.
Nonoccluded skin: beard, trunk.
Clinical manifestations | Large follicular pustules.
Diagnosis | Causative agent: *Candida albicans.*
KOH preparation showing pseudohyphae.
Fungal culture.

Viral
Herpes simplex
Location | Beard area, chest.
Clinical manifestations | Initially follicular vesicles, grouped or discrete, then later, erosions and crusting.
Seen in patients with HIV.
Diagnosis | Multinucleated giant cells in Tzanck smear.
Viral culture.
Multinucleated giant cells within epithelium in a skin biopsy specimen;
only for confirmation of diagnosis if culture or smear is negative.

Spirochetes
Syphilis (secondary)
Location | Scalp, beard.
Clinical manifestations | Dull red papules in oval groups.
Cause of nonscarring alopecia.
Diagnosis | VDRL test.
Skin biopsy.

Parasitic
Demodicidosis
Location | Face, scalp, eyelids.
Clinical manifestations | *Demodex folliculorum* (parasite of human hair follicle). Rosacea-like red,
papulopustular rash on a red background. Perifollicular scaling.
Diagnosis | Skin biopsy of hair follicle.

KOH, potassium hydroxide; HIV, human immunodeficiency virus; VDRL, Venereal Disease Research Laboratories.

Risk Factors

- *Hygiene.* Shaving, plucking, or waxing hair may be risk factors for infectious folliculitis.
- *Occlusions.* Occluding the hair-bearing skin areas also can facilitate the growth of bacteria, thus precipitating an occurrence of infectious folliculitis. Clothing, plastic wrap, prolonged pressure on an area of skin such as the buttocks or back, prostheses, and natural occlusions at intertriginous areas such as the axilla and inframammary and anogenital regions can also contribute to the development of infectious folliculitis.
- *Health.* Patients who have a chronic illness such as diabetes mellitus or are immunosuppressed may be at risk for folliculitis.
- Topical corticosteroids and, occasionally, systemic antibiotics may promote infectious folliculitis.

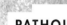

PATHOLOGY

Trauma, irritant chemicals, or infection (bacterial or fungal) causes an occlusion of the ostium of the hair follicle, sometimes resulting in an inflammatory (neutrophils) infiltrate within the superficial portion of the hair follicle and lymphocytic infiltrate deeper in the hair follicle.

Diagnosis

Diagnosis of infectious folliculitis is based on history and physical examination.

Differential Diagnosis

See Table 16.6.

Diagnostic Tests

- *Gram stain and culture* of the purulent discharge from the pustule may reveal a bacterial origin.
- A *potassium hydroxide (KOH) preparation* determines the presence of hyphae or multiple buds, which indicate a dermatophytic infection.
- Patients who have chronic or recurrent infectious folliculitis should be tested for diabetes mellitus or other immunocompromising disorders.

T ABLE 16.6. **Infectious Folliculitis: Differential Diagnosis**

HIV-associated (eosinophilic) folliculitis	Lesions are similar in appearance to staphylococcus folliculitis. Biopsy reveals eosinophils rather than neutrophils.
Keratosis pilaris	Nonbacterial folliculitis distributed symmetrically on the upper arm or anterior thighs.
Pseudofolliculitis barbae	Pseudofolliculitis barbae is most often seen in the beards of dark-pigmented men. Lesions are characterized by curved hair shafts piercing the skin, the tips of which, can be easily freed.

HIV, human immunodeficiency virus.

Referral

Referral may be indicated when the diagnosis is uncertain or the rash is unresponsive to treatment.

Management

- Management is focused on resolution of the rash and prevention of further occurrences.
- Most of the infections rapidly dissipate with treatment. However, *S. aureus* can progress to furuncles or abscesses, which may necessitate incision and drainage.
- Infectious folliculitis may occasionally become chronic unless certain risk factors (such as shaving, poor hygiene, or occlusion) are minimized.

Medications

See Table 16.7.

Other Treatment Modalities

- Warm compresses 3 to 4 times a day for 30 minutes are helpful in superficial folliculitis. Applying dry heat may "draw" the infection to the surface, thereby causing these lesions to drain spontaneously.
- Patients should stop shaving affected areas or use depilatory agents if hair removal is an occupational requirement.
- All contaminated objects such as combs, brushes, and razors should be disinfected in isopropyl alcohol or 2% Lysol solution.
- Washing with an antibacterial soap (e.g., pHisoDerm or Dial) or a mild antibacterial agent such as benzoyl peroxide 10% is useful in preventing the infections from occurring in the future.
- Large, painful lesions may need to be incised and drained. A description of the appropriate technique may be found in this chapter (Cellulitis Management).

Follow-up

Monitoring Patient Course

Close follow-up is usually unnecessary. However, patients should be told that if the infection does not resolve within 7 to 10 days, a return visit is indicated.

Potential Problems and Complications

Deeper infections such as carbuncles or infections involving muscles may cause sepsis, especially in diabetes or immunocompromised patients.

Patient Education

Compliance

- It is important for the patient to understand that most of these infections are contagious. Therefore treatment for 24 to 48 hours is necessary before the patient is no longer contagious.
- Patients should also be cautioned not to open or attempt to drain the pustules.
- It is not necessary to take the antibiotics longer than prescribed.

Lifestyle Changes

- Patients who develop bacterial or fungal folliculitis as a result of shaving should be advised to change blades often. Shaving equipment should be washed thoroughly in hot water after each use.
- Patients should be advised not to share razors with other individuals.

T ABLE 16.7.   Medical Treatment of Infectious Folliculitis[a]

Folliculitis
Staphylococcus Aureus
Topical antibiotics
Mupirocin 2% (Bactroban)

Availability:	Prescription.
Dosage:	Apply ointment topically to affected area twice daily.
Duration:	10 days.
Comments:	Effective against *Staphylococcus aureus*. First-line treatment for small, discrete lesions.

Oral antibiotics
Cephalexin (Keflex)

Availability:	Prescription.
Dosage:	*Adults:* 1 to 2 g/day orally in 4 divided doses.
	Children: 30 to 40 mg/kg per day orally in 4 divided doses (250 mg/5 mL).
Duration:	10 days.
Comments:	Alternate first-line treatment for larger or more extensive lesions.

Erythromycin

Availability:	Prescription only.
Dosage:	*Adults:* 250 to 500 mg orally 4 times daily.
	Children: 30 to 50 mg/kg per day orally in 4 divided doses.
Duration:	10 days.
Comments:	Use in penicillin-allergic patients. Some resistance associated with *S. aureus*.

Minocycline (Minocin)

Availability:	Prescription.
Dosage:	*Adults:* 100 mg orally twice daily.
	Children: N/A.
Duration:	10 days.
Comments:	Treatment of methacillin-resistant *S. aureus* (MRSA); **not for use** in children under 12 years of age or in pregnant women.

Oxacillin (Bactocill), **Dicloxacillin** (Pathocil)

Availability:	Prescription.
Dosage:	*Adults:* 1 to 2 g/day orally in 4 divided doses.
	Children: 50 to 100 mg/kg per day in 4 divided doses (125 to 250 mg/5 mL).
Duration:	10 days.
Comments:	First-line treatment for larger or more extensive lesions.

Pseudomonas species
Ciprofloxacin (Cipro)

Availability:	Prescription.
Dosage:	*Adults:* 500 mg orally twice daily.
	Children: N/A.
Duration:	10 days.
Comments:	Effective against *Pseudomonas* and gram-negative folliculitis. Rash usually regresses spontaneously within 7 days. Treat if symptomatic (pain). **Not for use** in children under 18 years of age or in pregnant women.

continued

TABLE 16.7.   *continued.*   **Medical Treatment of Infectious Folliculitis**[a]

Gram-negative organisms
Trimethoprim-sulfamethoxazole (TMP-SMX) (Bactrim)

Availability:	Prescription.
Dosage:	*Adults:* 1 double-strength tablet (160 mg TMP/800 mg SMX) orally twice daily.
	Children: 8 to 10 mg/kg per day of TMP orally (40 mg TMP/200 mg SMX/5 mL) in 2 divided doses.
Duration:	10 days.
Comments:	Effective against MRSA.

Dermatophyte
Topical antifungals
Clotrimazole 1% (Lotrimin), **miconazole 2%** (Micatin)

Availability:	Over the counter.
Dosage:	Apply topically to affected area twice daily.
Duration:	14 days.
Comments:	Effective against dermatophytosis. First-line treatment for small, discrete lesions with minimal side effects (see Table 17.4).

Ketoconazole 2% (Nizoral), **Econazole 1%** (Spectazole)

Availability:	Prescription.
Dosage:	Apply topically to affected area twice daily.
Duration:	14 days.
Comments:	Effective against dermatophytosis. First-line treatment for small, discrete lesions with minimal side effects (see Table 17.4).

Oral antifungals
Itraconazole (Sporanox)

Availability:	Prescription.
Dosage:	*Adults:* 100 to 200 mg/day orally.
	Children: N/A.
Duration:	14 days.
Comments:	First-line treatment for larger or extensive lesions. *Not approved* for pediatric use (see Table 17.5 for complete details on side effects).

Griseofulvin

Availability:	Prescription only.
Dosage:	*Adults:* N/A.
	Children: Microsize: 15 to 20 mg/kg per day orally (Grisactin).
	Ultramicrosize: 10 to 15 mg/kg per day orally (Gris-Peg).
Duration:	14 days.
Comments:	First-line treatment for children (see Table 17.5 for complete details on side effects).

continued

T ABLE 16.7.   *continued.*   **Medical Treatment of Infectious Folliculitis**[a]

Candida species
Topical Antifungals
Clotrimazole 1% (Lotrimin), Miconazole 2% (Monistat-Derm)
Availability:	Prescription.
Dosage:	Apply topically to affected area twice daily.
Duration:	14 days.
Comments:	First-line treatment for small, discreet lesions. Minimal side effects (see Table 17.4).

Ketoconazole 2% (Nizoral), econazole 1% (Spectazole), ciclopirox (Loprox)
Availability:	Prescription.
Dosage:	Apply topically to affected area twice daily.
Duration:	14 days.
Comments:	First-line treatment for small, discreet lesions. Minimal side effects (see Table 17.4).

Oral antifungals
Itraconazole (Sporanox)
Availability:	Prescription only.
Dosage:	*Adults:* 200 mg/day orally.
	Children: N/A.
Duration:	14 days.
Comments:	First-line treatment for larger or extensive lesions. *Not approved* for pediatric use (see Table 17.5 for complete details on side effects).

Fluconazole (Diflucan)
Availability:	Prescription.
Dosage:	*Adults:* 100 to 200 mg/day orally.
Duration:	14 days.
Comments:	Alternate first-line treatment for large or extensive lesions. *Not approved* for pediatric use (see Table 17.5 for complete details on side effects).

Pityrosporum
Oral antifungals
Itraconazole (Sporanox)
Availability:	Prescription.
Dosage:	*Adults:* 200 mg/day orally.
	Children: N/A.
Duration:	14 days.
Comments:	First-line treatment for pityrosporum. *Not approved* for pediatric use (see Table 17.5 for complete details on side effects).

Viral
Herpes simplex
Topical antivirals
Penciclovir 1% (Denavir)
Availability:	Prescription.
Dosage:	Apply topically every 2 hours.
Duration:	Until lesion resolves.
Comments:	For treatment of small discrete lesions.

continued

T ABLE 16.7. *continued.* **Medical Treatment of Infectious Folliculitis**[a]

Oral antivirals
Acyclovir (Zovirax)
Availability:	Prescription.
Dosage:	*Adults:* 400 mg orally 3 times daily.
	Children: N/A.
Duration:	7 days.
Comments:	First-line treatment for herpes simplex (see Table 4.4 for complete details on side effects).

Famcyclovir (Famvir)
Availability:	Prescription.
Dosage:	*Adults:* 125 mg orally twice daily.
	Children: N/A.
Duration:	5 days.
Comments:	See Table 4.4 for complete details on side effects.

Secondary syphilis
Intramuscular antibiotics
Benzathine penicillin G
Availability:	Prescription.
Dosage:	*Adults:* 2.4 million units.
	Children: 50,000 U/kg intramuscularly (maximum dose is 2.4 million units).
Duration:	Once intramuscularly.
Comments:	Preferred treatment of syphilis. In penicillin-allergic children, desensitize child to penicillin and use. May need to confer with an allergist.

Oral antibiotics
Doxycycline (Vibramycin)
Availability:	Prescription.
Dosage:	*Adults:* 100 mg orally twice daily.
	Children: N/A.
Duration:	2 weeks.
Comments:	Not for use in children less than 12 years of age or pregnant women.

Erythromycin
Availability:	Prescription.
Dosage:	*Adults:* 500 mg orally 4 times daily.
	Children: N/A.
Duration:	2 weeks.
Comments:	For use in penicillin-resistant adult patients.

Demodicidosis
Permethrim cream 5% (Elimite)
Availability:	Prescription.
Dosage:	Apply to face and scalp.
Duration:	8 to 14 hours, then rinse.
Comments:	See Table 19.4 for details on side effects.

N/A, not applicable.
[a]For side effects of antibiotics see Table 16.21.

- Contaminated brushes, combs, and the like should be disinfected in isopropyl alcohol or 2% Lysol solution.
- Patients should also refrain from swimming in pools or sitting in hot-tubs until the infections are cleared.
- Bed linens, towels, and other fabrics that come into contact with these infections should be washed and rinsed in hot water. Noninfected patients should avoid contact with these contaminated materials.

ERYSIPELAS AND CELLULITIS

- Cellulitis is an acute infection of the skin involving the dermal and subcutaneous tissues. Its hallmark is localized skin involvement, including warmth, redness, pain, and swelling.
- Periorbital cellulitis is often referred to as preseptal cellulitis, since the infection involves tissues anterior to the orbital septum, a structure that normally prevents these infections from penetrating the orbital or postseptal regions.
- Orbital cellulitis, with the inflammatory process and infection posterior to the orbital septum, is an uncommon but serious disease. This disorder is characterized by proptosis, which resists movement of the extraocular muscles and causes orbital pain.
- Erysipelas is an acute form of cellulitis involving dermal lymphatics. This disease is often referred to as "St. Anthony's fire" because of its fiery red appearance.

Chief Complaint

Patients with typical erysipelas or cellulitis complain of a localized area of skin involvement, which is generally painful, red, and swollen. In either disease patients may also complain of accompanying symptoms such as malaise and fever.

Clinical Manifestations

- Exposure to the bacteria typically occurs a few days before the actual onset of symptoms.
- Both erysipelas and cellulitis are preceded by a prodrome with symptoms of malaise, anorexia, fever, and chills, appearing 24 to 48 hours before the rash.
- Skin symptoms include pain, burning, tenderness, redness, and pruritus (Figure 16.4, see color insert following page 170; Figure 16.5).
- The local lesion may enlarge rapidly, often within a few hours.
- Associated physical findings of both erysipelas and cellulitis often include regional lymphadenopathy and red streaks moving toward regional lymph nodes, which is called lymphangitis.

Erysipelas
- The skin lesion in erysipelas is an erythematous, flat, macular rash with sharply demarcated borders.
- Vesicles may be observed at the advancing edge of the lesion. The edema and swelling of the lesion give it an "orange-peel" texture (peau d'orange).
- In erysipelas, which is most frequently caused by group A β-hemolytic streptococci (GABS), there is a more significant inflammatory response with lymphatic involvement demonstrating red, painful streaks of lymphangitis extending toward regional lymph nodes. This same type of lymphangitis can also be seen in cellulitis as well as erysipelas.
- Erysipelas may occur on the face, limbs, or abdomen; in scars; or on chronically edematous skin.

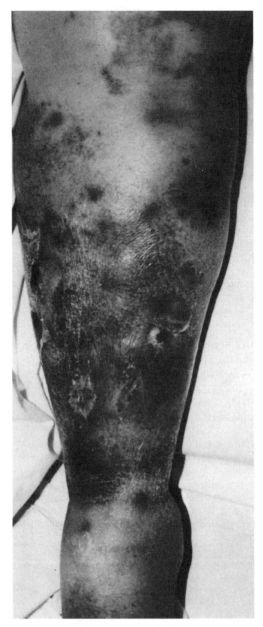

FIGURE 16.5. Cellulitis. From Roenigk HH. Psoriasis. In: Roenigk HH, ed. Office Dermatology. Baltimore: Williams & Wilkins, 1981:102, with permission.

Cellulitis

- Cellulitis appears as a localized area with erythema, warmth, edema, and tenderness.
- The lesions are usually flat to slightly elevated with definable but not sharply demarcated borders.
- Cellulitis generally occurs on the extremities as a result of local trauma, such as an abrasion, burn, laceration, puncture, or bite, which serves as a portal of entry for infection.
- Other points of entry include surgical wounds, incisions, venous access, chronic dermatosis, and skin lacerations.
- Cellulitis often is found on the lower legs of adults, the forearms of intravenous drug abusers, and the arms of women after mastectomy who have undergone lymph node resection.
- Cellulitis may also be found in areas of poor venous flow or lymphatic compromise.
- The infections may be spread through the blood to soft tissue.
- Cellulitis can be associated with systemic symptoms such as fever, chills, malaise, anorexia, and vomiting.
- In children from 6 months to 3 years of age, cellulitis, commonly caused by *H. influenzae,* may occur in the cheek or periorbital area. The lesions appear as a *violaceous* swelling and induration, usually without an obvious portal of entry. Children may also develop cellulitis in the extremities, which is generally caused by group A streptococci or staphylococci and usually has a portal of entry such as minor skin trauma or edema.
- Young children with cellulitis are usually febrile and irritable. A prodromal period of 1 to 2 days before the rash can be seen, with coughing, fever, sore throat, and malaise. About 68% of children with cellulitis caused by *H. influenzae* also have otitis media.
- *H. influenzae* cellulitis in adults is unusual, but can be seen in patients over age 50 years presenting with pharyngitis, high fever, and a red, edematous rash on the face or neck.
- Periorbital cellulitis is an acute inflammatory process characterized by fever, erythema, edema of tissue surrounding the eye, and conjunctivitis.
- Seventy-five percent of patients with *orbital cellulitis* demonstrate radiographic evidence of sinusitis, generally of the ethmoid or maxillary sinus. More than half of the infected individuals report visual disturbances.

Epidemiology

- Erysipelas and cellulitis may occur at any age.
- Periorbital cellulitis is more common in children.

Risk Factors

- *Dermatologic.* Risk factors for erysipelas and cellulitis include other illnesses, such as bullous pemphigoid, pemphigus vulgaris, sunburn, chronic lymphedema, herpes simplex, varicella zoster, atopic dermatitis, contact dermatitis, systemic lupus erythematosus, psoriasis, chronic venous insufficiency, stasis dermatitis, or dermatophytosis of the feet, head, or beard.
- *Trauma.* The infections may be caused by skin trauma or may occur following surgical wounds.
- *Health.* Other risk factors include cirrhosis, diabetes mellitus, human immunodeficiency virus (HIV), malnutrition, malignancy, immunocompromised states, renal failure, and treatment with chemotherapy. Predisposing factors for periorbital cellulitis include sinusitis, upper respiratory tract infections, and eye trauma.
- *Drugs.* Alcohol and drug abuse, particularly intravenous drug abuse, is a risk factor.

PATHOLOGY

Both cellulitis and erysipelas are characterized by dermal edema, marked vascular dilation, and an infiltration of the dermis and lymphatics with streptococci. Dermal infiltration of neutrophils may also be observed. The blood vessels are clear of bacteria.

Erysipelas is most commonly caused by GABS, but can be caused less often by *S. aureus* and groups B, C, or G streptococci.

Most cases of cellulitis are caused by GABS or *Staphylococcus* organisms. However, *H. influenzae, P. aeruginosa, Enterobacter* species, *Proteus mirabilis, Pasteurella multocida, E. coli, Pneumococcus* species, *Neisseria meningitidis, Acinetobacter* species, *Vibrio vulnificus, Mycobacterium fortuitum,* and *Cryptococcus neoformans* may also cause this infection. In children, common etiologic agents of cellulitis include *H. influenzae* type B, group A streptococci, and *S. aureus.*

Periorbital cellulitis is more common in children and is usually caused by *H. influenzae* type B (HIB). Adult periorbital cellulitis is usually caused by staphylococci and streptococci.

As with other forms of cellulitis, staphylococci and streptococci typically cause orbital cellulitis. *H. influenzae* is another common pathogen, particularly in children between the ages of 3 months and 4 years. Complications of this disorder can include abscess, impaired movement of the globe, and diplopia. Meningitis is a rare complication of this disorder, along with cavernous sinus thrombosis and brain abscess.

Diagnosis

Diagnosis of cellulitis is usually based on history and physical examination. Recognizing evidence of necrotic skin infections is essential to facilitate proper, quick treatment to prevent the progression of the infection to the fascia or muscle layers. Special vigilance is required for significant tissue necrosis, erythema, painful induration, eschar formation, and a lack of response to antibiotics.

Differential Diagnosis
See Table 16.8.

Diagnostic Tests
- Since blood culture, a leading-edge biopsy, or aspirate is positive in only 25% to 30% of cases, these tests are usually unnecessary.
- In children with facial cellulitis, causative organisms may be isolated from the throat, ear, wound, or blood cultures. Typically, needle aspiration of facial lesions in children is not attempted.

Referral

- *Consultation* should be considered for the treatment of cellulitis involving pain or in cases of orbital cellulitis.
- *Referral* may be indicated in cases of severe infection or involvement of fascia or muscle. It may also be indicated for cases of necrotizing skin infections that may require surgical debridement and exploration.
- *Hospitalization* is indicated for cases of unremitting fever, necrotic infection, or patients who are unresponsive to oral antibiotics within 24 to 48 hours of the initial dose.

T ABLE 16.8.   Erysipelas and Cellulitis: Differential Diagnosis

Erysipeloid	Lesions occur on the hands of patients who work with dead animal matter. Rash is less marginated than either erysipelas or cellulitis.
Herpes zoster	Lesions are characterized by severe neuralgic pain along the distribution of the affected nerve and groups of vesicles. Herpes zoster is usually unilateral and confined to a single or adjacent dermatome. Tzanck smear and viral culture are often positive.
Contact dermatitis	Contact dermatitis appears as a pruritic, red rash with fewer systemic signs than cellulitis.

Management

Before starting treatment, the borders of the lesion should be outlined with an ink marker. The lesions should be reevaluated 24 hours later, to determine whether there has been a response to treatment.

Medications

See Table 16.9.

Other Treatment Modalities

• Patients with recurrent erysipelas, particularly those with underlying venous insufficiency, should be treated with prophylactic antibiotics for about 2 years after the initial course of antibiotic treatment.
• Acetaminophen or ibuprofen may be recommended for pain relief.
• Surgical debridement and exploration in cases of necrotizing skin infections are recommended. Referral to a surgeon may be necessary.
• Warm compresses or a moist heating pad may also be of use for pain relief.

Follow-up

Monitoring Disease Course

Patients should be followed up 24 hours after initiation of therapy, with individualized follow-up thereafter depending on the severity of illness. Consider hospital admission in potential noncompliant patients, when close follow-up cannot be accomplished, or in patients with systemic symptoms.

Potential Problems and Complications

Complications of cellulitis and erysipelas are uncommon, but may occur if treatment is delayed (Table 16.10).

Patient Education

Compliance

• Patients should be advised that strict compliance with the recommended antibiotic treatment is essential for prompt resolution of the disorder, and to avoid disease progression.
• Cellulitis and erysipelas are highly contagious. Patients and caregivers should be cautioned about hand washing with antibacterial soap such as Dial after any contact with the site of infection.
• It is important that children with this infection remain home from school until they have been treated with antibiotics for 48 hours.

T ABLE 16.9. Medical Treatment of Erysipelas and Cellulitis[a]

Erysipelas and cellulitis
Intravenous antibiotics
Ampicillin/sulbactam (Unasyn)

Availability:	Prescription.
Dosage:	*Adults:* 1.5 to 3 g intravenously every 6 hours.
	Children: 150 to 300 mg/kg per day intravenously divided into four doses (maximum, 12 g daily).
Duration:	Until patient is less toxic, fever is decreasing, and infection is subsiding, then switch to oral antibiotics for 10 days.
Comments:	For the treatment of serious streptococci, staphylococci, *Haemophilus influenza,* and gram-negative infections. Also for use in patients with impaired immunity or decreased host defenses.

Cefazolin (Ancef)

Availability:	Prescription.
Dosage:	*Adults:* 1 g intravenously every 6 to 8 hours.
	Children: 25 to 50 mg/kg per day intravenously divided in 3 to 4 doses.
Duration:	Until patient is less toxic, fever is decreasing, and infection is subsiding; then switch to oral antibiotics for 10 days.
Comments:	For the treatment of serious streptococci and staphylococci infections. Also for use in patients with impaired immunity or decreased host defenses.

Ceftriaxone (Rocephin)

Availability:	Prescription.
Dosage:	*Adults:* 1 to 2 g intravenously or intramuscularly every 24 hours.
	Children: 50 to 75 mg/kg per day intravenously or intramuscularly every 24 hours.
Duration:	Until patient is less toxic, fever is decreasing, and infection is subsiding; then switch to oral antibiotics for 10 days.
Comments:	For the treatment of serious streptococci, staphylococci, *H. influenza,* and gram-negative infections. Also for use in patients with impaired immunity or decreased host defenses. Can also be used intramuscularly in ambulatory setting daily for 48 hours. If no response or worsening symptoms, hospitalize.

Ciprofloxacin (Cipro)

Availability:	Prescription only.
Dosage:	*Adults:* 400 mg intravenously every 12 hours.
	Children: N/A.
Duration:	Until patient is less toxic, fever is decreasing, and infection is subsiding; then switch to oral antibiotics for 10 days.
Comments:	Treatment of patients with serious infections and patients with impaired immunity or decreased host defenses. **Not for use** in children under 18 years of age or in pregnant women.

Vancomycin

Availability:	Prescription only.
Dosage:	*Adults:* 1 g intravenously every 12 hours.
	Children: 20 mg/kg per day intravenously in 4 or 6 divided doses.
Duration:	Until patient is less toxic, fever is decreasing, and infection is subsiding; then switch to oral antibiotics for 10 days.
Comments:	Treatment of serious MRSA infections.

continued

T ABLE 16.9. *continued.* **Medical Treatment of Erysipelas and Cellulitis***a*

Oral antibiotics
Azithromycin (Zithromax)
Availability: Prescription.
Dosage: *Adults:* 500 mg orally on day 1, then 250 mg daily for the next 4 days.
     Children: 10 mg/kg per day orally on day 1, then 5 mg/kg per day orally daily on days 2 to 5
          (100 and 200 mg/5 mL).
Duration: 5 days.
Comments: Alternate treatment for uncomplicated infection in penicillin-allergic patients.

Cephalexin (Keflex)
Availability: Prescription.
Dosage: *Adults:* 500 mg orally 4 times a day.
     Children: 30 to 40 mg/kg per day orally in 4 divided doses (125 to 250 mg/5 mL).
Duration: 10 to 14 days.
Comments: Alternate treatment for uncomplicated infection.

Ciprofloxacin (Cipro)
Availability: Prescription.
Dosage: *Adults:* 500 to 750 mg orally twice daily.
     Children: N/A.
Duration: 10 to 14 days.
Comments: Treatment of MRSA unresponsive to empiric treatment or culture proven;
          not for use in children under 12 years of age or in pregnant women.

Clarithromycin (Biaxin)
Availability: Prescription.
Dosage: *Adults:* 250 mg orally 2 times daily.
     Children: 7.5 mg/kg per day orally in 2 divided doses (125 or 250 mg/5 mL).
Duration: 7 days.
Comments: Alternate treatment for uncomplicated infection in penicillin-allergic patients.

Erythromycin
Availability: Prescription only.
Dosage: *Adults:* 250 to 500 mg orally 4 times daily.
     Children: 30 to 50 mg/kg per day orally in 4 divided doses.
Duration: 10 to 14 days.
Comments: Alternate treatment for uncomplicated infection in penicillin-allergic patients.

Minocycline (Minocin)
Availability: Prescription.
Dosage: *Adults:* 100 mg orally 2 times daily.
     Children: N/A.
Duration: 10 to 14 days.
Comments: Treatment of MRSA unresponsive to empiric treatment or culture proven;
          not for use in children under 12 years of age or in pregnant women.

continued

T ABLE 16.9.   *continued.*   **Medical Treatment of Erysipelas and Cellulitis**[a]

Oxacillin (Bactrocill), Dicloxacillin (Pathocil)

Availability:	Prescription.
Dosage:	*Adults:* 1 to 2 g/day orally in four divided doses.
	Children: 50 to 100 mg/kg per day in 4 divided doses (125 to 250 mg/5 mL).
Duration:	10 to 14 days.
Comments:	First-line treatment for uncomplicated infection.

Trimethoprim-sulfamethoxazole (TMP-SMX) (Bactrim)

Availability:	Prescription.
Dosage:	*Adults:* 1 double-strength tablet (160 mg TMP/800 mg SMX) orally twice daily.
	Children: 8 to 10 mg/kg per day of TMP orally (40 mg TMP/200 mg SMX/5 mL)
	in 2 divided doses.
Duration:	10 to 14 days.
Comments:	Treatment of MRSA unresponsive to empiric treatment or culture proven.

Orbital and periorbital cellulitis

Mild cases of periorbital cellulitis caused by *Staphylococcus* or *Streptococcus* species, or *Haemophilus influenzae*

Dosage and duration:	*Adults and children over 12 years of age:* Use oral antibiotics listed under cellulitis that cover staphylococci and streptococci for adults and staphylococci, streptococci, and *Haemophilus* infections in children.
	Children under 12 years of age: Cefprozil (Cefzil) 20 mg/kg per day orally in 2 divided doses for 10 days or *Cefuroxime* (Ceftin) 30 mg/kg per day orally in 2 divided doses for 10 days.
Comments:	Treatment of patients not having pain or moderate edema of the eyelids and an absence of fever.

Severe cases of orbital and periorbital cellulitis caused by *Staphylococcus* or *Streptococcus* species, or *H. influenzae*

Dosage and duration:	*Adults and children over 12 years of age:* Use parenteral antibiotics listed under cellulitis above for *Staphylococcus* and *Streptococcus* infections.
	Children under 12 years of age: Ceftriaxone use the same dose for children listed under cellulitis every 12 hours until patient is less toxic, fever is decreasing, and infection is subsiding; then switch to oral antibiotics for 10 days.
Comments:	Hospitalize in moderate to severe cases (fever, pain, or severe edema of the eyelids)

Suppressive therapy

Penicillin V, erythromycin, or dicloxacillin

Availability:	Prescription.
Dosage:	*Adults:* 500 mg orally daily.
	Children: 250 mg orally daily.
Duration:	Up to 2 years.
Comments:	Used as suppressive treatment for erysipelas and cellulitis. Dicloxacillin preferred for *S. aureus* infection, erythromycin for penicillin-allergic patients.

N/A, not applicable; MRSA, methacillin-resistant *Staphylococcus aureus.*
[a]For side effects see Table 16.21.

T ABLE 16.10.   Complications of Erysipelas and Cellulitis

Abscess
Gangrene
Necrotic cellulitis or fascitis
Thrombophlebitis (superficial and deep)
Venous stasis ulceration
Glomerulonephritis
Lymphedema (elephantiasis)
Septicemia
Endocarditis
Meningitis (especially in facial cellulitis)
Death

- If a limb is involved, elevation of the affected limb is important to prevent swelling, which helps the healing process.
- First-aid treatment of minor skin breaks or trauma can prevent the development or progression of cellulitis within these lesions.
- Parents should be strongly urged to have children younger than 3 years of age immunized with the HIB vaccine, which has greatly reduced the incidence of HIB cellulitis.

Lifestyle Changes
- The infection site should be protected from trauma (e.g., friction, rubbing, or pressure) and kept clean with antibacterial soap.
- If the top layer of skin falls off, the area should be kept clean by daily washing with water and antibacterial soap, kept dry otherwise, and covered with a dressing.

ERYSIPELOID

Erysipeloid is a specific form of cellulitis caused by the gram-positive bacteria *Erysipelothrix rhusiopathiae,* which is seen almost exclusively in patients who handle dead animal matter.

Chief Complaint
Patients complain of a painful, swollen, erythematous skin lesion of sudden onset.

Clinical Manifestations
- Erysipeloid first appears within a 1- to 7-day incubation period following exposure to the infectious agent.
- The lesions are tender, sharply defined, erythematous, swollen plaques that are sometimes diamond shaped, with irregular, raised borders.
- Erysipeloid lesions expand and extend around the initial site over 3 to 4 days, reaching a maximum diameter of approximately 10 cm.
- The lesions are often painful, with symptoms of throbbing or burning pain and pruritis.

- The infection is noted at the site of exposure, typically the hands or fingers, with sparing of the distal phalanges.
- A characteristic central fading may be observed within the lesions as the outer edges expand.
- Erysipeloid may cause edema in the skin.
- The lesions typically resolve in approximately 3 weeks.
- There is usually no deep extension into tendons of the hand.
- Lymphangitis or lymphadenitis, or both, may be associated findings.
- Systemic symptoms are rare, but may occur at the time of the skin lesion or 1 to 6 months after resolution of the skin lesion.

Epidemiology

Erysipeloid may occur following an abrasion, cut, or puncture to the skin.

Sex

The disease occurs more often among men, with a ratio of roughly 3:1.

Seasonal

Erysipeloid is more often seen in the summer and early autumn.

Regional

The disease occurs worldwide.

Risk Factors

Fishermen, butchers, meat processors, poultry workers, farmers, and veterinarians are at risk for erysipeloid.

PATHOLOGY

The etiologic bacterium *E. rhusiopathiae* is a ubiquitous organism capable of infecting vertebrates such as livestock and poultry, as well as invertebrates such as shellfish. Human infection by this organism occurs exclusively in individuals who are exposed to the meat, hides, or bones of infected dead animals.

Diagnosis

Diagnosis is based on physical examination and patient history of exposure.

Differential Diagnosis

See Table 16.11.

Diagnostic Tests

Diagnosis may be confirmed by a lesional biopsy or lesional aspirate of the advancing border demonstrating a positive culture for *E. rhusiopathiae*.

Referral

- Referral is indicated if the diagnosis is uncertain or the infection is unresponsive to the standard treatment modality.
- Referral is also indicated in the rare occurrence of a systemic complication such as septic arthritis or endocarditis causing severe cardiac symptoms such as malaise,

T ABLE 16.11. Erysipeloid: Differential Diagnosis

Allergic contact dermatitis	The patient does not have a history of contact with dead animal matter.
	Lesions appear as a red, vesiculopapular rash with sharply demarcated borders.
Erysipelas	The patient does not have a history of contact with dead animal matter.
	Lesions appear as a fiery red rash with sharply demarcated borders and tissue edema.

dyspnea, peripheral edema, and shortness of breath. Both can be hematogenously spread when the lesion is allowed to resolve spontaneously.

Management

Despite the self-limited nature of erysipeloid, patients should undergo a regimen of antibiotics to prevent systemic disease.

Medications

See Table 16.12.

Follow-up

Monitoring Disease Course

Follow-up is recommended on a weekly basis until complete resolution of symptoms is observed.

Potential Problems and Complications

• Potential problems and complications include bacteremia, septic arthritis, lymphadenitis, lymphangitis, and, rarely, endocarditis. These complications may occur without any noticeable skin changes.

T ABLE 16.12. Medical Treatment of Erysipeloid[a]

Intramuscular antibiotics
Benzathine penicillin G

Availability:	Prescription only.
Dosage:	*Adults:* 1.2 million units intramuscularly.
	Children over 6 years of age: 600,000 U intramuscularly.
	Children under 6 years of age: 300,000 U intramuscularly.
Duration:	Once.
Comments:	First-line treatment of erysipeloid.

Oral antibiotics
Erythromycin

Availability:	Prescription only.
Dosage:	*Adults:* 250 to 500 mg orally 4 times daily.
	Children: 30 to 50 mg/kg per day orally in 4 divided doses.
Duration:	7 days.
Comments:	Alternate treatment for erysipeloid; useful in penicillin-allergic patients.

[a]For side effects see Table 16.21.

- It is important to be vigilant for complications, since the mortality of endocarditis from *E. rhusiopathiae* is approximately 30% to 40%, despite appropriate antibiotic treatment.
- Relapses may occur from 4 days to 2 weeks after resolution of the skin lesions. The rash can appear at the same site as the initial infection or at another site by hematogenous spread.

Patient Education
Compliance
- Patients should be reassured that erysipeloid is not contagious.
- They must be cautioned to report cardiac symptoms or constitutional symptoms such as fever, night sweats, malaise, dyspnea, shortness of breath, or peripheral edema. Physical signs such as a heart murmur or splinter hemorrhages in the fingernails may represent early-stage endocarditis.

Lifestyle Changes
- Patients with recurrent infection should be advised to prevent these recurrences by wearing protective gloves and using proper hand-washing technique.
- The rash is not contagious by direct skin contact.
- Patients should be instructed to wash the site of exposure daily with an antibacterial soap.

ERYTHRASMA

Erythrasma is a chronic bacterial infection affecting the intertriginous areas of the body. Although erythrasma is caused by the bacteria *Corynebacterium minutissimum,* it is often mistaken for a dermatophytic infection.

Chief Complaint
Patients complain of a well-demarcated rash in the intertriginous regions of the body, such as the groin or axillary folds.

Clinical Manifestations
- Erythrasma is most often asymptomatic, although the rash may occasionally be accompanied by a burning sensation or pruritus.
- The rash is a sharply demarcated, erythematous, flat lesion that may be of considerable size.
- The rash is often the result of the coalescence of confluent patches, although some scattered discrete lesions may also be seen.
- The most common sites are the intertriginous areas of the skin, particularly the groin folds, axillae, intergluteal folds, inframammary areas, and the subpannicular areas. Erythrasma also occurs in toe-web spaces, where it becomes evident as an erosive, erythematous, scaly lesion.
- The rash can be present for months to years.

Epidemiology
Erythrasma generally affects adults.

Risk Factors
- *Endocrine.* Individuals with diabetes mellitus are at risk for erythrasma.
- *Environmental.* Patients who live in warm, humid climates are at risk for erythrasma.
- *Occlusion.* The rashes may occur at the site of macerated or occluded skin.

PATHOLOGY

Erythrasma is caused by the gram-positive rod *C. minutissimum*, which is part of the normal skin flora. Prolonged occlusion of the skin, maceration of the skin, and exposure to a warm, humid environment may trigger this superficial infection. On microscopic examination the skin scrapings or scale is devoid of fungal elements.

Diagnosis

Diagnosis is based on physical examination and patient history.

Differential Diagnosis

See Table 16.13.

Diagnostic Tests

- Diagnostic tests should include a KOH preparation of the skin lesions to rule out dermatophytic lesions by the absence of hyphae.
- Diagnosis may also be aided by the use of the Wood lamp, under which the lesion fluoresces to a coral-red color.
- In lesions with scale, Gram stain may also support the diagnosis by demonstrating the presence of *C. minutissimum*. This procedure, however, is often technically difficult and has a low yield.

Referral

Referral may be indicated if the diagnosis is uncertain or the rash is unresponsive to the standard treatment.

Management

Management is focused on the resolution of the rash through treatment with antibiotics.

T ABLE 16.13.   Erythrasma: Differential Diagnosis

Dermatophytic infestations, especially tinea cruris or tinea pedis	Lesions can be indistinguishable from erythrasma. When positioned under the Wood lamp, dermatophytic infections do not fluoresce to coral-red. A KOH preparation result is positive.
Candidiasis	Lesions occur in intertriginous areas and may appear indistinguishable from erythrasma. A KOH preparation shows pseudohyphae. When positioned under the Wood lamp, candidiasis does not fluoresce to coral-red.
Seborrheic dermatitis	Red plaques and greasy scales appear on the face, scalp, or groin. Both KOH preparation and Wood lamp results are negative.

KOH, potassium hydroxide.

Medications
See Table 16.14.

Other Treatment Modalities
Nonprescription diphenhydramine (Benadryl) may be used to control pruritus.

Follow-up
Monitoring Disease Course
Patients should be followed up at 1 to 2 weeks after the initiation of the treatment regimen.

Potential Problems and Complications
Erythrasma may recur if underlying conditions such as diabetes, occlusion, or maceration of the skin are not eliminated.

T ABLE 16.14.   Medical Treatment of Erythrasma [a]

Topical antibiotics
Benzoyl peroxide 2.5% gel (Benzac AC)
Availability:	Prescription.
Dosage:	Applied topically daily.
Duration:	7 days.
Comments:	Alternate treatment for erythrasma. Can cause redness, skin dryness, and allergic contact dermatitis.

Clindamycin gel or solution (Cleocin T)
Availability:	Prescription.
Dosage:	Applied topically twice daily.
Duration:	7 to 10 days.
Comments:	Alternate treatment for erythrasma. Can cause burning, redness, skin dryness, or itching.

Erythromycin 2% solution
Availability:	Prescription.
Dosage:	Apply topically twice a day.
Duration:	7 days.
Comments:	First-line treatment for erythrasma. Can cause burning, redness, itching, or skin dryness.

Oral antibiotics
Erythromycin
Availability:	Prescription.
Dosage:	*Adults:* 250 to 500 mg orally 4 times daily.
	Children: 30 to 50 mg/kg per day orally in 4 divided doses.
Duration:	2 weeks.
Comments:	Alternate treatment for erythrasma.

[a]For side effects see Table 16.21.

Patient Education

Compliance

- It is important for patients to take measures to prevent prolonged occlusion and maceration of the skin, as well as measures aimed at keeping the intertriginous areas of the skin cool and dry. These measures aid in the management of the disorder.
- Washing the lesions daily with a benzoyl peroxide 2.5% wash (such as Benzac AC Wash) is also beneficial in the prevention of this disorder.

Family and Community Support

Patients and family may be reassured that erythrasma is a superficial skin infection caused by normal skin flora. It does not represent a more serious illness, nor is it often accompanied by any systemic symptoms. Also, erythrasma is not contagious.

SCARLET FEVER

Scarlet fever is a characteristic exanthem caused by an erythrogenic exotoxin produced at the time of an acute infection of the tonsils, skin, or other sites by a strain of GABS.

Chief Complaint

Patients complain of headache, nausea, vomiting, and abdominal pain accompanied by sore throat or pain from other localized sites of infection.

Clinical Manifestations

- Classic symptoms of high fever, headache, nausea, vomiting, and pharyngitis typically begin after a 2- to 4-day incubation period following exposure to the causative agent, group A streptococci.
- The characteristic exanthem, a finely punctate, pink to deeply erythematous eruption noted first on the trunk, begins approximately 48 hours after the onset of the acute symptoms.
- The rash has a fine-sandpaper-like quality to the touch and blanches on pressure. This rash is the sole difference between scarlet fever and streptococcal pharyngitis or tonsillitis. The rash usually spares the palms and soles.
- The rash often demonstrates increased erythema or linear petechiae within the body folds, particularly of the neck, axillae, groin, and antecubital and popliteal fossae. This heightened erythema to the skin folds is known as Pastia lines.
- The exanthem is present for approximately 5 days; then it undergoes desquamation throughout the trunk, extremities, and, last, the palms and soles.
- The desquamation is generally complete in approximately 4 weeks, but may persist for up to 8 weeks. In cases with mild systemic symptoms and minimal exanthem, this desquamation of the hands and feet may be the most profound finding.
- The face, although usually spared from the typical or characteristic rash of scarlet fever, is often flushed and demonstrates the presence of a characteristic perioral pallor.
- The primary site of infection is usually the skin, pharynx, or tonsils.
- The mucosal membranes of the pharynx often reveal a beefy red appearance with cryptic exudative and hypertrophied tonsils.
- The tongue may also be covered by a thick, white coat with scattered red and swollen papillae (white, strawberry tongue). This hyperkeratotic white coating is sloughed within 4 to 5 days, leaving an intensely erythematous mucosa (red, strawberry tongue).

- The oral cavity may demonstrate punctate areas of erythema and petechiae occurring on the palate.
- Other physical findings associated with scarlet fever include anterior cervical chain lymphadenitis, particularly with pharyngitis and tonsillitis.
- Scarlet fever may also give rise to Beau lines, transverse grooves in the fingernails caused by a transient arrest in nail growth.

Epidemiology

Age

Scarlet fever may affect individuals of all ages, but is most common in children who lack immunity from prior exposure to the erythrogenic exotoxin. The maximum incidence of scarlet fever occurs in children ranging from 1 to 10 years of age. Scarlet fever is rare in newborns and infants.

Seasonal

The disease may occur at any time of the year, but its highest incidence is in late fall, winter, and early spring months.

Risk Factors

Recent exposure to an individual with known group A streptococcal infection is a risk factor for scarlet fever.

PATHOLOGY

The erythrogenic exotoxin causes an increased capillary fragility leading to petechiae. Gram stain of the throat, pharynx, or other sites most commonly reveals gram-positive cocci in chains, although less commonly, gram-positive cocci in clusters are evident, indicative of *S. aureus*.

Diagnosis

Diagnosis often can be made by physical examination, but should be confirmed by appropriate tests.

Differential Diagnosis

See Table 16.15.

Diagnostic Tests

- Gram stain, rapid antigen test, or cultures should be performed to confirm the presence of group A streptococci or *S. aureus*.
- Rapid, direct antigen tests are available to confirm the presence of group A streptococci.
- Cultures of the wound, pharynx, tonsils, or other sites of presumed infection can also be used to confirm the presence of group A streptococci or, rarely, *S. aureus*.
- Rising or elevated antistreptolysin O (ASO) titers are also useful in detecting and confirming antecedent streptococcal infections.

Referral

Referral is indicated if disease is unresponsive to standard treatment or when complications such as retropharyngeal or peritonsillar abscesses requiring surgical drainage are suspected.

T ABLE 16.15. Scarlet Fever: Differential Diagnosis

Toxic shock syndrome	Toxic shock syndrome is marked by a high fever, scarlet fever–like rash for 3 days, hypotension along with gastrointestinal and genitourinary tract and hematologic signs and symptoms.
Kawasaki syndrome	Pharyngitis is not evident but does have conjunctivitis, which is absent in scarlet fever. There is no evidence of a streptococcal or staphylococcal infection on Gram stain or culture.
Viral exanthems	The prodrome and distribution of rash for viral exanthems are different from those for scarlet fever. There is no evidence of a streptococcal or staphylococcal infection on Gram stain or culture.
Exanthematous drug eruptions	There is a history of medication use. There is no evidence of streptococcal or staphylococcal infection revealed on Gram stain or culture. A biopsy is useful to differentiate the two.

Management

- Management is focused on the eradication of group A streptococci via antibiotics to prevent the development of rheumatic fever or glomerulonephritis.
- Pain and fever may be relieved with ibuprofen or acetaminophen.

Medications
See Table 16.16.

Other Treatment Modalities
Good hand-washing technique and reduced contact with infected individuals are the best preventive measures.

Follow-up
Monitoring Disease Course
Patients with scarlet fever secondary to streptococci should be followed up within 7 to 10 days after the course of oral antibiotics, or 4 to 5 weeks after intramuscular injections of penicillin, for a repeat throat culture. If repeat cultures are positive, the patient should undergo a repeat treatment course. It is particularly important to consider reculturing the throat in individuals with a history of rheumatic fever.

Potential Problems and Complications
- Scarlet fever is not usually recurrent because patients usually develop an immunity to the infectious agent. However, other strains of group A streptococci, as well as *S. aureus,* can cause a scarlatiniform rash, theoretically raising the possibility of a recurrence.

T ABLE 16.16.   **Medical Treatment of Scarlet Fever** [a]

Intramuscular antibiotics
Benzathine penicillin G

Availability:	Prescription.
Dosage:	*Adults:* 1.2 million units intramuscularly.
	Children over 6 years of age: 600,000 U intramuscularly.
	Children under 6 years of age: 300,000 U intramuscularly.
Duration:	Once.
Comments:	First-line parenteral treatment for scarlet fever.

Oral antibiotics
Azithromycin (Zithromax)

Availability:	Prescription.
Dosage:	*Adults:* 500 mg orally on day 1, then 250 mg daily for the next 4 days.
	Children: 10 mg/kg per day orally on day 1, then 5 mg/kg per day orally daily on days 2 to 5 (100 and 200 mg/5 mL).
Duration:	5 days.
Comments:	Alternate treatment for scarlet fever; useful in penicillin-allergic patients.

Erythromycin

Availability:	Prescription.
Dosage:	*Adults:* 250 to 500 mg orally 4 times daily.
	Children: 30 to 50 mg/kg per day orally in 4 divided doses.
Duration:	10 days.
Comments:	Alternate treatment for scarlet fever; useful in penicillin-allergic patients.

Penicillin V

Availability:	Prescription.
Dosage:	*Adults:* 250 mg orally 4 times daily.
	Children: 25,000 to 50,000 U/kg per day orally in 4 divided doses. [b]
Duration:	10 days.
Comments:	First-line oral treatment for scarlet fever.

[a]For side effects see Table 16.21.
[b]250 mg = 400,000 U; 500 mg = 800,000 U.

- Potential sequelae from scarlet fever include rheumatic fever, glomerulonephritis, and erythema nodosum. These complications are generally secondary to an absence of antibiotic treatment or inadequate eradication of the causative organism. The incidence of rheumatic heart disease is about 3% in epidemics of group A streptococcal infection.
- Other possible complications include peritonsillar abscess, peritonsillar cellulitis, retropharyngeal abscess, otitis media, sinusitis, and suppurative cervical lymphadenitis.

Patient Education
Compliance
- Patients should be cautioned that compliance with antibiotic treatment is a necessity and that the entire course of antibiotics should be completed, even if symptoms seem to improve. Failure to comply with the entire treatment regimen can foster bacterial resistance to antibiotics.
- Patients should be informed that antibiotic treatment does not necessarily shorten the course of the disease process or decrease the severity of the symptoms. Antibiotics are given to prevent the development of possible future complications such as rheumatic fever and glomerulonephritis.
- Group A streptococci are highly contagious infectious agents. Patients are contagious until properly treated with antibiotics for at least 48 hours. Patients who have the desquamation of scarlet fever, but negative culture or antigen test result for group A streptococci are not considered contagious.

Lifestyle Changes
- During the contagious period, family members should be tested for group A streptococci with cultures or rapid antigen tests. They should avoid sharing toothbrushes and eating utensils. If the group A streptococcal infection occurs, sharing of towels and sleeping on infected linen should be avoided. Washing of these items in hot water eliminates the spread of infection.
- The etiologic organism responsible for scarlet fever is spread by mucosal contact via air, personal contact, aerosol, or fomite transmission. It is most commonly spread person to person by inhalation (coughing). Therefore risk reduction begins with good handwashing technique and reducing intimate contact with individuals who are known to be currently infected with these causative organisms.

LYME BORRELIOSIS

Lyme borreliosis is a tick-transmitted, spirochetal infectious disease characterized by an acute stage of systemic symptoms with a pathognomonic skin lesion called erythema migrans (EM), followed weeks to months later by intermittent and chronic stages typified by cardiac, central nervous system, and joint involvement. The chronic stage of Lyme borreliosis includes the cutaneous eruption called acrodermatitis chronica atrophicans (ACA).

Chief Complaint
Patients initially complain of fever, localized rash, joint pain, and muscle tenderness. Later complaints include headache, difficult concentration, fatigue, dementia, irritability, deafness, or ptosis.

Clinical Manifestations
- The initial skin lesion (EM) begins as a small red macule or papule that is located at or near the site of the tick bite. These macules expand within days and may be seen at more than one site (Figure 16.6, see color insert following page 170). EM can cause burning, itching, or pain, but is usually asymptomatic.
- The initial lesion gradually expands peripherally at a variable rate. Lesions may reach up to 12 × 17 cm within 2 weeks. Central clearing is often noted as the EM expands.

- As it expands, the center may demonstrate clearing or may become necrotic and indurated.
- In some patients secondary lesions may occur that are annular and multiple. These are usually smaller than the typical lesions of EM and fail to demonstrate central clearing or induration.
- The rim of erythema is approximately 1 cm wide and may be flat or raised.
- Lesions of EM are usually found on the buttocks, thigh, or axillary areas.
- The tick bite itself is asymptomatic.
- Symptoms include malaise, fatigue, fever, chills, nausea, vomiting, arthralgias, and headaches that often accompany or precede the cutaneous manifestations by a few days.
- Lyme borreliosis occurs without the cutaneous manifestation of EM in roughly 25% of cases; only 14% of patients are able to distinctly report a history of being bitten at that site by a tick. Conversely, the EM lesion may occur without systemic symptoms.
- Lymphocytoma cutis, a benign pseudolymphoma, may be observed during stage 1 of Lyme borreliosis. These red, purple, or brown nodules or plaques may be grouped, but are most often solitary and range from 3 to 5 cm in diameter. The lesions, typically located on the head (particularly on the earlobe) or the areola, scrotum, or extremities, are usually asymptomatic.
- Cutaneous findings of ACA may be seen in chronic cases of Lyme borreliosis. The early inflammatory phase of ACA may occur months to years after the initial onset of Lyme disease and includes discrete or diffuse erythematous, mildly edematous lesions that commonly affect the periarticular areas, usually the extensor surface of one extremity. After this initial phase, plaques (most notably on the extremities) progress centrifugally over several months to years, leaving central areas of atrophy in their wake. As the process progresses, the skin becomes increasingly atrophic. The resultant atrophy leaves an altered violoceous epidermis with prominent subcutaneous tissue and veins that has a tissue-paper–like texture.
- Subcutaneous nodules on the knees and elbows may develop from localized fibrosis. The fibrotic manifestations may extend to the joint capsule, resulting in pain and limitation of movement of the involved joints.
- Within weeks to months after the development of the initial lesion, central nervous system (CNS) abnormalities such as frank neurologic abnormalities can occur, including meningitis, cranial neuropathies, sensory and motor neuropathies, and Bell palsy, which may be bilateral. The CNS involvement usually resolves completely, but may persist for months.
- Cardiac abnormalities occur in approximately 8% of patients, typically within 4 weeks after the appearance of EM. Cardiac abnormalities include various degrees of atrioventricular block including first-degree, Wenckebach; or third-degree heart block. Less common cardiac abnormalities include myopericarditis with resultant reduction in the left ventricular ejection fraction, and cardiomyopathy.
- In more than 50% of untreated cases of Lyme borreliosis, arthritis develops 4 to 6 weeks after a tick bite, although intervals of nearly 2 years have been reported.
- Joint involvement includes intermittent pain and swelling, generally affecting only a few large joints, especially the knee. Although knee involvement occurs in nearly 90% of cases of arthritis, shoulder, hip, ankle, and elbow joints are also commonly affected. Episodes of arthritis typically occur over a period of several years and may be preceded or accompanied by malaise, fatigue, and low-grade fevers.

Stages of Lyme Borreliosis
See Table 16.17.

T ABLE 16.17. Stages of Lyme Borreliosis

Stage 1: Acute (early localized infection)	Stage 2: Intermediate (disseminated infection)	Stage 3: Chronic (late infection or tertiary neuroborreliosis)
Fever, headache, myalgia, arthralgia, lymphadenopathy, and EM An alternate presentation with flulike symptoms without EM	Carditis, meningitis, arthralgia or myalgia, cranial neuritis (cranial nerve palsy), and radiculoneuropathy Can see recurrence of EM	Arthritis Acrodermatitis chronic atrophicans Encephalomyelitis

EM, erythema multiforme.

Epidemiology
Age and Sex
Lyme borreliosis may occur at any age or in either sex, although there is a slightly higher incidence in male patients from 10 to 19 years of age and in female patients from 30 to 39 years of age.

Seasonal
The disease generally occurs in the spring and summer, when the temperature remains consistently over 45°F.

Regional
- Lyme borreliosis in the United States occurs primarily in the northeastern and north central regions.
- Patients usually reside in or have recently visited an endemic area.

Risk Factors
- Individuals living in or visiting Wisconsin, Minnesota, or the northeastern coast from Massachusetts to Maryland are at increased risk for Lyme borreliosis.
- Camping, hunting, or hiking in wooded areas where ticks are endemic are risk factors for this disease.

PATHOLOGY
The etiologic agent responsible for Lyme disease is the spirochete *Borrelia burgdorferi,* which is transmitted by hard-bodied, or ixodid, ticks, such as the deer tick *(Ixodes scapularis)*. These ticks are found primarily in the northeastern and north central regions of the United States. The tick *Ixodes pacificus* is seen in the western coastal states.

The spirochete enters the skin through the bite of the infected tick. After an incubation period of approximately 3 to 32 days the organism migrates toward the skin, creating the pathognomonic cutaneous finding of the disease. There is an infiltration of mononuclear cells around the blood vessels and skin appendages at all layers of the epidermis.

In the center of the EM lesion the epidermis demonstrates a thickened keratin layer and intracellular and extracellular edema. These histologic findings in the skin biopsy of an EM lesion resemble those of an insect bite.

Diagnosis

Diagnosis is based on physical examination and history and confirmed by laboratory testing.

Differential Diagnosis

See Table 16.18.

Diagnostic Tests

- Serologic testing such as the enzyme-linked immunosorbent assay (ELISA) should be performed to confirm the diagnosis.

TABLE 16.18.   Lyme Borreliosis: Differential Diagnosis

Differential diagnoses for stage 1

Tinea corporis	Lesions appear as a rash with central clearing that may resemble erythema migrans. There are no systemic symptoms. KOH preparation is positive for hyphae.
Insect bites (arthropods)	There is pain and ulceration at the site of the bite, and the rash is usually gone in several days.
Cellulitis	Cellulitis is marked by localized erythema and tenderness; however, there is no evidence of erythema migrans. A skin culture or Gram stain result is often positive.
Erythema multiforme	Lesions are small and targetlike and are seen more on the extremities or mucosa.
Drug eruptions	There is a history of medication use. Biopsy is useful to differentiate the two.
Pityriasis rosea	Lesions are distributed differently than in erythema migrans.

Differential diagnosis for stage 2

Secondary syphilis	Papulosquamous eruptions appear on the trunk, palms, and soles. There is arthralgia of the knees or ankles. VDRL test may have a positive result.
Bell palsy	Bell palsy may mimic cranial nerve palsy of Lyme disease, which can be bilateral, whereas Bell palsy is usually unilateral.
Meningitis	Meningitis can be indistinguishable from the neurologic symptoms of Lyme disease. CSF evaluation is helpful to differentiate the two.

Differential diagnoses for adults with arthritis

Reiter syndrome	Peripheral arthritis is associated with urethritis and uveitis, which are not present in Lyme disease. Can have a positive HLA-B27 result.
Rheumatoid arthritis	Rheumatoid arthritis is marked by chronic pain and soft tissue swelling. Rheumatoid factor may be positive and, therefore, may be useful to differentiate the two.
Acute rheumatic fever	Acute rheumatic fever should also be considered in a patient with migratory polyarthritis.

KOH, potassium hydroxide; VDRL, Venereal Disease Research Laboratory; CSF, cerebrospinal fluid; HLA-B27, human leukocyte antigen-B27.

- Although *B. burgdorferi* can be cultured from skin lesions and rarely from the blood and cerebrospinal fluid, the process is far too difficult and slow to be used in the routine diagnosis of Lyme borreliosis. Within the first few weeks of the appearance of EM, one may detect significant titers of specific antispirochetal antibodies. Immunoglobulin M (IgM) is the first antibody present, followed by immunoglobulin G (IgG) 6 weeks after the onset of the disease. These findings may last for months to years. The sensitivity and specificity of these tests vary depending on the type of test used.
- Any positive or equivocal specimens should be tested by a standardized Western blot test. Individuals with disseminated or late-stage Lyme borreliosis almost always have a strong IgG response to *B. burgdorferi* antigens. Seronegative results can be seen if treatment occurs before antibodies have developed. Three percent to 5% of the population, including patients with syphilis, leptospirosis, rheumatoid arthritis, systemic lupus erythematosus, malaria, endocarditis, or mononucleosis, may have a false-positive serology test result. Patients with a positive finding on ELISA but a negative finding on Western blot test are considered to have a false-positive test result.
- Other useful laboratory values include an elevated erythrocyte sedimentation rate (ESR), most notably highest when the patient is feeling ill. White blood cell count with differential cell count is generally within normal limits. In addition, aspartate aminotransferase (AST) and lactate dehydrogenase (LDH) levels may be slightly abnormal when the cutaneous manifestations of EM are present.
- Forty percent of skin biopsy specimens from sites of EM demonstrate spirochetes.

Referral

Referral may be indicated if the diagnosis is uncertain, complications are present, or the disease is unresponsive to standard treatment modalities.

Management

- Prophylactic treatment of patients with a recognized tick bite is not recommended; only patients with a recognized tick bite *and* systemic flu-like symptoms or EM should be treated.
- No treatment is necessary for asymptomatic individuals who are seropositive.
- Transmission of bacteria rarely occurs if the tick is on the human host for less than 48 hours. Remove recognized ticks as soon as possible to reduce the chance of infection.

Medications

See Table 16.19.

Other Treatment Modalities

- Avoidance of endemic areas known to be infected with ticks and taking precautions to avoid being bitten by ticks when exposed to endemic areas, particularly, wooded areas, is the key to prevention of Lyme borreliosis.
- Tick and mosquito repellents containing 20% to 30% N, N′-diethylmetatoluamide (DEET), such as Deep Woods Off or Cutter spray, should be applied to exposed skin and hair before any outdoor activities. These sprays should not be used on the face. Concentrations higher than 30% should not be used because of risk for toxicity, especially in children and pregnant women.
- Permethrin 0.5% spray (A-200 spray, nonprescription) should be sprayed on clothing to kill ticks on contact. Each application of this clothing spray will last 2 days.
- Light-colored, long-sleeved shirts and long pants tucked into the shoes should be worn to prevent tick bites.

T ABLE 16.19.   Medical Treatment of Lyme Borreliosis[a]

Stage 1 (3 days to 4 weeks after tick bite)
Amoxicillin
Availability:	Prescription.
Dosage:	*Adults:* 500 mg orally 3 times daily.
	Children: 25 to 50 mg/kg per day orally in 3 divided doses (250 mg/5 mL)
Duration:	14 to 21 days.
Comments:	Alternate treatment in children and pregnant women.

Azithromycin (Zithromax)
Availability:	Prescription.
Dosage:	*Adults:* 500 mg orally daily for 2 days, then 250 mg daily for days 3 to 10.
	Children: 10 mg/kg per day orally daily for 2 days, then 5 mg/kg per day daily for days 3 to 10.
Duration:	10 days.
Comments:	Alternate treatment in penicillin-allergic patients.

Cefuroxime (Ceftin)
Availability:	Prescription.
Dosage:	*Adults:* 500 mg orally twice daily.
	Children: 30 mg/kg per day orally in 2 divided doses.
Duration:	14 to 21 days.
Comments:	Alternate treatment for Lyme borreliosis.

Doxycycline (Vibramycin)
Availability:	Prescription.
Dosage:	*Adults:* 100 mg orally twice daily.
	Children: N/A.
Duration:	14 to 21 days.
Comments:	First-line treatment in adults; *not for use* in children under 12 years of age and pregnant women.

Stage 2 (weeks to months after bite)
Clinical manifestations:	*Dermatologic:* recurrent EM.
Medications:	Use same oral treatment as in stage 1.
Duration:	30 days.
Clinical manifestations:	*Joints:* periarticular arthritis.
Medications:	Doxycycline, amoxicillin.
Availability:	Prescription.
Dosage and duration:	*Doxycycline.* *Adults:* 100 mg orally twice daily for 30 days.
	Children: N/A.
	Amoxicillin. *Adults:* 500 mg orally 3 times daily for 30 days.
	Children: 50 mg/kg per day orally in 3 divided doses for 30 days.
Clinical manifestations:	*Cardiac:* carditis, first-degree A-V block <0.3 milliseconds.
Medications:	Use same oral treatment as in stage 1.
Duration:	30 days.

continued

T ABLE 16.19.   *continued.*   **Medical Treatment of Lyme Borreliosis**[a]

Clinical manifestations:	*Cardiac:* First degree A-V block >0.3 milliseconds, second- and third-degree A-V block.
Medication:	Cefotaxine, ceftriaxone, penicillin G.
Availability:	Prescription.
Dosage and duration:	*Cefotaxime.* *Adults:* 2 g intravenously every 4 hours for 14 to 21 days.
	Children: 100 to 200 mg/kg per day intravenously in 3 to 6 divided doses for 14 to 21 days.
	Ceftriaxone. *Adults:* 2 g intravenously every 24 hours for 14 to 21 days.
	Children: 75 to 100 mg/kg per day intravenously every 24 hours for 14 to 21 days.
	Penicillin G. *Adults:* 20 to 24 million units/day intravenously in 4 divided doses for 14 to 21 days.
	Children: 300,000 U/kg per day intravenously in 4 divided doses for 14 to 21 days.
Comments:	Hospitalize and monitor, may need cardiology consultation. Ceftriaxone is first-line treatment with penicillin G and cefotaxime as the alternates. Use with caution since high doses of penicillin can cause seizures.
Clinical manifestations:	*Neurologic:* Bell palsy, cranial nerve palsies, peripheral neuropathy, meningitis or encephalitis.
Medications:	Cefotaxime, ceftriaxone, penicillin G.
Availability:	Prescription.
Dosage and duration:	Same intravenous treatment as for carditis, and hospitalize patient.

Stage 3 (weeks, months, or years after bite)

Clinical manifestations:	*Arthritic and neurologic*
Medications:	Amoxicillin, doxycycline, ceftriaxone, penicillin G
Availability:	Prescription.
Dosage and duration:	*Amoxicillin.* *Adults:* 500 mg orally 3 times daily for 30 days.
	Children: 25 to 50 mg/kg per day orally in 3 divided doses (250 mg/5 mL) for 30 days.
	Doxycycline. *Adults:* 100 mg orally twice daily for 30 days.
	Children: N/A.
	Ceftriaxone. *Adults:* 2 g intravenously every 24 hours for 14 to 21 days.
	Children: 75 to 100 mg/kg per day intravenously every 24 hours for 14 to 21 days.
	Penicillin G. *Adults:* 20 to 24 million units/day intravenously in 4 divided doses for 14 to 21 days.
	Children: 300,000 U/kg day intravenously in 4 divided doses for 14 to 21 days.
Comments:	Optimal treatment is not well established in stage 3 disease. Doxycycline is **not for use** in children under 12 years of age or pregnant women. High doses of penicillin can cause seizures. Use with caution.

[a]For side effects see Table 16.21.

N/A, not applicable; EM, erythema multiforme; A-V, atrioventricular.

- A careful total-body search for ticks should be performed daily following any trip outdoors in an endemic tick area.
- Removing a tick within the first 48 hours after biting is crucial to decrease the incidence of Lyme disease. To remove these insects, grasp the tick gently with a pair of tweezers and remove it with a constant pulling motion; do not twist. Do not use hot materials or fingernail polish to kill the tick; these will cause the insect to inject more bacteria into the bite.

Follow-up
Monitoring Disease Course
Patients should be followed closely at regularly scheduled intervals during the treatment regimen to monitor for stage II or III manifestations of Lyme borreliosis. Monitoring serologic values via comparison of convalescent titers to titers taken during the acute disease phase is also recommended.

Potential Problems and Complications
- Both the primary and secondary lesions of EM can fade and recur over a period of 1 to 14 months.
- Fatigue from the early stages of Lyme borreliosis may persist for several weeks after treatment.

Patient Education
- Patients should be cautioned to watch for stage I signs and symptoms for 4 to 6 weeks following a recognized tick bite.
- The Jarisch-Herxheimer type of reaction can occur within the first 2 days of therapy, causing a worsening of rash and systemic symptoms.
- Patients should be educated about the typical disease course of Lyme disease and reassured that this disease is not contagious.
- Ticks do not need to be carried from one live animal to another. Hard-bodied ticks, that is *Ixodes* species, may be found on grass or other plant material waiting for a host to come within reach. These ticks seek carbon dioxide sources and can travel up to 30 feet to find a host. Spraying an insecticide inside a house alone will not be effective; the area surrounding the house should be sprayed as well.
- Table 16.20 describes other tick-borne diseases in North America.
- Table 16.21 lists the antibiotics used in treatment and their side effects.

T ABLE 16.20.   Other Tick-borne Diseases in North America

Disease	Etiology	Vector
Babesiosis	*Babesia microti*	*Ixodes* species
Rocky Mountain spotted fever	*Rickettsia rickettsii*	*Dermacentor* species
Tularemia	*Francisella tularensis*	*Dermacentor, Amblyomma* species
Ehrlichiosis	*Ehrlichia chaffeensis*	*Dermacentor, Amblyomma* species
Colorado tick fever	Orbivirus	*Dermacentor* species
Relapsing fever	*Borrelia* species	*Ornithodoros* species
Q fever	*Coxiella burnetti*	*Dermacentor, Amblyomma* species
Powassan encephalitis	*Flavivirus* species (arbovirus)	*Ixodes* species

T ABLE 16.21.   Side Effects and Precautions of Antibiotics

Generic	Brand name	Formation	Side effect/precaution
Mupirocin	Bactroban	Topical ointment	• Can cause burning, stinging, pain, and pruritus.
Penicillins			
• Penicillin G & V	—	• Oral 250–500 mg and 250 mg/5 mL	• Can see all types of hypersensitivity reactions (urticaria, angioedema, pruritus, anaphylaxis, Stevens-Johnson syndrome, erythema multiforme, serum sickness, and toxic epidermal necrolysis).
• Benzathine Penicillin G	Bicillin LA	• IM 300,000, 600,000, 1.2 million, 2.4 million U	
• Oxacillin	Bactocill	• Oral 250–500 mg and 250 mg/5 mL	
• Dicloxacillin	Pathocil		• Can see nausea, vomiting, diarrhea, and epigastric distress.
			• About 6% cross-over hypersensitivity to cephalosporins.
			• High doses of penicillin can cause seizures, hemolytic anemia, and thrombocytopenia infrequently.
• Amoxicillin	—	• Oral 250–500 mg and 125–250 mg/5 mL	• Hypersensitivity reactions.
			• Causes nausea, vomiting, and diarrhea.
			• Avoid use in mononucleosis— may cause rash.
• Amoxicillin/ clavulanate	Augmentin	• Oral 250, 500, 875 mg and 125, 200, 250, 400 mg/5 mL	• Hypersensitivity reactions.
			• Can see diarrhea, nausea, skin rash, vomiting, and vaginitis.
			• Avoid use in mononucleosis— may cause rash.
• Ampicillin/ sulbactam	Unasyn	• IV 1.5, 3 g	• Hypersensitivity reactions.
			• Can see diarrhea, skin rash.
			• Avoid use in mononucleosis— may cause rash.
Cephalosporins			
• Cephalexin	Keflex	• Oral 250, 500 mg and 125 and 250 mg/5 mL	• Hypersensitivity reactions.
			• Can see a 6% cross-over hypersensitivity to penicillin.
			• Can see diarrhea and rash.
• Cefazolin	Ancef	• IV 500 mg, 1 g	• Hypersensitivity reactions.
			• Can see a 6% cross-over hypersensitivity to penicillin.
			• Can see diarrhea, oral candidiasis, vaginitis, stomach cramps.

continued

T ABLE 16.21. *continued.* Side Effects and Precautions of Antibiotics

Generic	Brand name	Formation	Side effect/precaution
• Ceftriaxone	Rocephin	• IV or IM 250, 500 mg; 1, 2 g	• Hypersensitivity reactions. • Can see a 6% cross-over hypersensitivity to penicillin. • Can see eosinophilia, diarrhea, rash, thrombocytopenia, leukopenia, and pain at injection site.
• Cefprozil	Cefzil	• Oral 250, 500 mg and 125 and 250 mg/5 mL	• Hypersensitivity reactions. • Can see 6% cross-over hypersensitivity with penicillins. • Can see diarrhea, nausea, pruritus, vaginitis, and diaper rash.
• Cefuroxime	Ceftin	• Oral 125, 250, 500 mg and 125 and 250 mg/5 mL	• Hypersensitivity reactions. • Can see 6% cross-over hypersensitivity with penicillins. • Can see diarrhea, nausea, vomiting, and eosinophilia.
• Cefotaxime	Claforan	• IV or IM 500 mg, 1, 2 g	• Hypersensitivity reactions. • Can see 6% cross-over hypersensitivity with penicillins. • Can see pain with injection, rash, pruritus, fever, eosinophilia, colitis, and diarrhea.
Macrolides			
• Erythromycin	—	• Oral 250, 333, 500 mg and 200 and 400 mg/5 mL	• Some hypersensitivity reactions. • Mainly GI tract side effects— nausea, vomiting, abdominal pain, diarrhea, and anorexia.
• Clarithromycin	Biaxin	• Oral 250, 500 mg and 125 and 250 mg/5 mL	• Some hypersensitivity reactions. • Can see diarrhea, nausea, abnormal taste, dyspepsia, abdominal pain, and headache. • Fewer GI tract side effects than with erythromycin.
Azalides			
• Azithromycin	Zithromax	• Oral 250 mg and 100 and 200 mg/5 mL	• Some hypersensitivity reactions. • Can see diarrhea, nausea, and abdominal pain. • Usually well tolerated.

continued

TABLE 16.21. *continued.* Side Effects and Precautions of Antibiotics

Generic	Brand name	Formation	Side effect/precaution
Sulfonamides			
• TMP-SMX	Bactrim, Septra	• Oral 80 mg TMP/400 mg SMX, DS 160 mg TMP/800 mg SMX, and 40 mg TMP/200 mg SMX per 5 mL	• Do not use in children under 2 months of age, in pregnancy, or in nursing mothers. • Hypersensitivity reactions. • Can see nausea, vomiting, anorexia, and skin rash.
Tetracyclines			
• Minocycline	Minocin	• Oral 50, 100 mg	• Do not use in children under 12 years of age or in pregnancy. • Hypersensitivity reactions. • Anorexia, nausea, photosensitivity, vomiting, diarrhea, rash, pseudotumor cerebri, and vertigo.
• Doxycycline	Vibramycin	• Oral 50, 100 mg	• Do not use in children under 12 years of age or in pregnancy. • Hypersensitivity reactions. • Can see anorexia, nausea, vomiting, diarrhea, skin rash, and photosensitivity.
Floroquinolones			
• Ciprofloxacin	Cipro	• Oral 250, 500, 750 mg	• Some hypersensitivity reactions. • Can see nausea, diarrhea, vomiting, abdominal pain, headache, restlessness, and rash. • Do not use in children under 18 years of age or in pregnancy.
• **Vancomycin**	Vancocin	• IV 500 mg, 1 g	• Hypersensitivity reactions. • Can see neutropenia, phlebitis at injection site, and ototoxicity.
• **Rifampin**	Rifadin	• Oral 150, 300 mg	• Some hypersensitivity reactions. • Can see liver dysfunction, epigastric distress, anorexia, nausea, vomiting, flatulence, abdominal cramps, diarrhea, headache, fever, and fatigue. • Avoid in pregnancy and in patients with liver disease.

LA, long-acting; U, units; TMP, trimethoprim; SMX, sulfamethoxazole; DS, double strength; GI, gastrointestinal.

BIBLIOGRAPHY

Bratton RL, Nesse RE. St. Anthony's fire: diagnosis and management of erysipelas. *Am Fam Physician* 1995;51(2):401-404.

Jorup-Ronstrom C, Britton S. Recurrent erysipelas: predisposing factors and cost of prophylaxis. *Infection* 1987;15:105-106.

Levine J. The cellulitides from minor to catastrophic. *Emerg Med* 1997;29(5):60-71.

McHugh CP. Arthropods: vectors of disease agents. *Lab Med* 1994;25(7):429-437.

O'Dell ML. Skin and wound infections: an overview. *Am Fam Physician* 1998;57(10): 2424-2432.

Rahn DW, Felz MW. Lyme disease update. *Postgrad Med* 1998;103(5):51-70.

Reagan DR, Doebbeling BN, Pfaller MA, et al. Elimination of coincident *S. aureus* nasal and hand carriage with intranasal application of mupirocin calcium ointment. *Ann Intern Med* 1991;114(2):101-106.

Sigal LH. Lyme disease. In: Klippel JH, Weyand CM, Wortmann RL, eds. *Primer on the rheumatic diseases,* 11th ed. Atlanta: Arthritis Foundation, 1997:204-207.

Spach DH, Liles WC, Campbell GL, Quick RE, Anderson DE, Fritsche TR. Tick-borne diseases in the United States. *N Engl J Med* 1993;329(13):936-947.

Verdon ME, Sigal LH. Recognition and management of Lyme disease. *Am Fam Physician* 1997;56(2):427-436.

CHAPTER 17

Superficial Fungal Infections

DERMATOPHYTOSIS

Dermatophytes are a group of fungi that are capable of infecting nonviable keratinized skin, which includes the stratum corneum, nails, and hair. These infections are also known as tinea infections with a second modifier according to the anatomic site of infection. The most common genera of fungi involved are *Trichophyton, Microsporum,* and *Epidermophyton.*

Transmission occurs from person to person by fomites (called anthrophilic infections), from animals such as puppies and kittens (called zoophilic) and, least commonly, from the soil (called geophilic). Zoophilic infections cause more inflammation than those from anthrophilic transmission.

Chief Complaint

Patients report an itching, burning, red rash that is expanding peripherally.

Clinical Manifestations

The dermatophytic infections are compared in Table 17.1 by offending organism, patient complaints, and clinical manifestations (Figures 17.1–17.3, see color insert following page 170).

Epidemiology
Age

Children are more likely to have scalp infections, whereas young adults have more intertriginous infections.

Race

African American adults have a lower incidence of dermatophytosis.

Sex

The infections occur equally among male and female patients.

Risk Factors

An individual can become infected from contact with other infected individuals, animals, or sometimes even from the soil.

PATHOLOGY

Biopsy specimens reveal hyperkeratosis, acanthosis, sparse perivascular infiltrate and, occasionally, epidermal neutrophils.

T ABLE 17.1. Comparison of History and Physical Findings of Dermatophytic Infections

Dermatophytosis	Organism	Patient complaints (history)	Clinical manifestations	Comments
1. Tinea Barbae	*Trichophyton* species	• Usually very pruritic • Tenderness and pain in beard and moustache area • Occurs mainly in adult men	• Red inflammatory papules or pustules • Papules may coalesce on face (Kerion) • Scaling can occur • Can cause regional lymphadenopathy • Hair shafts involved with infection can be easily removed	• Can be acquired through animal exposure • Seen commonly in farmers
2. Tinea Capitis	*Trichophyton* (90% of cases) or *Microsporum* species	• Takes weeks to months to evolve • Seen predominately in children 6–10 years of age • Pain and tenderness can occur in inflammatory disease (Kerion) • More common in African-Americans than in whites • Common modes of transmission include barbershop, hats, protective head-gear, theater seats, pets, or other children (playmates)	• Ectothrix infection invades outside part of hair shaft—hyphae leads to hair cuticle destruction • Patchy hair loss in scalp with scale formation ("gray patch" tinea capitis) hair shaft becomes brittle, breaking off at scalp line • Wood's lamp testing can exhibit green fluorescence • Endothrix infection occurs within hair shaft without cuticle destruction ("black dot" tinea capitis, which are broken-off hairs near the scalp surface) • Can develop a boggy inflammatory tumor of the scalp associated with hair loss, multiple pustules, and tenderness (Kerion) • Can cause cervical and occipital lymphadenopathy	

3. Tinea Corporis (Ringworm)	*Epidermophyton, Trichophyton,* or *Microsporum* species	• Can occur in any age group • Weeks to years to develop • Often asymptomatic • Mild pruritus can occur • Often **coexists** with **tinea pedis** or **cruris** • More common in tropical and subtropical regions	• Seen on the trunk • Small to large, scaling, sharply marginated plaques • Pustules or vesicles can be seen at the periphery of the rash • Bullae can also occur • Usually a central clearing with peripheral erythema	• Can be transmitted by frequent contact between cats or dogs and children, veterinarians, and animal handlers
4. Tinea Cruris (Jock itch)	*Trichophyton* or *Epidermophyton* species	• Usually seen in adults • Men predominate over women • Months to years to evolve • **Associated** with **long standing tinea pedis** • Usually asymptomatic • Can cause pruritus or burning • Warm, humid environment, obesity, and tight clothing are predisposing factors	• Large scaling plaques with well-demarcated borders • Sometimes has central clearing • Papules and pustules can be present at the margin of the rash • Can be seen in the groin, anterior and lateral portions of the thighs, and buttocks • Rarely involves the penis and scrotum	• Can see post-treatment hyperpigmentation, especially in darker-skinned individuals • Chronic scratching can lead to lichen simplex chronicus • Can be directly transmitted by infected scale in bed linens, towels, and clothing
5. Tinea Facialis	*Trichophyton* or *Microsporum* species	• Usually asymptomatic, but pruritus and photosensitivity can be seen • Common in children	• Well-circumscribed macules or plaques of varying size with elevated borders and central clearing • Minimal scaling, but can be pronounced in some patients • Asymmetric rash • Occurs on glabrous facial skin	• Can be acquired by animal contact

continued

TABLE 17.1. *continued.* **Comparison of History and Physical Findings of Dermatophytic Infections**

Dermatophytosis	Organism	Patient complaints (history)	Clinical manifestations	Comments
6. Tinea Manuum	*Trichophyton* or *Epidermophyton* species	• Takes months to years to evolve • Frequently symptomatic with pruritus and pain • Usually associated **with tinea pedis** and sometimes associated **with tinea cruris** • If rash becomes secondarily infected, deep skin fissures can cause pain • Can be unilateral	• Dyshidrotic-type: papules, vesicles, and sometimes bullae around margin of lesion can be seen • Hyperkeratotic-type: well-demarcated scales with hyperkeratosis and fissures on the palmar surface of the hand • Well-demarcated border with central clearing • Rash can extend onto dorsum of the hand with papules, nodules, and pustules	• Can be associated with immunosuppression, topical corticosteroid use, diabetes, atopic dermatitis, excessive sweating and warm, humid climates
7. Tinea Pedis	*Trichophyton* or *Epidermophyton* species	• Most commonly seen between 20–50 years of age • Men predominate over women • Takes months to years to evolve • Usually asymptomatic, but can cause pruritus and pain, especially with secondary bacterial infection	• Four types • Interdigital-type: maceration, peeling skin and fissuring between the toes. Underlying skin can be red and sometimes weep • Moccasin-type: well-demarcated erythema with minute papules on the plantar and lateral aspects of the foot, thick keratin layer, arciform scaling	• Walking barefoot on floors contaminated by trichophyton spores (which can survive up to 12 months on desquamated human skin) can lead to tinea pedis infections

- Predisposing factors include occlusive foot wear, hot and humid environments, and communal baths or pools

- Inflammatory or bullous-type: vesicles or bullae filled with clear fluid. Can sometimes become secondarily infected with *Staphylococcus aureus*. After spontaneous rupture of bullae, erosions with ragged borders can occur
- Ulcerative-type: interdigital rash extends into the dorsum and plantar aspects of the foot due to maceration and secondary bacterial infection

8. Onychomycosis *Trichophyton, Epidermophyton or Candida species or Scopulariopsis brevicularis*

- Commonly seen between 20 to 50 years of age
- Dermatophyte infections are often preceded by nail trauma and **are often accompanied by tinea pedis**
- Predisposing factors include positive family history, trauma, abnormal nail anatomy, psoriasis, immunosuppressed condition (HIV) or impaired peripheral circulation such as caused by diabetes

- Starts as white patch in nail plate that changes to brown/black
- Infection more commonly seen in the great toenails
- Thickened nails with distal subungual debris and hyperkeratotic scale
- Can see onycholysis (separation of the nail from the nail bed) caused by the subungual debris
- Nail is dystrophic and crumbling with increased friability
- Can be seen on any nail, but more common in the toe nails

- Tinea unguium refers to a dermatophyte infection that accounts for 80%–90% of all nail infections, the remainder are caused by Candida Spp. (6%) and molds (Scopulariopsis) 4%

continued

TABLE 17.1. *continued.* **Comparison of History and Physical Findings of Dermatophytic Infections**

Dermatophytosis	Organism	Patient complaints (history)	Clinical manifestations	Comments
8. Onychomycosis *(continued)*	*Trichophyton, Epidermophyton* or *Candida* species or *Scapulariopsis brevicularis*	• In candidal infection, history of frequent immersion of the feet or hands in water • Dermatophytic infections more common in men and candidal infections more common in women • Dermatophytic infections transmitted by direct or fomite contact. *Candida,* since part of the normal flora, becomes pathogenic because of altered local host resistance (immunosuppression, diabetes or corticosteroid use) • Molds are transmitted by direct contact with the soil		

Diagnosis

Diagnosis is based on physical examination, history, and appropriate tests.

Differential Diagnosis

See Table 17.2.

Diagnostic Tests

- *Wood lamp.* For some dermatophytoses the diagnosis can be made by Wood lamp examination. Hairs infected with *Microsporum* species usually fluoresce green. The endothrix type of tinea capitis caused by *Trichophyton* species does not fluoresce. However, the Wood lamp examination is only useful in about 20% of cases of tinea capitis. Therefore a negative Wood lamp examination in the scalp does not rule out tinea capitis.
- *Potassium hydroxide preparation.* The potassium hydroxide (KOH) test is useful in making a presumptive clinical diagnosis in all dermatophytic infections. Sampling of the lesion should begin by using a No. 15 scalpel blade to collect the scale at the periphery of a dermatophyte infection, causing the scale to drop onto a glass microscope slide. In tinea unguium, cut the toenail back to reveal the hyperkeratotic debris, scrape, then place on a slide. The coverslip is applied, and a drop of KOH solution (5% to 10%) placed next to the coverslip will be drawn underneath by capillary action. The slide is heated with a match or Bunsen burner, but not to the point of boiling. Dermatophytes can be recognized as septated, tubelike structures, which represent hyphae. For tinea capitis, hairs can be removed with a needle holder or forceps, then processed in the same manner to look for hyphae (Figure 17.4).
- *Fungal cultures.* Although useful in confirming dermatophyte infections (e.g., hair or nail infections that often have a negative KOH preparation result), fungal cultures are rarely used in dermatophytic infections of the skin because of the long time in receiving final culture results. Scale and hair from suspected fungal infections are removed and cultured on Sabouraud medium, which then takes 4 to 8 weeks to grow. This is the slower method of identifying fungal infections, but with great specificity.
- *Bacterial cultures.* Bacterial cultures are useful to rule out secondary bacterial infections. The origin of these infections is usually *Staphylococcus aureus* or group A streptococci.
- *Punch biopsy.* Dermatopathology also can be used to diagnose fungal infections. A small, 4-mm punch biopsy or shave biopsy specimen can be obtained from the leading edge of the infection. Physicians should always alert the pathologist that they are looking for fungal infections so that the pathologist may apply the correct stains to these slides. A punch biopsy is usually not needed for most dermatophytic infections of the skin that have a positive finding on KOH preparation. A biopsy may also be useful in diagnosing a kerion.

Referral

Referral may be indicated if diagnosis is uncertain or disease is unresponsive to standard treatment modalities.

Management

Current antifungal therapy is very effective for the treatment of dermatophytosis. Two types of therapy, topical and systemic, are available. The topical agents are especially useful for dermatophytes that reside in the epidermis. However, systemic agents are probably more useful when the infection occurs in the hair, palm, or nails.

T ABLE 17.2.   Differential Diagnosis of Dermatophytic Infections

Tinea barbae

Staphylococcus folliculitis	Lesions are characterized by crustules and pustules with scaling. Result of KOH preparation is negative. Bacterial culture is positive for *Staphylococcus* species.
Furuncle or carbuncle	Painful, red abscess on the face with scales that can involve the regional lymph nodes. Result of KOH preparation is negative.
Acne vulgaris	Rash involves the entire face and shoulder areas of both male and female patients. KOH preparation result is negative.
Rosacea	Telangiectasia involving the nose and cheeks. Result of KOH preparation is negative.
Pseudofolliculitis barbae	Infection occurs primarily in patients of African descent. It is usually characterized by painless bumps with hair shafts coming out of the papules. KOH preparation result is negative.

Tinea capitis

Alopecia areata	Patient presents with discrete, nonscaling hair loss. KOH preparation result is negative.
Seborrheic dermatitis	Seborrheic dermatitis is rare in children. KOH preparation result is negative.
Bacterial cellulitis or abscess	Lesions may resemble severe infections such as kerion. KOH preparation result is negative. Bacterial culture is usually positive.
Psoriasis	Rash is characterized by plaques with silver scale on the scalp. KOH preparation result is negative.

Tinea corporis

Nummular eczema	Diffuse, small coin-shaped lesions that are scaly and very pruritic. KOH preparation result is negative.
Pityriasis rosea	There is an acute onset of multiple systemic papules and plaques with peripheral scale. KOH preparation result is negative.
Granuloma annulare	Lesions have a lack of scale. KOH preparation result is negative.
Lyme disease	Erythema migrans is without scale. KOH preparation result is negative.

Tinea cruris

Erythrasma	Rash is characterized by symmetric red patches with fine scales. KOH preparation is negative. Wood lamp examination reveals coral to red fluorescence.
Candidiasis	Beefy, red infection that has poorly defined borders and satellite papules or pustules. It may also involve the scrotum. KOH preparation result may be positive for pseudohyphae.
Psoriasis	Lesions are thick, silvery scales without central clearing. KOH preparation result is negative.
Seborrheic dermatitis	Lesions usually involve the scalp, face, ears, and chest. The rash is an ill-defined, red, scaling rash. KOH preparation result is negative.

continued

TABLE 17.2. *continued.* **Differential Diagnosis of Dermatophytic Infections**

Intertrigo	Rash is usually characterized by red, sometimes weepy lesions in skin folds. KOH preparation result is usually negative unless caused by candidiasis.

Tinea facialis

Seborrheic dermatitis	Rarely occurs in children. Rash usually involves nonglabrous skin and is a red, scaly rash without central clearing. KOH preparation result is negative.
Erythema migrans (Lyme disease)	Lesions lack scale. KOH preparation result is negative.
Lupus erythematosus	Symmetric facial rash that does not have scale. ANA test result is positive. KOH preparation result is negative.
Photosensitivity rash	Rash involves the entire face or sun-exposed skin. KOH preparation result is negative.

Tinea manuum

Eczema	Bilateral rash that appears on hand as well as on other areas of body. KOH preparation result is negative.
Contact dermatitis	Patient presents with a very pruritic rash appearing on both hands and has a history of contact with an offending agent. KOH preparation result is negative.
Granuloma annulare	Lesions do not have any scale. KOH preparation result is negative.
Psoriasis	Lesions are characterized by a thick, silvery rash. There is also nail pitting. KOH preparation result is negative.

Tinea pedis

Eczema	Rash involves other areas of the body. KOH preparation result is negative.
Contact dermatitis	Patient presents with a symmetric rash that usually appears on the plantar surface or dorsum of the foot and has a history of contact with an offending agent. KOH preparation result is negative.
Psoriasis	Lesions are characterized by thick, silvery scale, and there are signs of rash elsewhere on body. KOH preparation result is negative.
Bacterial or yeast infection	There is maceration in the space between toes. KOH preparation result may be positive for pseudohyphae in candidal infections and negative in bacterial infections. Bacterial cultures may be positive.

Onychomycosis and tinea unguium

Psoriasis	There is nail pitting. KOH preparation result is negative.
Eczema	There is nail dystrophy with crumbling or friability and no subungual hyperkeratotic debris. KOH preparation is usually negative, but onychomycosis may coexist.

KOH, potassium hydroxide; ANA, antinuclear antibody.

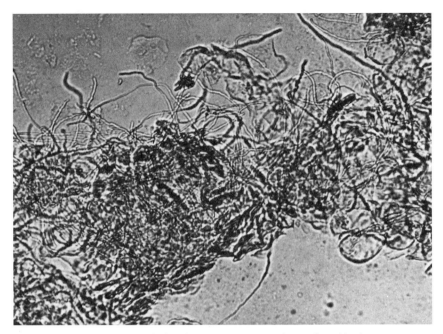

FIGURE 17.4. Potassium hydroxide (KOH) preparation slowing fungal hyphae. From Zuger-man C. Procedures and techniques in dermatology. In: Roenigk HH, ed. *Office dermatology.* Balti-more: Williams & Wilkins, 1981:15, with permission.

Medications
See Table 17.3.

Other Treatment Modalities
- In kerions, incision and drainage are often necessary to drain the purulent mater-ial, to facilitate the healing process.
- Burrow solution (over the counter) helps dry moist or weeping lesions, such as those seen in interdigital tinea pedis. Solution should be mixed in water according to manufacturer's directions and used to lightly saturate gauze, which is applied to weeping area. Gauze should be removed when dry. Burrow solution may dry or burn the lesion if used for more than 2 to 3 days.
- Prevention of the dermatophytic infections, especially tinea pedis and tinea cruris, can be achieved by applying miconazole (Micatin) or tolnaftate powder (Tinactin) to areas that are prone to fungal infections, especially immediately after bathing. Cornstarch should not be used, since it promotes these infections.
- In secondary bacterial infections that are seen with tinea capitia, tinea manus, and tinea barbae, the staphylococcal and streptococcal infections can be controlled with cephalexin, dicloxacillin, or erythromycin (see Chapter 16, Cellulitis, Table 16.9, for dosage).

Follow-up
Monitoring Disease Course

For the more serious infections requiring a longer time for treatment (e.g., tinea capi-tis), monitor the infections closely and continue treatment until results of both the

TABLE 17.3. Medical Treatment of Superficial Fungal Infections

Tinea barbae, tinea capitis, tinea corporis, tinea cruris, tinea manuum, tinea pedis

Medication:	*Griseofulvin* microsize (Grisactin) or ultramicrosize (Gris-Peg)
Dosage:	*Adult:* Microsize: 500 to 1000 mg orally daily.
	Ultramicrosize: 330 to 660 mg daily or 375 to 750 mg daily.
	Children: Microsize: 15 to 20 mg/kg daily orally (maximum, 500 mg/day).
	Ultramicrosize: 10 to 15 mg/kg daily orally.
Duration:	*Tinea barbae, tinea capitis:* 8 weeks.
	Tinea cruris, tinea manuum, tinea pedis: 4 to 8 weeks.
Comments:	For adult patients; may be used for children with tinea capitis.
	Use for extended disease in tinea manuum and tinea pedis.

Tinea barbae, tinea capitis, tinea corporis, tinea cruris, tinea manuum, tinea pedis, tinea unguium, onychomycosis

Medication:	*Terbinafine* (Lamisil)
Dosage:	250 mg orally daily for all infections.
Duration:	*Tinea barbae, tinea capitis:* 4 to 6 weeks.
	Tinea corporis, tinea cruris: 2 to 4 weeks.
	Tinea manuum, tinea pedis, tinea unguium, onychomycosis:
	6 weeks on fingernails and 12 weeks on toenails.
Comments:	For use in adult patients. Only approved for tinea unguium, but used for other tineas; monitor with CBC.

Tinea barbae, tinea capitis, tinea corporis, tinea cruris, tinea manuum, tinea pedis, tinea unguium, onychomycosis

Medication:	*Itraconazole* (Sporanox)
Dosage:	*Tinea barbae, tinea capitis*
	Adults: 100 to 200 mg daily orally.
	Children: Tinea capitis, 5 mg/kg daily.
	Tinea corporis, tinea cruris: 200 mg orally daily.
	Tinea manuum, tinea pedis: 200 mg orally twice daily.
	Tinea unguium, onychomycosis: 200 mg twice daily for the first 7 days of each month, or (more expensive) 200 mg orally daily.
Duration:	*Tinea barbae, tinea capitis:* 4 to 6 weeks.
	Tinea cruris, tinea corporis, tinea manuum and tinea pedis: 1 week.
	Tinea unguium and onychomycosis: 2 months for fingernails or 3 months for toenails.
Comments:	For adult patients; may be used for children with tinea capitis.
	For tinea unguium and onychomycosis: Nail may still look abnormal at end of treatment; confirm resolution with fungal culture or KOH preparation.

continued

T ABLE 17.3. *continued.* **Medical Treatment of Superficial Fungal Infections**

Tinea barbae, tinea capitis, tinea corporis, tinea cruris, tinea pedis, tinea unguium, onychomycosis

Medication:	Ketoconazole (Nizoral)
Dosage:	*Adults:* 200 mg orally daily and up to 400 mg daily for tinea capitis.
	Children with tinea capitis: 5 mg/kg per day.
Duration:	*Tinea capitis:* Use for 6 to 8 weeks.
	Tinea corporis, tinea cruris: 2 to 3 months.
	Tinea pedis: 4 to 6 months.
	Tinea unguium: 4 to 18 months.
Comments:	Alternative therapy for adult patients; may be used for children with tinea capitis.

Tinea corporis, tinea cruris, tinea manuum, tinea pedis, tinea unguium, onychomycosis

Medication:	Fluconazole (Diflucan)
Dosage:	150 mg orally once weekly.
	Tinea unguium, onychomycosis: 300 mg weekly.
Duration:	Use for up to 4 weeks.
	Tinea unguium, onychomycosis: 3 to 5 months in fingernails and 9 to 12 months for toenails.
Comments:	Alternative treatment when disease is recalcitrant or recurrent.

Tinea facialis, tinea pedis, tinea manuum, tinea corporis (limited to small area or single lesion)

Medication:	Use any topical fungal agent listed in Table 17.4.
Dosage:	Applied topically once or twice daily.
Duration:	Until lesion is gone.
Comments:	First-line treatment in tinea facialis.
	Must eradicate associated fungal infection in feet and/or hands.

CBC, complete blood cell count; KOH, potassium hydroxide.

KOH preparation and fungal cultures are negative. Often, long-term use of systemic antifungal agents requires liver or hematologic monitoring (Table 17.5).

Potential Problems and Complications

- *Kerions.* Some dermatophytic infections may progress to the development of a kerion, which may lead to a secondary bacterial infection. Close follow-up is appropriate to monitor the success of the treatment. Scalp kerions can lead to scarring alopecia with permanent hair loss.
- *Hair loss* is a complication of tinea capitis. Alopecia is usually poorly circumscribed, multiple, and scattered and can be scarring or nonscarring.
- *Nail loss.* Tinea unguium can lead to onycholysis (separation of the nail plate from the nail bed) resulting in total nail loss. The nail usually returns, and prophylactic topical antifungal treatment is needed to prevent the new nail from becoming infected.
- *Bacterial superinfection.* Superficial fungal infections such as tinea capitis and tinea pedis are susceptible to bacterial superinfection. The local host defenses of the skin are sometimes decreased by the superficial fungal infection leading to a bacterial overgrowth.

TABLE 17.4. Topical Antifungal Agents[a]

Medication	Dosage	Availability	Organisms indicated				
			Candida albicans	Tricho-phyton species	Epidermo-phyton species	Micro-sporum species	Pityro-sporum species
Sulconazole nitrate 1% (Exelderm)	qd–bid	Cream, solution		X	X	X	X
Terbinafine HCL 1% (Lamisil)[b]	qd–bid	Cream		X	X	X	
Clotrimazole 1% (Lotrimin)[b]	bid	Cream, lotion, solution	X	X	X	X	X
Ciclopirox 1% (Loprox)	bid	Cream, lotion,	X	X	X	X	X
Miconazole nitrate[b] 2% (Monistat)	bid	Cream	X	X	X	X	X
Ketoconazole 2% (Nizoral)	qd	Cream	X	X	X	X	X
Oxiconazole 1% (Oxistat)	qd–bid	Cream, lotion	X	X	X	X	X
Econazole 1% (Spectazole)	qd–bid	Cream	X	X	X	X	X
Butenafine 1% (Mentax)	qd	Cream		X	X	X	
Naftifine HCL 1% (Naftin)	qd	Cream, gel		X	X	X	
Nystatin (Mycostatin)	bid	Cream	X				
Tolnaftate (Tinactin)[b]	bid	Cream, solution, spray, powder		X	X	X	
Undecylenic acid[b] (Desenex)	bid	Cream, powder, ointment		X	X	X	

[a]Side effects of topical antifungal agents are minimal and include pruritis, burning, dryness, skin irritation, allergic contact dermatitis, erythema, and stinging.

[b]Available over the counter.

T ABLE 17.5. Oral Antifungal Agents

Generic name	Brand name	Strength	Side effects
Griseofulvin			• Better absorption when taken with a fatty meal.
Microsize	• Grifulvin V		• Monitor CBC and liver function monthly if using
	Tablets	250 and 500 mg	for more than 3 months because leukopenia
	Suspension	125 mg/5 mL	and granulocytopenia can be seen with
	• Grisactin		prolonged use.
	Capsules	250 and 500 mg	• Can see photosensitivity, GI tract upset,
			and headache.
			• Interferes with phenobarbital,
			warfarin (Coumadin) (lowered effect), and
			other medications metabolized by liver.
Ultramicrosize	• Fulvicin P/G		• Do not use in patients who have liver disease,
	Tablets	125 and 250 mg	pregnancy, or porphyria.
		165 and 330 mg	• Do not use with alcohol.
	• Gris-Peg Tablets	125 and 250 mg	
	• Grisactin		
	Ultratabs	250 and 330 mg	
Itraconazole	• Sporanox		• Requires an acid pH in stomach for absorption;
	Tablets	100 mg	therefore avoid concomitant use with
	Solution	10 mg/mL	antacids or H_2-blockers.
			• Contraindicated with coadministration of terfenadine
			(Seldane), cisapride (Propulsid), triazolam
			(Halcion),and astemizole (Hismanal), because
			of life-threatening ventricular arrythmias.
			• Can cause GI tract upset, rash, pruritis, peripheral
			edema, liver toxicity, and hypokalemia.
			• Monitor liver function periodically if taking this
			for more than 1 month in all patients with
			preexisting liver disease or who are taking
			the drug chronically.
			• Can increase level of digoxin or cyclosporine
			(Sandimmune).
Ketoconazole	• Nizoral		• Requires an acid pH for absorption; therefore avoid
	Tablets		concomitant use with antacids or H_2-blockers.
	200 mg		• Can cause GI tract upset, rash, and allergic reactions.
			• Can cause liver toxicity.
			• Should monitor liver function at initiation of
			and at frequent intervals treatment
			thereafter (once every 4 to 6 weeks).
			• Contraindicated with coadministration of terfenadine,
			cisapride, triazolam, and astemizole because of
			life-threatening ventricular arrhythmias.

continued

T ABLE 17.5. *continued.* **Oral Antifungal Agents**

Generic name	Brand name	Strength	Side effects
Terbinafine	• Lamisil Tablets	250 mg	• Can cause headache, GI tract upset, rash, abdominal pain, loss of taste, rare liver toxicity, and severe neutropenia. • Must monitor liver function if patient has preexisting liver disease, liver symptoms that develop during therapy, or if treatment lasts longer than 1 month. Monitor every 4 to 6 weeks. • Must monitor CBC every 4 weeks if treatment lasts longer than 1 month.
Fluconazole	• Diflucan	50, 100, 150, 200 mg 10 mg/mL 40 mg/mL	• Monitor liver function tests when using in patients with serious underlying medical illnesses (HIV, etc.). • Can cause rare cases of lymphopenia, thrombocytopenia,and hypokalemia. • Can cause skin rash—discontinue if rash progresses. • Avoid use with astemizole, terfenadine, oral hypoglycemics, phenytoin (Dilantin), cyclosporines, rifampin (Rifadin), cisapride, and warfarin because they can cause significant drug interactions. • No absorption problems when used concomitantly with antacids. • Decreased absorption of fluconazole when used with cimetidine.

CBC, complete blood cell count; GI, gastrointestinal; H_2, histamine type 2; HIV, human immunodeficiency virus.

- *Fungal recurrence.* Superficial fungal infections can be recurrent in patients who are predisposed to these infections (see Table 17.1 for these predisposing factors), patients who have diabetes, or patients who are immunocompromised [e.g., human immunodeficiency virus (HIV)]. Topical corticosteroid use can also cause recurrence.
- *Id reaction.* Severe fungal infections that are associated with inflammation can lead to an id reaction. The id reaction is a severe inflammatory reaction occurring at a distant site other than the original fungal infection and represents an immunologic reaction to the fungus and the associated severe inflammation. Treating the original fungal site successfully causes the id reaction to dissipate.

Patient Education
Compliance
- Dermatophytosis requires, in some instances, a longer time to treat than the standard 10 days patients are commonly accustomed to with bacterial infections. Sometimes these infections require months to be eradicated. Therefore patients should

be educated about the length of time it takes to correctly treat these infections. Adherence problems can lead to recurrence or inadequate treatment.

- Minimizing or eliminating contact with infected individuals prevents the transmission of these infections.
- Fomites such as hats, protective head gear, and other items that come in contact with the infected hair should be washed in hot water and detergent. Contaminated objects such as combs and brushes should also be cleaned.
- Folds of the skin should be kept as dry as possible. Avoid vigorous rubbing of the skin with a towel; pat dry instead.
- Shower shoes should always be worn while bathing, both at home and in public facilities. Washing the feet with benzoyl peroxide soap directly after the shower is also useful to prevent recurrence.
- Patients should be encouraged to aerate the feet by going barefoot or wearing sandals whenever this is possible. Cotton socks, as well as shoes made from natural materials such as leather or cotton, should be worn instead of synthetic materials that virtually seal in moisture and prevent its drying. Changing socks several times a day also reduces the retention of moisture in the feet.

Lifestyle Changes

Avoiding hot, humid environments such as saunas, indoor pools, and subtropical and tropical climates helps decrease the chances for contracting a dermatophytosis.

ONYCHOMYCOSIS

Onychomycosis is a fungal infection of the fingernail or toenail. A subtype of onychomycosis is tinea unguium, which is caused by the dermatophytes. Dermatophytes cause 90% of onychomycotic infections. The remainder are derived from molds (4%) and from yeasts including *Candida* species (6%).

Chief Complaint

Patients usually report disfigured fingernails or toenails with nail distrophy, discoloration, nail plate thickening, friability of the nails, and subungual hyperkeratotic scale and debris.

Clinical Manifestations

See Table 17.1.

Epidemiology

See Table 17.1.

Risk Factors

See Table 17.1.

PATHOLOGY

Under periodic acid–Schiff (PAS) staining, fungal elements can be seen within the nail.

Diagnosis

The diagnosis of onychomycosis is best made by clinical findings (e.g., hyperkeratotic debris and a friable nail).

Differential Diagnosis

See Table 17.2.

Diagnostic Tests

KOH preparation or a fungal culture may be used to diagnose onychomycosis. The best material to sample is obtained by cutting back the nail or nail bed, or both, to obtain the debris. The same nail scrapings can be sent for fungal culture, which are then placed in Sabouraud medium. Nail clippings may also be sent for histopathologic diagnosis.

Referral

Referral may be indicated if diagnosis is uncertain, which is uncommon, or disease is unresponsive to standard treatment modalities.

Management

- To prevent recurrence, topical antifungal agents [sulconazole (Exelderm), econazole (Spectazole), clotrimazole (Lotrimin), terbinafine (Lamisil), naftifine (Naftin), oxiconazole (Oxistat), ketoconazole (Nizoral), and ciclopirox (Loprox)) can be applied twice daily to the nail and subungual area.
- Antifungal sprays or powders such as undecylenic acid (Desenex), miconazole, and tolnaftate are useful to prevent recurrence and should be applied twice daily.

Medications

See Table 17.3.

Other Treatment Modalities

Nail avulsion. Surgical nail avulsion is indicated if there is pronounced nail dystrophy or onycholysis, especially if just one nail is involved. It is also useful in patients who are taking medications that may interact with systemic antifungal agents, thereby contraindicating their use. Surgical avulsion should begin with a digital nerve block with lidocaine 1% without epinephrine. Once the nail is removed, topical antifungal agents should be applied to the nail bed twice daily.

Follow-up

Patients with onychomycosis do not need close follow-up. KOH preparations or fungal cultures may confirm the eradication of the onychomycosis after the appropriate treatment period.

Patient Education

- Patients should be counseled that treatment will take a long time (2 to 4 months) and that recurrence can occur with any treatment regimen selected. Sometimes, no treatment is better.
- Topical antifungal creams or powders need to be applied daily to the affected nails as a preventive measure.
- Patients should also be warned that onychomycosis caused by dermatophytes can be transmitted by fomites or direct contact with someone who is infected.
- There is no special diet or vitamin proven to be effective in the prevention of onychomycosis.

CANDIDIASIS

Candidiasis of the skin is a superficial infection occurring on moist skin surfaces or mucous membranes. *Candida* species often inhabit the normal flora of the oral cavity, gastrointestinal tract, and vagina without any signs or symptoms of disease. However, candidiasis develops in a setting of lowered host defenses, such as HIV or other immunocompromised states, diabetes, bacterial infection, during use of medications such as antibiotics or corticosteroids, or in cases of skin occlusion.

Chief Complaint

- Patients report a painful, burning, or itching rash that appears in the skin folds of various parts of the body (e.g., axilla, inframammary area, the web spaces between the fingers and toes, and the intergluteal region).
- Uncircumsized male patients may present with a discharge from the foreskin.
- Lesions appear as a diaper rash on infants (Figure 17.6, see color insert following page 170).

Clinical Manifestations

- Candidiasis appears as a red, moist, papular rash that may develop a white exudate. Pruritis, burning, or pain may accompany these lesions (Figure 17.5, see color insert following page 170).
- See Table 17.6 for a comparison of candidal infections by location, offending organism, patient complaints, and clinical manifestations.

Epidemiology

Age

Candidiasis may occur at any age.

Sex

The infections occur equally among male and female patients.

Risk Factors

- Individuals who immerse their hands in water a great deal, such as homemakers, health care workers, bartenders, florists, and individuals who reside in a tropical climate with high heat and humidity are at risk for candidiasis.
- Other risk factors include systemic illnesses such as diabetes, obesity, endocrinopathies, and hyperhidrosis, as well as systemic immunocompromised states (e.g., HIV).
- Long-term use of systemic or topical corticosteroids may lead to the development of candidiasis.
- Tight, occlusive undergarments can also cause candidiasis.
- *Candidiasis* can also be transmitted through sexual contact in both men and women.

PATHOLOGY

Candida albicans is a normal inhabitant of mucosal surfaces such as the oral pharynx and the gastrointestinal tract. However, individuals with altered local or systemic immunity can develop an increase in *C. albicans,* leading to candidiasis.

Candida spores and hyphae are present in the stratum corneum with subcorneal neutrophils noted. PAS or methenamine silver staining best demonstrates the organism.

Diagnosis

Diagnosis is based on history and physical examination and confirmed by direct microscopy or fungal culture.

Differential Diagnosis

See Table 17.7.

Diagnostic Tests

- Direct microscopy using a 10% to 30% KOH preparation is helpful in demonstrating pseudohyphae and spores.
- A fungal culture is also helpful in the identification of *Candida* species.
- In any situation where a secondary bacterial infection is suspected, a bacterial culture is warranted.

Referral

Referral may be indicated if the diagnosis is uncertain or if the rash is unresponsive to the standard treatment modalities.

Management

Management is focused on elimination of the rash through the use of antifungal medications.

Medications

See Table 17.8.

Other Treatment Modalities

- Irritation, inflammation, and pruritus can be relieved with 1% hydrocortisone cream alternated twice per day with antifungal creams. The cream should be applied in a thin layer and worked into the skin thoroughly. Thicker layers of antifungal cream may cause skin maceration.
- Patients who develop candidiasis in intertriginous or interdigital regions because of heavy perspiration can prevent recurrences by using benzoyl peroxide soap or miconazole powder as a prophylactic agent.

Follow-up

Patients should be followed up 1 to 2 weeks after treatment if the rash does not resolve. Recurrent or recalcitrant candidal infections should prompt the physician to consider testing glucose levels or consider HIV testing. If the rash is on the penis, vulva, or vagina and does not dissipate in 4 to 6 weeks, skin cancer should be considered.

Patient Education

- Patients should be counseled on the appropriate treatment and prevention techniques for candidiasis. Often, sexual contact can cause a recurrence of balanitis and vaginitis.
- Avoid constant exposure to water (hand washing). Use absorbent powder daily to reduce moisture. Use benzoyl peroxide soap daily when washing to reduce candidal infection.
- Wearing shoes, socks, and clothing made from natural fibers and avoiding tight, occlusive clothing (e.g., pantyhose), are helpful measures to prevent recurrences.
- Patients should be advised to avoid cornstarch because it can promote recurrences of candidiasis.

TABLE 17.6.   Candidiasis

Location	Organism	Patient complaints		Comments
		History	Clinical manifestations	
Intertriginous	*Candida albicans*	Soreness, burning, and itching. Located in body folds of axilla, web spaces between fingers and toes, inframammary area, scrotum, groin, and intergluteal region. Predisposing factors: hot, humid environments; tight underclothing; diabetes; immunocompromised states (HIV).	Papules/pustules on erythematous base. Can become eroded and confluent with other lesions. Can develop satellite lesions (smaller, red papules/pustules at periphery of main lesion). Can see skin maceration and fissuring with weeping (exudate). Can cause scaling.	KOH preparation from the exudate shows pseudohyphae.
Balanitis	*C. albicans*	Soreness and skin irritation. Discharge from foreskin in uncircumcised men. Predisposing factors: diabetes, sexual exposure with infected partner.	Multiple, discrete, red papules/plaques on the glans penis or inner aspect of foreskin. Lesions can be umbilicated. Can see skin edema, ulcerations, and white exudate. Can also see scaling and skin erosions. White plaques can also be seen on inner aspect of foreskin.	KOH preparation of scraping of exudate shows pseudohyphae. Can be transmitted sexually; treat both partners simultaneously.
Vulva	*C. albicans*	Soreness, burning, and itching. Occasionally, dysuria. Predisposing factors: diabetes; hot, humid environments; tight underclothing; immunosuppressed patients.	Red papules/pustules with erythema and swelling. Can have a whitish vaginal or vulvar discharge. Can see erosions.	KOH preparations of discharge can show pseudohyphae. Can be transmitted sexually; treat both partners simultaneously.

Diaper rash	Secondary infection with *Candida* species.	Irritant dermatitis secondarily infected with *Candida* organisms or, less commonly, staphylococci and streptococci. Irritable child. Crying after urination or defecation.	Red papules with edema. Erosions with wetness and exudate. Marginal scaling. Satellite papules/pustules noted. Lesions can be umbilicated. Can see ulcerations. Usually spares inguinal creases but can spread to lower abdomen and inner thighs.	KOH preparation of exudate can show pseudohyphae.
Paronychia	*C. albicans*	Painful swelling of nail folds. Frequent washing of hands or frequent immersion of hands into water. Predisposing factors: diabetes.	Redness and swelling of nail folds. Swelling can lift nail fold away from nail plate. Pus can be seen from nail fold secondary to bacterial infection (usually staphylococci).	KOH preparation can show pseudohyphae.
Mucosal Oral and vaginal	*C. albicans* most commonly, but other *Candida* species as well.	Vaginal: discharge, pain or soreness, pruritus, burning, dyspareunia; occasionally, dysuria. Can be transmitted sexually. Oral: usually asymptomatic; occasionally, burning and diminished taste; pain on swallowing in esophageal disease. Predisposing factors (oral and vaginal): immunocompromised patients (HIV, cancer), diabetes, antibiotic therapy (vaginal). Systemic or topical corticosteroids, pregnancy, and acquisition from maternal genital tract (neonatal). Oral disease: can occur on dorsum of tongue, buccal mucosa, hard/soft palate, pharynx, and commissures of lips (cheilitis).	In oral lesions: Nonremovable white plaques in mouth When plaques removed, can leave red or bleeding mucosal surface. In cheilitis: Red fissures at corners of mouth. In vaginal lesions: Red vaginal mucosa with white "curdish" discharge. White plaques on vaginal mucosa. Edematous mucosa.	KOH preparation of plaques or discharge can show pseudohyphae. Since vaginal candidiasis can be transmitted sexually, treat both partners simultaneously.

KOH, potassium hydroxide; HIV, human immunodeficiency virus.

T ABLE 17.7.   Differential Diagnosis for Candidiasis

Intertriginous

Psoriasis	Lesions appear as thick, silvery scales with signs of psoriasis elsewhere. KOH preparation result is negative for pseudohyphae.
Erythrasma	Rash is characterized by asymmetric velvet patches with fine scales in the groin and upper thighs. KOH test result is negative, but Wood lamp examination may show coral-red fluorescence.
Seborrheic dermatitis	There is red, scaling plaque with discrete borders or satellite lesions. KOH preparation result is negative.
Dermatophytosis	Tinea cruris, tinea corporis, and tinea pedis infections have well-demarcated borders, no satellite lesions, and do not involve scrotum as does candidiasis. KOH preparation shows hyphae rather than pseudohyphae.

Balanitis

Erythroplasia of Queyrat (in situ squamous cell skin cancer)	Lesions are characterized by velvet, red plaques on penis. KOH preparation result is negative. Biopsy may be helpful in differentiating the two.
Fixed drug eruption	Patient presents with hyperpigmented plaques on penis and has history of the rash recurring when using a particular medication. KOH preparation result is negative.
Contact dermatitis	Lesions are characterized by pruritic vesicles on penis with edematous skin. KOH preparation result is negative.
Psoriasis	There is thick, silvery scale that could resemble the white exudate of candidiasis on penis. KOH preparation result is negative.
Lichen planus	There are red papules/plaques with scales and erosions on penis. KOH preparation result is negative.
Seborrheic dermatitis	The rash is characterized by red, scaling plaques with discrete borders on satellite lesions. KOH preparation result is negative.
Molluscum contagiosum	Lesions are red papules with central umbilication. KOH preparation result is negative.

Vulva

Lichen planus	There are red papules/plaques with scale and erosions with white lacelike patterns on the papules/plaques (Wickham striae). KOH preparation result is negative.

Diaper rash

Seborrheic dermatitis	Lesions are red, scaling plaques involving the inguinal creases. KOH preparation result is negative.
Kawasaki syndrome	Early sign is diffuse erythema of groin. Other signs to look for are fever, lymphadenopathy, and erythema of palms and soles. KOH preparation result is negative.

continued

T ABLE 17.7. *continued.* **Differential Diagnosis for Candidiasis**

Psoriasis	Thick, silvery scale have well-demarcated areas and involve the inguinal creases. Other signs should be looked for elsewhere. KOH preparation result is negative.
Molluscum contagiosum	Lesions are red papules with central umbilication. KOH preparation result is negative.

Paronychia

Tinea unguium	Characterized by friable nail plate with subungual keratin debris. However, it spares the nail folds. KOH preparation result may show hyphae rather than pseudohyphae. Fungal cultures may also be useful in differentiating the two.
Bacterial paronychia	There is an acute infection of nail folds with red pustules and edema. It may also develop into an abscess. Bacterial cultures are positive for *Staphylococcus* species.
Herpetic whitlow	There is a painful, vesicular, red rash of the nail fold with pustules and edema. KOH preparation is negative. Tzanck smear may be positive.

Muscosal
Oral

Oral hairy leukoplakia	Lesions are characterized by white plaques on the lateral tongue margins; cannot be scraped off; sparing the rest of the oral mucosa. KOH preparation is negative.
Lichen planus	There are red papules/plaques with scale and erosions with white lacelike patterns on the papules/plaques (Wickham striae). KOH preparation result is negative.
Leukoplakia	Patient presents with white plaque on buccal mucosa, tongue and hard palate, which cannot be scraped off. KOH preparation result is negative.

Cheilitis

Vitamin B deficiency	Angular cheilitis can be indistinguishable from vitamin B deficiency. KOH preparation result is negative for pseudohyphae.

Vaginitis

Bacterial vaginitis	Patient presents with discharge that is curdlike and not white and can be malodorous. KOH preparation result is negative for pseudohyphae but may have clue cells or bacteria.

KOH, potassium hydroxide.

T ABLE 17.8. **Medical Treatment of Candidiasis**

Castellani paint

Availability:	Over the counter.
Dosage:	Applied to affected areas twice daily.
Duration:	Until rash is resolved.
Area of infection:	Intertriginous, balanitis, paronychia, or vulva.
Comments:	Can stain skin or clothing. A combination of fuschin, resorcin, 3.5% phenol, boric acid, acetone, and isopropyl alcohol, may also be of use.

Clotrimazole 1% vaginal cream, Mycelex-7, Gyne-Lotrimin cream

Availability:	Over the counter.

Mycelex-G, suppository

Availability:	Prescription.
Dosage:	One applicator (5 g) or one suppository intravaginally.
Duration:	7 days.
Area of infection:	Vagina.
Comments:	Minimal side effects.

Clotrimazole troche (adults) (Mycelex, 10mg)

Availability:	Prescription.
Dosage:	Allow troche to dissolve in mouth 5 times daily.
Duration:	14 days.
Area of infection:	Oral mucosal lesions.
Comments:	First-line treatment. No significant side effects.

Fluconazole (Diflucan) (adults)

Availability:	Prescription.
Dosage:	150 mg orally.
Duration:	One time only.
Area of infection:	Oral mucosal lesions. Vagina.
Comments:	See Table 17.5 for side effects.

Nystatin ointment/cream (Mycostatin)

Availability:	Prescription.
Dosage:	Apply to rash twice daily (for diaper rash, apply after each diaper change).
Duration:	14 days.
Area of infection:	Intertriginous, balanitis, or paronychia; vulva, diaper rash, or oral mucosal lesions.
Side effects:	Minimal.
Comments:	First-line treatment.

Oral nystatin suspension (adults or children) or pastille (adults) (Mycostatin)

Availability:	Prescription.
Dosage:	Swish 2 mL 4 times daily, or allow one pastille to dissolve daily.
Duration:	14 days.
Area of infection:	Oral mucosal lesions.
Comments:	First-line treatment. No significant side effects. In frequent recurrences of diaper rash use orally as well for 7 to 10 days to eliminate candidal overgrowth of gastrointestinal tract.

continued

T ABLE 17.8. *continued.* **Medical Treatment of Candidiasis**

Gentian violet

Availability:	Over the counter.
Dosage:	Applied topically 2 to 3 times daily.
Duration:	12 days.
Area of infection:	Vulva.
Comments:	Will stain clothes.

Ketoconazole (adults)

Availability:	Prescription.
Dosage:	200 mg orally daily.
Duration:	1 to 2 weeks.
Area of infection:	Intertriginous, balanitis, paronychia, vulva.
Side effects:	See Table 17.5.
Comments:	For extensive (macerated, exudative) or recurrent infection.
also	
Dosage:	200 mg orally.
Duration of use:	One time only.
Area of infection:	Oral mucosal lesions; cheilitis.
Comments:	See Table 17.5 for side effects and cautions.

Butoconazole nitrate 2% vaginal cream (Femstat)

Availability:	Over the counter.
Dosage:	One applicator (5 g) daily intravaginally.
Duration:	3 days.
Area of infection:	Vagina.
Comments:	Minimal side effects.

Miconazole nitrate 1% vaginal cream (Monistat)
Monistat 3 vaginal suppositories

Availability:	Vaginal cream: Over the counter.
	Suppositories: prescription.
Dosage:	One applicator (5 g) daily intravaginally or 1 suppository daily intravaginally.
Duration of use:	Use cream for 7 days or suppository for 3 days.
Area of infection:	Vagina.
Comments:	Minimal side effects.

Terconazole 0.8% vaginal cream (Terazol 3)

Availability:	Prescription.
Dosage:	One applicator (5 g) daily intravaginally.
Duration of use:	Use for 3 days.
Area of infection:	Vagina.
Comments:	Broad-spectrum agent effective against several *Candida* species.

continued

T ABLE 17.8. *continued.* **Medical Treatment of Candidiasis**

Terconazole 0.4% cream or suppository (Terazol-7)

Availability: Prescription.
Dosage: One applicator (5 g) or one suppository daily intravaginally.
Duration: 7 days.
Area of infection: Vagina.
Comments: Minimal side effects.

Tioconazole 6.5% vaginal cream (Vagistat 1)

Availability: Prescription.
Dosage: One applicator (4.6 g) intravaginally.
Duration: One time only.
Area of infection: Vagina.
Comments: Broad-spectrum agent effective against several *Candida* species. Minimal side effects.

Itraconazole tablets (Sporanox)

Availability: Prescription.
Dosage: 200 mg orally.
Duration of use: One time only.
Area of infection: Vagina.
Comments: See Table 17.5 for side effects and cautions.

Topical anticandidial agents
Clotrimazole 1% cream: Over the counter.
Ciclopirox 1% cream (Loprox): Prescription.
Miconazole nitrate 2% cream: Prescription.
Ketoconazole 2% cream: Prescription.
Oxiconazole 1% cream (Oxistat): Prescription.
Econazole 1% cream (Spectazole): Prescription.

Dosage: Applied topically once or twice daily (for diaper rash, after each change).
Duration: 14 days.
Area of infection: Intertriginous, balanitis, paronychia, vulva, diaper rash and cheilitis.
Side effects: Minimal.
Comments: See Table 17.4 for details on use. First-line treatment.

- For diaper rash, parents should be counseled regarding changing soiled diapers as soon as possible and using mild soap and water or fragrance-free infant wipes, allowing the skin to dry before applying medication, and avoiding the use of rubber or plastic diaper pants that keep moisture in against the skin. Apply moisture barriers to the skin like zinc oxide, A & D, or Desitin ointment. Avoid lanolin-containing products and cornstarch. If using cloth diapers, parents should rinse them in a washing machine half-filled with water and a $^1/_2$ cup of white distilled vinegar added to it for 30 to 45 minutes, then spin dry them as usual. This helps to counteract the alkaline environment, which can be irritating to children's skin.

PITYRIASIS VERSICOLOR

Pityriasis versicolor is a chronic, asymptomatic, scaling, superficial fungal infection caused by *Pityrosporum ovale* (formerly known as *Pityrosporum orbiculare* or *Malassezia furfur*) that commonly occurs on the trunk. This disease was formerly known as tinea versicolor. The opportunistic organism causes an overgrowth when favorable conditions are achieved.

Chief Complaint

Patients report an erythematous or hypopigmented "summertime" rash appearing on the sun-exposed surfaces of the body. Patients may express cosmetic concerns when many hypopigmented or hyperpigmented areas are noticed on the trunk or sun-exposed skin surfaces.

Clinical Manifestations

- Pityriasis versicolor appears as a sharply marginated macule with fine scaling that is apparent when the lesion is gently scraped (Figure 17.6, see color insert following page 170).
- In tanned skin these macules are usually whitish, in untanned skin the macules are usually light brown, and in darker-pigmented individuals the macules tend to be dark brown or off-white.
- Lesions may occasionally become confluent.
- Pityriasis versicolor may involve the upper trunk, upper arms, neck, abdomen, axilla, groin, thigh, and genitalia but is very uncommon on the face.
- The infection is usually asymptomatic but may occasionally cause mild pruritus, and the rash may persist for months to many years.

Epidemiology

Age

Pityriasis versicolor is usually seen in young adults; occurrence tends to decrease in the fifth and sixth decades of life.

Seasonal

In the temperate zones of the United States the rash usually appears in the summer and fades over the cooler months, but for individuals who are physically active and perspire a great deal, the rash may persist year-round.

Regional

- The incidence of the rash is approximately 2% in temperate zones and up to 40% in tropical zones.
- *Pityrosporum* infections are not contagious.

Risk Factors

- Patients with a high production of sebum on the skin are at risk for pityriasis.
- Individuals living in geographic locations that are high in humidity are at risk to develop pityriasis versicolor.
- The application of high-fat tanning preparations, especially those containing cocoa butter, can lead to pityriasis versicolor.
- Topical corticosteroid use or high doses of systemic corticosteroids may also predispose patients to pityriasis.

PATHOLOGY

Hyphae and spores are noted in the stratum corneum with little inflammatory reaction.

Diagnosis

Diagnosis is based on direct microscopic examination of the scales under KOH preparation.

Differential Diagnosis

See Table 17.9.

Diagnostic Tests

- *KOH preparation.* The slide should be prepared with a 15% to 20% KOH solution. For a detailed description on preparing the slide, see Dermatophytosis. The result is positive if hyphae and globular yeast forms are found. This is commonly known as the spaghetti and meatball distribution under the microscope.
- *Wood lamp examination.* Wood lamp examination of pityriasis versicolor may occasionally show blue-green fluorescence of the scales; however, Wood lamp examination may be negative, especially in individuals who have recently showered or who have no scale.
- *Direct biopsy* specimens of the lesions can also show budding yeast and hyphae under PAS stain. Biopsy may be indicated if the rash is unresponsive to treatment or if the KOH preparation result is negative, making the diagnosis uncertain.

TABLE 17.9.   Pityriasis Versicolor: Differential Diagnosis

Vitiligo	Lesions are characterized by hypopigmentation without scaling. KOH preparation result is negative.
Postinflammatory hypopigmentation	There is a history of preceding infection or rash with no scaling. KOH preparation result is negative.
Leprosy	Lesions are characterized by hypopigmented macules/plaques on the face or trunk. KOH preparation result is negative.
Tinea corporis	An erythematous rash than has central clearing and scaling. KOH preparation is positive for hyphae.
Seborrheic dermatitis	Rash is characterized by red, greasy, scaling plaques on the face, scalp, and chest. KOH preparation result is negative.
Pityriasis rosea	There are red papules that have central scaling on the trunk and upper extremities. KOH preparation result is negative.
Psoriasis	Red plaques/papules that have silver scale appearing on the extensor surfaces. There is also evidence of nail pitting. KOH preparation result is negative.
Nummular eczema	Red scaling plaques that are located on the extremities and are quite pruritic. KOH preparation result is negative.

KOH, potassium hydroxide.

Referral

Referral may be indicated if the diagnosis is uncertain or the disease is unresponsive to standard treatment modalities.

Management
Medications

See Table 17.10 and Table 17.11.

T ABLE 17.10.   Medical Treatment of Pityriasis Versicolor

Selenium sulfide 2.5% lotion [Selsun (prescription); not Selsun Blue (OTC), which is only 1% selenium]
Dosage:	Apply daily to affected areas, leave on for 10 to 15 minutes and rinse.
Duration of use:	Continue for 7 days.
Side effects:	Minimal.
Comments:	First-line therapy.

Oral antifungal agents
Ketoconazole (Nizoral)
Availability:	Prescription.
Administration:	400 mg orally initially, repeat in 7 days or 200 mg daily for 7 to 10 days.
Comments:	For use in extensive (larger area) or recalcitrant disease. See Table 17.5 for side effects.

Fluconazole (Diflucan)
Availability:	Prescription.
Administration:	400 mg orally daily.
Duration:	3 days.
Comments:	For use in extensive or recalcitrant disease. See Table 17.5 for side effects.

Itraconazole (Sporanox)
Availability:	Prescription.
Administration:	200 mg orally daily.
Duration:	7 days.
Side effects:	See Table 17.5 for side effects.
Comments:	For use in extensive or recalcitrant disease.

Topical anticandidial agents
Clotrimazole 1% cream (Lotrimin): OTC.
Ciclopirox 1% cream (Loprox): Prescription.
Miconazole nitrate 2% cream (Monistat): Prescription.
Ketoconazole 2% cream (Nizoral): Prescription.
Oxiconazole 1% cream (Oxistat): Prescription.
Econazole 1% cream (Spectazole): Prescription.
Sulconazole nitrate 1% cream, solution (Exelderm): Prescription.
Dosage:	Applied topically once or twice daily.
Duration:	14 days.
Side effects:	Minimal side effects.
Comments:	First-line treatment for limited disease (isolated lesions).

OTC, over the counter.

T ABLE 17.11. Medical Prevention of Pityriasis Versicolor

Ketoconazole shampoo (Nizoral) 2%

Availability:	Prescription.
Dosage:	Applied to affected areas once or twice weekly; leave on overnight.
Duration:	Use during warm, humid months.

Selenium sulfide 2.5% lotion (Selsun)

Availability:	Prescription.
Dosage:	Apply to affected areas monthly; leave on overnight.
Duration of use:	Use during warm, humid months.

Pyrithione zinc shampoo

Availability:	Over the counter.
Administration:	Applied to affected areas monthly; leave on overnight.
Duration of use:	Use during warm, humid months.

Follow-up

Close follow-up is not necessary; however, patients should be counseled to return for follow-up if the rash does not resolve within 1 month.

Patient Education

- Patients may be reassured that pityriasis versicolor is not contagious and that the yeast causing this rash resides only in the superficial layers of the skin and will leave no scarring after the rash has resolved.
- They should also be advised to avoid the use of tanning oils that may promote the growth of the yeast.
- Skin with the rash of pityriasis versicolor does not tan because of the yeast's ability to block out the sun's effect on the melanocytes. This results in a stark difference between the two areas, making them cosmetically unpleasant. Patients should be reminded that the hypopigmented areas will take several months to resolve after the infection is treated. In the meantime, there are skin-tanning agents and cosmetic cover-ups available to make the hypopigmented rash look more like the surrounding skin.

BIBLIOGRAPHY

Bergus GR, Johnson JS. Superficial tinea infections. *Am Fam Physician* 1993;48(2): 259-268.

Brodell RT, Elewski BE. Clinical pearl: systemic antifungal drugs and drug interactions. *J Am Acad Dermatol* 1995;33:259-260.

Brodell RT, Hels SE, Snelson ME. Office dermatologic testing: the KOH preparation. *Am Fam Physician* 1991;43(2):2061-2065.

De Doncker P, Decroix J, Pierard GE, et al. Antifungal pulse therapy for onychomycosis. *Arch Dermatol* 1996;132:34-41.

Gupta AK, Sauder DN, Shear NH. Antifungal agents: an overview. Part II. *J Am Acad Dermatol* 1994;30(6):9211-9233.

Radentz WH. Fungal skin infections associated with animal contact. *Am Fam Physician* 1991;43(4):1253-1256.

Roberts DT. Oral therapeutic agents in fungal nail disease. *J Am Acad Dermatol* 1994; 31(3, pt 2):S78-S81.

Savin R. Diagnosis and treatment of tinea versicolor. *J Fam Pract* 1996;43(2):127-132.

Sires UI, Mallory SB. Diaper dermatitis: how to treat and prevent. *Postgrad Med* 1995; 98(6):79-86.

Tobin MJ. Vulvovaginal candidiases: topical vs. oral therapy. *Am Fam Physician* 1995; 51(7):1715-1720.

Topical butenafine for tinea pedis. *Med Lett* 1997;39(1004):63-64.

Zaias N, Glick B, Rebell G. Diagnosing and treating onchomycosis. *J Fam Pract* 1996; 42(5):513-518.

CHAPTER 18

Viral Infections Affecting the Skin

VIRAL EXANTHEMS

The rashes precipitated by viruses, including rubella, measles, adenovirus, echovirus, roseola, infectious mononucleosis, and erythema infectiosum, all appear similar, and only a small difference in physical findings and history may be noted to make a diagnosis (Table 18.1). Since there are no special treatments for these viruses, their management and follow-up would be better addressed by an infectious disease textbook. Rubella, measles, and erythema infectiosum all require special treatment and follow-up for exposed pregnant women, which is also beyond the scope of this book.

HUMAN PAPILLOMAVIRUS

Human papillomavirus (HPV) is a double-stranded DNA virus that has more than 65 numbered types. Each number is associated with a particular clinical presentation (Table 18.2). The four most common presentations of HPV are common, plantar, flat-type, and genital warts.

Chief Complaint

Patients report common external warts in the genital region or elsewhere. Female patients may have an abnormal Pap smear.

Clinical Manifestations

- HPV lesions can be placed into one of five categories: common, plantar, filiform, flat-type, or genital warts.
- The incubation period for warts is 2 to 6 months, and warts may persist for years if left untreated.
- Warts can occur singly or in clusters.
- The lesions may be located on face, hands, nose, eyelids, soles, palms, and genital tract.
- If found on the face or hands, warts can be cosmetically disfiguring.
- Warts also obscure normal skin lines.
- Although usually asymptomatic, some warts (e.g., plantar warts) can be painful (Figure 18.1, see color insert following page 170).
- Mucosal and genital lesions are contagious both nonsexually and sexually, but the most common mode of transmission is through sexual contact.
- The lesions can develop secondary bacterial infection.
- See Table 18.2 for physical characteristics of each wart.

Epidemiology

Age

- Occurrences peak in the third decade of life, but warts can occur at any age.
- Common warts are most prevalent in children and young adults.

TABLE 18.1. Common Viral Exanthems

Virus	Disease	Clinical presentation	Comments
Adenovirus	—	Occurs under age 20. Incubation period under 3 weeks. Prodrome with fever, malaise, coryza, sore throat, nausea, vomiting, diarrhea, abdominal pain, and headache. Red macular/papular rash centrally located (i.e., head, trunk, neck, proximal extremities). Rash resolves in 10 days.	Supportive treatment with antipyretics and hydration.
Coxsackieviruses A and B	Hand-foot-mouth disease	See Chapter 18 for full details.	—
Echovirus	—	Incubation of 3 to 7 days. Sudden onset of fever, pharyngitis, gastroenteritis, cervical adenopathy, and myalgia. Red, macular rash that begins on the face and spreads to trunk and limbs lasting 2 to 7 days.	Supportive treatment with antipyretics and hydration.
Herpesviruses 6 and 7	Roseola	3 to 5 days of high fever greater than or equal to 40°C accompanied by mild constitutional symptoms. Discrete, 2-5-mm pink/rose macules and papules occurring on the trunk and neck, appearing right after defervescence. Rash disappears in 1 to 3 days. Occurs in children under 3 years of age.	No specific treatment. Use antipyretics to reduce fever, since 10% of patients can develop febrile seizures.
Epstein-Barr virus (herpesvirus)	Infectious mononucleosis	Begins with fever, exudative tonsillitis/pharyngitis, fatigue, posterior cervical adenopathy, and occasionally, hepatosplenomegaly. Rarely see rash unless patient given amoxicillin or ampicillin. Diagnosis confirmed by complete blood cell count and serology tests. Illness can last 30 to 60 days.	Supportive treatment. Avoid contact sports and physical education until well, because of hepatosplenomegaly (avoid rupture).

continued

T ABLE 18.1. *continued.* **Common Viral Exanthems**

Virus	Disease	Clinical presentation	Comments
Paramyxovirus	Measles (rubeola)	Highly contagious illness. Incubation period of 9 to 14 days. Prodromal symptoms include cough, coryza, conjunctivitis, photophobia, and fever for 2 to 4 days. Can get blue/gray papules of 1 to 3 mm on buccal mucosa, called Koplik spots. Rash starts on the head and spreads downward. Red macular rash lasting 3 to 6 days, no pruritus. Can cause otitis media, pneumonia, or encephalitis as complications.	Symptomatic treatment including antipyretics and hydration. Prevention with live vaccine is important.
Parvovirus B19	Erythema infectiosum (Fifth disease)	Moderately contagious affecting children 3 to 12 years of age. 2-week incubation period. Sudden appearance of red macular rash on cheeks, appearing as a "slapped cheek." Rash fades in several days as another rash begins on exterior surfaces of the proximal extremities appearing lacelike or reticulated. This rash can last 1 to 14 days. Usually asymptomatic. Not contagious after onset of rash.	No specific treatment is necessary. Pregnant women need to avoid children with this disease, since it can cause hydrops fetalis.
Togavirus	Rubella	Most infections (80%) are subclinical. Incubation period of 14 to 21 days. Prodromal stage of mild upper respiratory tract and constitutional symptoms. Rash seen as pink macules and papules beginning on the face, then progressing to the trunk and lower extremities. Rash usually disappears by third day. Tender retroauricular and suboccipital adenopathy.	Supportive treatment. Prevention with live vaccine is important. Can cause problems with pregnancy: congenital rubella syndrome.

T ABLE 18.2.   Types of Human Papillomavirus

Type	Presentation	Physical examination
1, 2, 4, 26–29	Common warts	Fleshy papules 1 to 10 mm in size, hyperkeratotic, may be skin-colored or pink and may appear anywhere.
1, 4, 63	Plantar warts	Translucent, tender, yellow, round nodules that may progress to having a hyperkeratotic plaque. Predilection for sole of foot.
2, 3, 10, 26–29, 41	Flat warts	Flat, pink papules with sharp borders, minimal hyperkeratosis; these typically appear on dorsum of hand.
2, 3, 10, 26–29, 41	Filiform warts	Multiple wart projections on a narrow stalk situated on a pedunculated papule typically appearing on the face (nares, eyelids, and lips) or mucous membranes.
6, 11, 30, 43, 44, 55	Genital warts (not associated with dysplasia)	Varies from fleshy papules that coalesce to flat, tan, erythematous plaques occurring in genital tract of either sex.
16, 18, 31, 32, 33, 35, 39, 42, 51–54	Cancer-associated genital warts	Flesh-colored papules, plaques, or nodules occurring in the anogenital region, vulva, vagina, penis, or cervix.

Sex
Warts occur in equal proportions among male and female patients.

Risk Factors
- Risk factors include atopic dermatitis, immunosuppression [acquired immunodeficiency syndrome (AIDS)], or meat handlers.
- Some warts are inherited (autosomal recessive).
- Oral warts are associated with oral genital sex.
- Warts are usually spread by skin-to-skin contact.

PATHOLOGY
HPV usually enters through a break in the skin with viral replication occurring in the upper levels of the epithelium. See Koilocytosis and foci of keratohyaline granules in cells.

Diagnosis
Diagnosis of warts is based on physical examination and history.

Differential Diagnosis
See Table 18.3.

Diagnostic Tests
- A *Pap smear* is indicated for female patients with genital warts. If the Pap smear is abnormal or if examination of the cervix reveals an obvious lesion, colposcopy should be performed.

T ABLE 18.3.   Human Papillomavirus: Differential Diagnosis

Genital warts

Condyloma lata	Flesh-colored papules caused by secondary syphilis located in genital region. VDRL test result is positive.
Molloscum contagiosum	Pearly papules with umbilicated center; should be able to differentiate based on clinical appearance.
Squamous cell carcinoma	Can present as genital ulcer or erosion, or appear as a wart in anogenital region. Biopsy is needed to differentiate the two.

Common and flat warts

Lichen planus	Flat papules of lichen planus can be indistinguishable from flat warts, but usually have symmetric distribution and Wickham striae.
Seborrheic keratosis	Stuck-on appearance with an occasional horny cyst on surface; usually pigmented in contrast to flesh-colored or yellow pigment of wart.
Squamous cell carcinoma	Can present as an ulcer or an irregular growth refractory to wart therapy. Biopsy is needed to differentiate the two.

VDRL, Venereal Disease Research Laboratory.

- Cutting a common or flat-type wart with a No. 15 scalpel blade exposes thrombosed capillaries (appearing as black dots) or "seeds," thereby confirming the diagnosis. A wart bleeds more profusely than other types of lesions when incised.
- *Acetic acid test.* A 5% acetic acid solution (white vinegar) is painted on the penis, labia, or perianal area, causing metaplastic or dysplastic squamous epithelium to opacify. Causes of parakeratosis, such as HPV, psoriasis, lichen planus, and candidiasis, become white when painted by acetic acid, thus indicating the area to be treated. Sexual partners of women with abnormal Pap smears should be examined. Well-circumscribed papular or macular lesions are observed.
- *Screening for GC (gonorrhea or gonococcus), Chlamydia organisms, hepatitis,* and *human immunodeficiency virus (HIV)* should be performed, since patients with genital warts are also at risk for other sexually transmitted diseases.
- *Virus typing.* Tests for typing the virus present in genital warts will soon be available for use. These tests will facilitate aggressive treatment of cancer-associated types 16, 18, 31, 32, 33, 35, 39, 42, and 51–54.

Referral
Referral is usually unnecessary.

Management
- Over-the-counter preparations with salicylic acid and lactic acid are appropriate initially for the treatment of warts (*not* genital warts) for several months.
- If untreated, 20% to 30% of genital warts resolve within 3 months. However, the possibility of contagion and the association of many of these virus types with cancer make treatment essential.

Medications
See Table 18.4.

T ABLE 18.4.   Medical Treatment of Human Papillomavirus

Common or flat-type warts
Salicylic acid 17%
Availability: Over the counter.
Dosage: Applied topically to wart daily.
Duration: Until wart disappears.
Comments: Treatment is useful for common, flat, plantar and palmar warts and for
                      multiple warts; can cause burning, erosion, pain, or inflammation.

Salicylic acid 40% plaster (Mediplast, Sal-Acid plaster, Duofilm plaster)
Availability: Prescription.
Dosage: Cut a section of the sheet to cover the wart only; sticky surface adheres firmly,
                      but may be occluded with tape. Remove after 48 to 72 hours. Pare away
                      dead skin with a scalpel between treatments.
Duration: Weekly until wart disappears.
Comments: Treatment of choice for single plantar warts. Burning, erosion, pain,
                      or inflammation can occur.

5-Fluorouracil 5% cream (Efudex)
Availability: Prescription.
Dosage: Applied topically to warts twice daily.
Duration: 3 to 5 weeks.
Comments: Treatment is useful for multiple, flat warts. Use sunblock to avoid photosensitivity.
                      Medication can cause burning, pain, ulcerations, blistering, pruritus, and
                      allergic contact dermatitis.

Tretinoin .05% or 0.1% cream (Retin-A)
Availability: Prescription.
Dosage: Applied topically to warts once or twice daily.
Duration: 2 to 3 weeks.
Comments: Treatment is useful for multiple, flat warts. For best results, use highest concentration
                      tolerated. Use sunblock to avoid photosensitivity. Tretinoin can cause erythema,
                      dryness, burning, and tingling of skin.

Genital warts
Podofilox 0.5% (Condylox)
Availability: Prescription.
Dosage: Applied topically twice daily to affected areas for 3 days followed by no treatment
                      for 4 days, then repeat the cycle for 4 weeks. In other words, treat for 3 days,
                      then off for 4 days, then treat for 3 days, off for next 4 days, etc.
Duration: Treatment cycle up to 4 weeks, or stop when no wart is visible.
Comments: Patients may apply this medication—after the proper method is demonstrated by
                      physician—as long as the total area of the wart does not exceed 10 cm^2 or involve
                      using more than 0.5 mL of solution per day. Burning, pain, inflammation,
                      pruritus, and skin erosion may occur. *Do not use* during pregnancy.

continued

T ABLE 18.4. *continued.* **Medical Treatment of Human Papillomavirus**

Podophyllin resin 10% to 25% (mixed with tincture of benzoin to help the resin adhere to the wart)

Availability:	Prescription.
Dosage:	Physician should apply once per week. Burning or pain can occur in 1 to 4 hours; the resin should be washed off at first signs of pain, or 4 hours after application. The strength used should be individualized to the patient.
Duration:	6 weeks.
Comments:	Treatment is for use on areas smaller than 10 cm^2; do not use more than 0.5 mL of this solution. Be sure the solution dries, to avoid contact with normal skin. Burning, inflammation, pain, pruritus, and skin erosion can occur. *Do not use* during pregnancy.

Trichloroacetic acid 80% to 90%

Availability:	Prescription.
Dosage:	Physician should apply weekly.
Duration:	Up to 6 weeks; change treatments if unresponsive.
Comments:	Burning, pain, inflammation, pruritus, skin erosion, and scarring can occur.

Imiquimod 5% cream (Aldara)

Availability:	Prescription.
Dosage:	Patient may apply 3 times per week before sleep; leave on for 6 to 10 hours, then wash thoroughly with mild soap and water.
Duration:	Continue until the warts are completely gone, but do not exceed 16 weeks.
Comments:	Imiquimod is an immune-response modifier. Erythema, erosion, excoriation, edema, pruritus, burning, and pain can occur.

Other Treatment Modalities

Secondary bacterial infections are rarely a problem; however, patients may be advised to be observant of possible signs of infection.

Physical and environmental

- *Common and flat-type warts*
  Cryosurgery (see Appendix B). After scraping off the outermost keratotic layer of skin of the wart, apply liquid nitrogen, using a cotton-tipped applicator to freeze the wart and a 1- to 2-mm ring of surrounding normal tissue. Repeat freeze may be performed if needed every 1 to 4 weeks until warts resolve. Scarring is minimal. This is first-line therapy for common and isolated flat-type warts.
- *Resistant warts*
  Electrosurgery (see Appendix B). After induction of local anesthesia, electrocautery removes the wart. Scarring is a risk of this treatment. This treatment is best for large warts or cases in which application of topical medication would exceed dosage restrictions, other treatments would take many weeks, or repeated cryotherapy procedures would be required before the wart regressed.
  CO$_2$ laser surgery. This is the recommended treatment for recalcitrant warts. This procedure should be performed by a physician who is experienced in this type of surgery.

- *Filiform warts.* Filiform warts may be removed by snip excision (see Appendix B).
- *Genital warts.* Genital warts may be removed by cryotherapy if topical treatment fails or if the patient is pregnant. Electrosurgery may also be performed in some cases. Interferon may be indicated for some patients with genital warts. Both procedures should be performed by a physician trained in their use.

Psychological

- *Common and flat-type warts.* The stigma associated with warts is tremendous, particularly to children and teenagers, who find these lesions very upsetting. Psychological support for these patients may ease the stress inherent in this cosmetically disfiguring disease. Some warts can spontaneously regress after the patient undergoes hypnotic suggestion.
- *Genital warts.* Patients may require psychological support to ease the stress resulting from a diagnosis of a sexually transmitted disease.

Follow-up

- Common and flat-type warts may be self-monitored by the patient, who should be advised to return for follow-up if nonprescription treatments prove ineffective.
- Genital warts should be followed closely every 3 to 4 months; if any suspect change is noted, a biopsy specimen should be taken.
- Annual Pap smears are strongly advised for women with genital warts and in female partners of men with genital warts, unless colposcopy dictates otherwise. Men should be followed up if penile warts are not receding following treatment.

Patient Education

Common and Flat-Type Warts

- Compliance is normally not a problem with these patients because most individuals find warts to be bothersome and cosmetically unattractive.
- They should be advised that warts can be transmitted to another person through skin-to-skin contact; usually the virus is transmitted to a site of recent trauma or broken skin.
- For simple, single warts there are many good over-the-counter medications containing salicylic acid that patients can use themselves to remove warts.
- Patients may be reassured that the viruses that cause common, flat-type, filiform, and plantar warts do not cause cancer.
- To prevent further occurrences, patients may be advised to avoid coming in contact with the HPV virus by wearing sandals or shower slippers when walking in hot, humid environments.

Genital Warts

- Patients should be informed that virus types 16, 18, 31, 32, 33, 35, 39, 42, and 51-54 are cancer associated, making treatment for these warts essential.
- In addition, they should understand that these warts are contagious and the use of condoms is strongly advised during sexual intercourse for protection from this virus that can go unrecognized.
- Patients should be informed that treating the visible signs of the infection does not ensure that the virus has been totally eradicated; therefore recurrences are possible.
- Genital warts caused by certain virus types can lead to genital tract cancer. Female patients with genital warts and partners of male patients with genital warts should be advised to have an annual Pap smear and genital examination. For any penile,

vaginal, or vulva lesions that are treated as genital warts and do not respond in several weeks biopsy should be performed to rule out malignancy.

- The virus causing genital warts can be transmitted by the delivery process to the newborn infant. The virus may be dormant in the infant until skin conditions become right for clinical manifestation.
- In some cases patients may be able to apply medication on genital warts themselves, once they have received the physician's instruction on correct application. It should be stressed, however, that the instructions must be followed closely because these medicines can cause painful side effects.

HAND-FOOT-AND-MOUTH DISEASE

Hand-foot-and-mouth disease is a systemic infection characterized by ulcerative oral lesions and a vesicular rash on the distal extremities.

Chief Complaint

Patients report a blisterlike rash, most commonly beginning in the mouth, along with lesions on the hands and feet.

Clinical Manifestations

- The incubation period for hand-foot-and-mouth disease is 3 to 6 days, with a 12- to 24-hour prodrome that includes low-grade fever, malaise, abdominal pain, or respiratory tract symptoms such as cough. Following the prodrome, 5 to 10 painful, ulcerative oral lesions can appear, which may prevent some children from eating (Figure 18.2, see color insert following page 170).
- In some patients high fever, diarrhea, joint pain, and severe malaise may be apparent.
- Shortly after the appearance of the oral lesions, as many as 100 cutaneous lesions may appear on the distal extremities. These cutaneous lesions can be asymptomatic or painful and usually heal without scarring.
- Lesions can be seen on the palms and soles and on the sides of fingers and toes and are usually 2- to 8-mm papules or macules that quickly evolve to vesicles.
- The papules can be pink to red, with a characteristic dark red ring around the edge.
- Vesicles usually have clear fluid inside, and those located on the palms and soles do not rupture.
- The mucosal lesions are 5- to 10-mm, punched-out ulcerations that are preceded by macules, leading to grayish vesicles. They are usually distributed on the hard palate, tongue, or buccal mucosa.
- Cervical and submandibular lymphadenopathy may also be present.

Epidemiology

- The *etiologic agent* is usually coxsackievirus A16 or enterovirus 71. Other types of coxsackievirus have been implicated, including A4–A7, A9, A10, B2, and B5.
- Hand-foot-and-mouth disease is *highly contagious* and is spread by oral-to-oral and fecal-to-oral transmission.

Age

Hand-foot-and-mouth disease usually occurs in children under 10 years of age, but may sometimes occur in young and middle-aged adults.

Sex

Hand-foot-and-mouth disease occurs in equal proportions among male and female patients.

Seasonal

Epidemic outbreaks occur about every 3 years. In temperate zones these outbreaks usually occur during the warmer months of May to August and into the autumn months.

Risk Factors

Epidemics can occur in day care centers or among family members.

PATHOLOGY

Biopsy specimens reveal epidermal reticular degeneration with intraepidermal vesicles filled with neutrophils and mononuclear cells. The dermis reveals a perivascular mixed-cell infiltrate.

Diagnosis

Diagnosis is based on history and physical examination. Diagnostic testing is unnecessary.

Differential Diagnosis

- See Table 18.5.
- Other illnesses that occur predominately on the palms and soles are Kawasaki disease, syphilis, and Rocky Mountain spotted fever. However, these diseases usually have more severe constitutional symptoms and may involve older individuals. Venereal Disease Research Laboratory or antibody tests for *Rickettsia rickettsii* can be useful to differentiate.

Diagnostic Tests

- For cases in which the diagnosis is in doubt, histopathologic determination of the lesions from a *biopsy specimen* or an *acute and convalescent viral titer* may be performed.
- *Tzanck preparation* may be useful to rule out varicella zoster virus or herpesvirus, which have multinucleated giant cells.

Referral

Referral is rarely indicated unless the diagnosis is uncertain or the patient does not show improvement within 7 to 10 days. If this is the case, the patient should be referred to a pediatrician or pediatric infectious disease specialist.

T ABLE 18.5. Hand-Foot-Mouth Disease: Differential Diagnosis

Varicella	Widespread lesions beginning on trunk with the rash lasting longer than the hand-foot-mouth rash.
Herpes simplex	Oral or genital lesions only; history and age of the patient differentiate the two.
Aphthous stomatitis	Spares the hard palate, and there are no palmar or plantar lesions.
Herpangina	Limited to the back of throat, soft palate, tonsils, and uvula. There are no lesions on extremities.
Erythema multiforme	Target lesions darkened with halo of pallor, and there are no oral lesions.

Management

- Because hand-foot-and-mouth disease is self-limited, no antiviral or systemic medication is required.
- In rare instances prolonged or recurrent cases have been reported.

Medications

See Table 18.6.

Other Treatment Modalities

Because the oral lesions make eating and drinking painful, dehydration may occur. It is important to maintain adequate fluid intake in these patients. Ice cubes or popsicles may be easier for patients to tolerate, and the cold may help to dull the pain of the lesions.

Follow-up

Monitoring Disease Course

Patients should be followed up 2 to 3 days after the initial diagnosis, observing for signs of dehydration.

Potential Problems and Complications

Sequelae rarely occur in hand-foot-and-mouth disease; however, reports have been published of myocarditis, meningioencephalitis, and aseptic meningitis developing. Parents should be advised to look for any problems that may arise, including high fever or central nervous system disturbances.

T ABLE 18.6.   Medical Treatment of Hand-Foot-Mouth Disease

Acetaminophen

Availability:	Over the counter.
Dosage:	*Children:* 10 to 15 mg/kg every 4 hours.
Duration:	Until symptoms resolve.
Comments:	Use to reduce pain and fever of the disease.

Ibuprofen

Availability:	Over the counter.
Dosage:	*Children:* 5 to 10 mg/kg every 6 to 8 hours.
Duration:	Until symptoms resolve.
Comments:	Use to reduce pain and fever of the disease.

Topical dyclonine hydrochloride or viscous lidocaine 2% or carafate suspension

Availability:	Prescription and over the counter.
Dosage:	Rinse mouth and expectorate before eating or drinking.
Duration:	Until symptoms resolve.
Comments:	May reduce discomfort of painful oral lesions. *Do not* swallow, because of potential paralysis of the gag reflex (viscous lidocaine).

Patient Education

- Parents should be advised that children with hand-foot-and-mouth disease must be watched closely to avoid dehydration and nutritional compromise.
- Patients should be informed that this is a highly contagious illness transmitted by oral-to-oral or fecal-to-oral routes. Children who have this virus should be removed from school or daycare.
- When the lesions crust over and no longer weep, patients are no longer contagious; children may then return to school or daycare.

MOLLUSCUM CONTAGIOSUM

Molluscum contagiosum is a self-limited viral infection causing umbilicated papules; this disease occurs mainly in children and sexually active adults.

Chief Complaint

Patients report small, circular growths on skin, usually in clumps, with waxy material in the center of the papule.

Clinical Manifestations

- Molluscum contagiosum is an asymptomatic skin infection that can be pruritic if the rash develops a secondary bacterial infection (Figure 18.3, see color insert following page 170).
- Lesions usually occur on the face, eyelids, trunk, axilla, and anogenital region; however, the mucous membranes are spared.
- Lesions are typically 1- to 2-mm papules or 5- to 10-mm nodules, usually round or oval, and there may be a single lesion or multiple, scattered lesions.
- There is a central keratotic plug in the papule or nodule, giving it an umbilication.
- General pressure on the nodule or papule can cause the central plug to be expressed.
- Initially the lesions are pearly white. In darker-pigmented individuals, hyperpigmentation may follow treatment or spontaneous regression.
- Some lesions have a red halo, particularly when regressing.
- Secondary bacterial infection or abscess may sometimes be observed.
- The rash can persist up to 6 months, but usually regresses spontaneously except in patients with HIV, who require treatment.
- In HIV-infected patients, the lesions can be very widespread, numbering from hundreds to thousands and most often occurring on the face, where shaving causes the lesions to spread. The lesions may also be larger, sometimes up to 1.5 cm. Severe infections in patients with HIV may signal advanced immunodeficiency.

Epidemiology

- The cause or origin is the molluscum contagiosum virus (MCV), a pox virus, of which there are two clinically indistinguishable types. Neither have been cultured.
- Molluscum contagiosum is usually transmitted via skin-to-skin contact with an infected person.

Age

The virus is usually seen in children and sexually active adults.

Sex

The infection occurs more often among male than among female patients.

Risk Factors

Sexual contact with an infected individual is a risk factor.

PATHOLOGY

Epidermis contains intracytoplasmic inclusion bodies (molluscum bodies).

Diagnosis

Diagnosis of molluscum contagiosum is usually based on clinical examination.

Differential Diagnosis

See Table 18.7.

Diagnostic Tests

Histopathologic examination of biopsy specimens may be indicated if the diagnosis is uncertain.

Referral

Referral may be indicated for patients whose diagnosis is uncertain or in cases that are unresponsive to treatment.

Management

Molluscum contagiosum usually regresses spontaneously within 6 months except in patients with HIV.

Medications

See Table 18.8.

Other Treatment Modalities

- Some patients may prefer to have the lesions removed via *curettage or cryosurgery* rather than waiting for spontaneous regression.
- *Curettage* with a small curette may be performed to remove the central keratinous plug in molluscum contagiosum, thereby causing the lesion to regress.
- *Cryosurgery* may also be used to freeze the lesions for 10 to 15 seconds, followed by removal via curettage.
- Either of the above is first-line therapy.

T ABLE 18.7.   Molluscum Contagiosum: Differential Diagnosis

Simple flat warts	There is no keratotic plug or central umbilication.
Condyloma accumulata	Lesions have a rough surface and are wart-like with sharp borders.
Keratoacanthoma	Darker pigmentation is sometimes indistinguishable from molluscum. Biopsy may be necessary to differentiate the two.
Squamous cell carcinoma	Darker pigmentation is sometimes indistinguishable from molluscum. Biopsy may be necessary to differentiate the two.

TABLE 18.8. Medical Treatment of Molluscum Contagiosum

Cantharidin 0.7% (Canthacur)

Availability:	Prescription.
Dosage:	Apply single drop to each lesion.
Duration:	Blister will form in 1 day, and the lesion usually sloughs off; repeat every 2 to 3 weeks until lesions resolve.
Comments:	Cantharidin is the first-line treatment in children. Follow up in 2 to 6 weeks to see if new lesions have developed. Skin may have to be anesthestized with lidocaine 2.5% and prilocaine 2.5% (EMLA cream) approximately 1 hour before treatment. Do not apply near eyes or mucous membranes.

Retinoic acid .05% (Retin-A)

Availability:	Prescription.
Dosage:	Apply topically at bedtime.
Duration:	Until erythematous response occurs.
Comments:	Follow up in 2 to 6 weeks to see if new lesions have developed. Do not apply near eyes or mucous membranes. Burning, stinging, or erythema may occur.

Trichloroacetic acid 25% to 50% (Tri-Verzone)

Availability:	Prescription.
Dosage:	Apply topically daily.
Duration:	Until erythematous response occurs.
Comments:	Follow up in 2 to 6 weeks to see if new lesions have developed. Do not apply near eyes or mucous membranes.

Salicylic acid 17%

Availability:	Over the counter.
Dosage:	Applied topically at bedtime.
Duration:	Until irritation occurs and lesions peel off.
Comments:	Follow up in 2 to 6 weeks to see if new lesions have developed; can cause burning, erosion, pain, or inflammation.

- Patients who are unresponsive to cryosurgery or curretage may be treated with electrocautery. EMLA cream (lidocaine 2.5% and prilocaine 2.5%) is applied topically to each lesion at a dose of 2.5 g of cream over 20 to 25 cm^2 of skin 1 hour before the procedure. In larger lesions a local infiltration of 1% lidocaine may be used. The lesions may then be cauterized and curetted to remove the bulk of the lesion.

Follow-up

- Close follow-up is unnecessary in most patients, since this rash regresses spontaneously.
- Molluscum contagiosum in patients with HIV progresses rapidly. Aggressive treatment is necessary to prevent the number of disfiguring lesions.

Patient Education

- The lesions usually spontaneously regress in approximately 6 months, but patients with HIV do not have spontaneous regression.
- Patients with HIV should be advised to shave sparingly or to grow a beard to prevent the spread of this infection.
- Small children should be isolated from other children until these lesions disappear.
- Cases of molluscum contagiosum should not prompt patients to be tested for HIV. However, patients with hundreds of lesions or lesions that do not regress after being treated should be counseled about HIV testing.
- Patients may be reassured that molluscum contagiosum causes minimal scarring.
- Lesions may become more erythematous (inflamed) during regression. They may then resemble staphylococcal disease but are not necessarily infected. Patients should be advised of the difference between normal inflammation and possible infection.
- The rash can be transmitted sexually; sexual partners should be examined and treated, if necessary.
- Patients should be advised to prevent further occurrences of molluscum contagiosum by avoiding skin-to-skin contact with individuals who already have the virus. No transmission has been noted when patients come into contact with towels or other linens that have been exposed to these lesions.

KAWASAKI DISEASE

Kawasaki disease, also called mucocutaneous lymph node syndrome, is an acute febrile illness of infants and children.

Chief Complaint

Parents report prolonged fever, painful swelling of the extremities, red eyes, and rash in infants and children.

Clinical Manifestations

- Kawasaki disease does not have a prodrome (Figure 18.4, see color insert following page 170).
- The disease initially manifests with a sudden onset of fever and constitutional symptoms consisting of diarrhea, joint pains, arthritis, ear pain, and photophobia.

Phases of Kawasaki Disease

Phase 1

- Phase 1 is characterized by erythema that is noted on the palms and soles spreading to the trunk and extremities 2 days later.
- Lesions usually appear 1 to 3 days after the onset of fever and last for approximately 12 days.
- Initial lesions are red macules that become larger and more numerous.
- The most commonly seen macules are urticaria-like. The second most common macule is of the morbiliform type. The scarlatiniform and erythema multiforme–like macules are seen in less than 5% of patients.
- Macules on the perineum coalesce to form plaques. These plaques persist after the other skin findings resolve.
- There is a great deal of edema on the hands and feet, at first, erythematous, but turning into a violaceous color.
- Skin lesions are tender to palpation.

- Mucous membranes, including bulbar conjunctivitis and conjunctival injection, are also involved. This involvement occurs 2 days after the onset of fever and lasts approximately 1 to 3 weeks. The lips become red, dry, and fissured, occasionally becoming hemorrhagic—a condition that may last 1 to 3 weeks. The oropharynx can become red. The tongue can develop a typical "strawberry tongue" appearance.
- There may be generalized findings, such as cervical lymphadenopathy, diarrhea, and in more severe cases, hepatic dysfunction and aseptic meningitis.

Phase 2

- Desquamation follows soon after the resolution of the exanthem. It begins on the tips of the fingers and toes at the junction of the nails and skin. The desquamating sheets of epidermis are progressively shed.
- Generalized findings can be seen, such as meningeal irritation, pneumonia, and cervical lymphadenopathy; arthritis and arthralgia of the knees, hips, and elbows are evident.
- Pericardial tamponade, cardiac arrhythmia, heart rubs, congestive heart failure, and left ventricular dysfunction can also be present.

Phase 3

- Beau lines can be seen in the fingernails.
- The patient can sometimes develop telogen effluvium.

Epidemiology

The disease can occur in epidemics; however, there is no evidence or mention of it being contagious.

Age

The peak incidence for Kawasaki disease is approximately 12 months of age; occurrence is uncommon after 8 years of age.

Sex

In the United States the incidence is higher in individuals of Asian origin than in lighter- or darker-skinned patients.

Race

Occurs more often in male than in female patients, with a ratio of 1.5:1.

Seasonal

Kawasaki disease is usually seen in the winter and spring months.

PATHOLOGY

There is a generalized vasculitis with endarteritis of the vasa vasorum of the coronary arteries involving the intimal lining with ectasia, aneurysmal dilation, and obstruction. Etiology is idiopathic, although an infectious origin has been theorized.

Diagnosis

Diagnosis is made by a careful history and physical examination. Diagnosis is aided by obtaining a liver profile, complete blood cell count (CBC), and sedimentation rate.

Electrocardiogram (ECG) is necessary to rule out any possibility of QT-interval changes or ST-segment and T-wave changes indicative of infarction or coronary artery involvement.

Centers for Disease Control and Prevention Diagnostic Criteria for Kawasaki Disease

See Table 18.9.

Differential Diagnosis

See Table 18.10.

Diagnostic Tests

- In Kawasaki disease, patients should have a *liver function panel* performed initially. Often, abnormal liver function is seen. A *CBC* shows a leukocytosis of more than 18,000 µL. A mild anemia and polycythemia may also be evident.
- As the patient develops into Phase 2, an elevated sedimentation rate is apparent.
- By the time the patient is in Phase 3, the sedimentation rate is returning to normal. *Urinalysis* often indicates pyuria. *Electrocardiograms* are also important in the diagnosis of Kawasaki disease. Prolongation of the PR and QT intervals is often evident, and sometimes ST-segment and T-wave changes are apparent. Because 25% of patients can develop coronary artery aneurysms, an echocardiogram is necessary. Ultimately, cardiac angiography may be necessary to definitively diagnose a coronary artery aneurysm.

Referral

- Patients with Kawasaki disease should be hospitalized.
- Cardiovascular complications occur in 25% to 30% of patients, making consultation with a pediatric cardiologist essential.
- Referral to a specialist in the management of Kawasaki disease may also be appropriate.

T ABLE 18.9.   Centers for Disease Control and Prevention Diagnostic Criteria for Kawasaki Disease

Fever (38.3° C or higher) lasting longer than 5 days, plus at least four of the following:
Bilateral conjunctival injection
Mucous membrane changes (one or more):
    Red or fissured lips
    Red pharynx
    "Strawberry" tongue
Lower extremity changes (one or more):
    Erythema of palms or soles
    Edema of hands or feet
    Desquamation (generalized or periungual)
Rash: erythematous exanthem
Cervical lymphadenopathy: at least 1 node larger than 1.5 cm

Velez-Torres R, Callen JP. Acute febrile mucocutaneous lymph node (Kawasaki) syndrome: an analysis of 24 cases. *Int J Dermatol* 1987;26:96–102.

T ABLE 18.10.   Kawasaki Disease: Differential Diagnosis

Infectious mononucleosis	Disease is characterized by exudative tonsillitis or pharyngitis, red macular rash, fatigue, posterior cervical lymphadenopathy, and hepatosplenomegaly. Monospot test result can be positive.
Rocky Mountain spotted fever	There is a history of tick exposure.
Toxic shock syndrome	Characterized by a generalized rash with hypotension, fever, and shock.
Staphylococcus scalded skin syndrome	Large areas of desquamation and superficial blisters that rarely involve the mucous membranes.
Stevens-Johnson syndrome (erythema multiforme)	Rash is characterized by target lesions, bullae, and/or erosions in mucous membranes.
Measles	Conjunctival discharge and a cough are present. Koplik spots may also be present.
Scarlet fever	There is exudative pharyngitis but no conjunctivitis. Throat culture is positive for streptococci.

Management

Patients should be hospitalized and monitored closely for cardiovascular complications. Echocardiogram should be performed to rule out coronary aneurysm, which occurs in 25% of cases.

Medications

See Table 18.11.

Other Treatment Modalities

- *Corticosteroids are contraindicated* in these patients because of the association with a higher rate of coronary aneurysms.
- *Monitor sedimentation rate* to judge when patient is improving.
- Patients should be closely monitored for secondary infections in the skin.
- *Close cardiac monitoring,* as well as *close monitoring of vital signs,* is essential.
- Patients should be well hydrated with intravenous fluids.

Follow-up

Monitoring Disease Course

The patient will be hospitalized, and close monitoring for the previously mentioned cardiovascular complications is essential. Follow-up echocardiogram is needed 2 to 8 weeks after onset of disease to check for the development of coronary artery aneurysms.

Potential Problems and Complications

- There appear to be no long-lasting complications of Kawasaki disease unless coronary artery disease develops, and the parents of patients with Kawasaki disease should be made well aware of these major complications.
- Coronary artery aneurysms can occur within 2 to 8 weeks after the onset of the illness. Kawasaki disease is also associated with carditis, cardiac ischemia and infarction, pericarditis, peripheral vascular occlusion, stroke, and small bowel obstruction. It is important that echocardiograms be performed initially and 2 to 8 weeks

T ABLE 18.11.   Medical Treatment of Kawasaki Disease

Aspirin therapy

Availability:	Over the counter.
Dosage:	100 mg/kg per day orally every 4 hours in 6 divided doses.
Duration:	Until fever resolves, or until day 14 of the illness; then reduce to 5 to 10 mg/kg daily until platelet count and sedimentation rate return to normal.
Comments:	Can cause gastric irritation.

Intravenous gamma globulin

Availability:	Prescription.
Dosage/Duration:	400 mg/kg per day over a 2-hour infusion for 4 days, or 2 g/kg per day, infused over 10 hours, for 1 day.
Comments:	Helps reduce the risk of coronary aneurysm and myocardial infarction.

after the onset of the illness to monitor for potential cardiac complications. Parents should also be advised that the patient runs a 1% mortality risk from Kawasaki disease, primarily from myocardial infarction.

Patient Education

- Parents often want to know where the child would have contracted this illness. The origin is essentially unknown, but is possibly an infectious origin that leads to an immune-mediated syndrome in genetically predisposed patients.
- There seems to be no contagious component with Kawasaki disease. Therefore household members or close contacts do not need to worry about contracting this illness from the patient.
- It is unlikely that a child will have this disease more than once.

BIBLIOGRAPHY

Bligard CA. Kawasaki disease and its diagnosis. *Pediatr Dermatol* 1987;4(2):75-84.

Cobb MW. Human papillomavirus infection. *J Am Acad Dermatol* 1990;22:547-566.

Drake LA, Ceilley RI, Cornalison RI, et al. Guidelines of care for warts: human papillomavirus. *J Am Acad Dermatol* 1995;32:98-103.

Goldfard MT, Gupta AK, Gupta MA, Sawchuk WS. Office therapy for human papillomavirus infection in nongenital sites. *Dermatol Clin* 1991;9:287-296.

Imiquimod for gential warts. *Med Lett* 1997;39(1016):118-119.

Miller DM, Brodell RT. Human papillomavirus infection: treatment options for warts. *Am Fam Physician* 1996;53(1):135-143.

Velez-Torres R, Callen JP. Acute febrile mucocutaneous lymph node (Kawasaki) syndrome: an analysis of 24 cases. *Int J Dermatol* 1987;26(2):96-102.

CHAPTER 19

···

Insects and Parasites Affecting the Skin

PEDICULOSIS

Lice are small (approximately 2 mm), six-legged insects that are obligate human parasites. Infestation of lice in humans is caused by one of three species of lice: *Pediculis humanis capitis,* or head louse; *Pediculis humanis corporis,* or body louse; or *Pediculis humanis pubis,* or pubic louse (or "crab").

Chief Complaint

Patients report matting of the hair or severe pruritus at the affected areas of the body. However, many patients are asymptomatic, complaining only of louse infestation, such as lice eggs, or nits, in the hair. Affected individuals may also report localized redness and pain associated with secondary bacterial infection and lymphadenopathy.

Clinical Manifestations

- Pediculosis may initially involve only 10 or less lice, making it sometimes difficult to isolate a live louse. However, nits are invariably observed on examination. The nits themselves are generally an oval-shaped, grayish-white egg capsule, approximately 1 mm long (Figure 19.1, see color insert following page 170).
- Pruritis affects the scalp, the pubic area, or a larger body area, depending on the type of infestation.
- Pruritus involving the eyelashes or eyebrows may occur secondary to blepharitis, causing scaling, crusting, and even a purulent discharge. Infestations of the eyelashes occur almost exclusively in children, usually from head lice transmitted by other children.
- Scratching and excoriation associated with pruritis may lead to secondary bacterial infections with lymphadenopathy.
- Some patients may have a hypersensitivity from the saliva and the fecal matter of lice.

Pediculosis corporis

These lice or nits live within the clothing, usually in the seams or folds of fabric. Body lice are found on the host body only while feeding.

Pediculosis capitis

- In pediculosis capitis the live adult lice and the nits are large enough to be seen by the naked eye.
- Distribution of the infestation is primarily to the scalp.
- Given that the average hair grows approximately 0.5 mm per day, it can be assumed that nits seen further from the scalp represent a longer period of infestation.
- Secondary physical findings of excoriations and secondary bacterial infections, leading ultimately to cervical or occipital lymphadenopathy, may be observed.

Pediculosis pubis
- Pediculosis pubis infestation appears in the pubic area, but may also include the axilla, perineum, thighs, lower legs, chest, eyelids, and rarely, the beard.
- Brown specks in underwear representing louse feces may be seen.
- Maculae caeruleae, gray-bluish macules located at a distant site from the infestation, are occasionally seen in cases of pediculosis pubis. The cause of maculae caeruleae is largely unknown, although it has been hypothesized that they represent a secondary inflammatory reaction to the irritating saliva injected into the skin by feeding lice.
- Children may receive eyelash infestation from adults infested with pubic lice.

Epidemiology
Pediculosis Corporis
Pediculosis corporis infestation can occur among individuals of all ages, races, and gender (but is commonly seen in older individuals) who practice poor personal hygiene habits, such as bathing and changing clothing infrequently.

Pediculosis Capitis
- *Age.* Pediculosis capitis affects all ages, but most commonly occurs in children. In the United States, approximately 6 to 10 million children will become infested annually.
- *Race.* In the United States, white or light-skinned individuals are more commonly infested than darker-skinned individuals, such as those of African descent.
- *Sex.* Head lice generally occur in female more often than in male patients.

Pediculosis Pubis
- *Age.* Pediculosis pubis may occur at any age; however, it is most common among sexually active young adults.
- *Race.* Pubic lice generally affect persons of all races or ethnic origins equally.
- *Sex.* These lice infest male more often than female patients.

Risk Factors
- Risk factors for pediculosis includes close personal contact with anyone who is currently infested with lice.
- Sharing of hats, combs, clothing, or bedding also increases the risk of infestation.
- The risk of infestation with pubic lice following only one exposure to an infected individual is greater than 90%.
- Children who are victims of sexual abuse are at risk for eyelash infestation of pubic lice.

PATHOLOGY
Lice range from 1 to 4 mm in length. Of the three types of lice that infest humans, *Pediculis humanis corporis* is the largest; the smallest is *Pediculis humanis pubis,* or crab.

Lice observed immediately after feeding may have a slightly red appearance under the microscope.

Lice feed by piercing the skin with their jaws, injecting an irritating saliva, and sucking blood, a process that occurs approximately 5 times per day. Lice do not demonstrate complete body enlargement with engorgement of blood, as do ticks.

The female louse may lay approximately six eggs or nits a day, which take approximately 8 to 10 days to hatch. The nit is initially cemented firmly near the scalp for purposes of incubation.

Diagnosis

- Diagnosis is based on history and physical examination, including the presence of lice or nits.
- Pediculosis capitis infestation requires a close inspection of the individual hair strands of the scalp. A magnifying glass may aid in this process.

Differential Diagnosis

See Table 19.1.

Diagnostic Tests

- Live nits fluoresce a pearly color under Wood lamp, which may be of diagnostic use.
- Other diagnostic tests are unnecessary.

Referral

Referral may be indicated when the diagnosis is uncertain or the disorder is unresponsive to conventional treatment modalities.

Management

- Management of pediculosis is focused on elimination of the lice and nits.
- Up to 30% of patients with pubic lice, or crabs, have at least one other concomitant sexually transmitted disease. Therefore these patients should be screened for other sexually transmitted diseases, including human immunodeficiency virus (HIV), Venereal Disease Research Laboratory (VDRL), *Chlamydia* species, and gonorrhea.

Medications

See Table 19.2.

- Lindane is a potentially neurotoxic substance and can cause seizures in patients with a history of seizures or in children under 2 years of age. It is *not* recommended for use in small children and is contraindicated in pregnant and lactating women.

T ABLE 19.1.   Pediculosis: Differential Diagnosis

Pediculosis capitis

Seborrheic dermatitis	Greasy-appearing scales on scalp and debris in the hair that is attached less firmly than nits.
Impetigo	No nits visible on hair shaft; localized erythema with crusts.
Lichen simplex chronicus	No nits visible on hair shaft.

Pediculosis corporis

Scabies	Typical burrowing lesions; distributed differently.
Senile or winter's itch	Evidence of dry skin, usually aggravated by bathing.

Pediculosis pubis

Scabies	Typical burrowing lesions; no nits visible on hair shafts.
Pyoderma secondary to contact dermatitis	History of reactivity or sensitivity to condoms, spermicidal jellies, underwear, or douches.
Seborrheic dermatitis	Absence of nits; greasy scales easily removed from hair shaft.

T ABLE 19.2.   Medical Treatment of Pediculosis

Pyrethrin 0.33% (Rid, A-2000)

Availability:	Over the counter.
Dosage:	Apply to scalp and lather for 10 minutes; rinse out.
Duration:	Repeat every 3 to 7 days until signs of infestation resolve.
Comments:	For treatment of pediculosis capitis and pediculosis pubis.
	Probably the least toxic.
	Avoid contact with eye and mucous membranes.
	Contraindicated in patients who are allergic to ragweed.

Permethrin (Nix 1%, Elimite 5%)

Availability:	Nix, over the counter; Elimite, prescription.
Dosage:	Apply and leave in hair for 10 minutes; rinse out.
Duration:	Repeat every 3 to 7 days until signs of infestation resolve.
Comments:	For treatment of pediculosis capitis and pediculosis pubis.
	5% Elimite is useful for resistant cases.
	Can cause transient burning or stinging on initial application.
	Use as rinse after shampooing affected areas

Lindane 1% lotion or shampoo (Kwell)

Availability:	Prescription.
Dosage:	*Shampoo:* Lather and comb into hair; leave in for 5 minutes, rinse out.
	Lotion: Apply lotion to body from neck down; leave in place for 8 to 10 hours, then shower off.
Duration:	Repeat every 3 to 7 days until signs of infestation resolve.
Comments:	For pediculosis capitis, pediculosis pubis, pediculosis corporis.
	Potent pesticide; most toxic treatment.
	May cause seizures in patients with a history of seizures or in children under 2 years of age.
	Contraindicated for pregnant or lactating women, or children.

Physostigmine ophthalmic ointment 0.25% (Eserine)

Availability:	Prescription.
Dosage:	Apply twice per day.
Duration:	1 to 2 days.
Comments:	For persistent infestations of the eyelashes.
	Causes dilation of the pupils.

- It is recommended that a reapplication of medication be performed after the initial treatment. Sometimes some of the nits can survive the initial treatment, and it takes an incubation period of 7 to 10 days for a nit to hatch. Reapplication should occur approximately 1 week after initial treatment.

Other Treatment Modalities

Physical

- Treatment for eyelash infestations, especially in children, includes the use of petroleum jelly (Vaseline) applied to the eyelashes three times daily for 5 days, rubbing it into the eyelids, eyelashes, and eyebrows as necessary.

Physostigmine ophthalmic ointment 0.25% (Eserine) should be administered twice daily for 1 to 2 days in persistent eyelash infestation.
- The area may also be swabbed with Johnson & Johnson's baby shampoo three times daily for 5 days.
- Calamine lotion may be applied twice daily for relief of pruritus associated with pediculosis corporis.
- Nit removal is necessary, since dead nits may remain firmly attached to hair shafts after treatment, and for removal of any surviving nits. Modalities for nit removal include over-the-counter commercial products containing 8% formic acid, which loosen the bond between the hair and the nit. This is generally a cream rinse that is applied to the hair after a pediculocidal shampoo is used. These products usually come with a fine-toothed nit comb, which can be used to remove the nits.
- White vinegar compresses applied at 15-minute intervals may be useful to loosen the bond between the nit and the hair, allowing removal by a fine-toothed nit comb.

Environmental
- Lice are obligate human parasites and cannot survive off the host longer than 10 days for adult lice and longer than 3 weeks for fertile eggs. Therefore environmental measures should include thoroughly vacuuming areas inhabited by those infested, as well as laundering or dry cleaning all clothing, bedding, and headwear exposed to individuals with active pediculosis.
- Bedding and furniture may be sprayed with permethrin 0.5% (A-2000 lice control spray, nonprescription).
- Storing infested clothing, bedding, or headwear in an airtight container for 30 days without human contact eradicates both nits and lice.
- Items such as combs and brushes should be soaked in a 2% Lysol solution or rubbing alcohol for 1 hour or in hot water for 5 to 10 minutes to guarantee eradication and prevent the spread of lice.

Follow-up
Monitoring Disease Course
- Patients should be followed up in 7 to 10 days, since it may be necessary to repeat the initial treatment.
- If the infestation remains unresponsive after a second treatment, additional follow-up is necessary to determine whether family members or other contacts are infected and in need of treatment.

Potential Problems and Complications
The most likely potential problem or complication is that of a secondary bacterial infection caused by excoriations attributable to persistent pruritus. This is usually easily treated with topical or oral antibiotics as necessary.

Patient Education
- Patients should be reminded that lice are contacted through close personal contact with someone already infested or through contact with bedding, linens, hats, or towels that have been in contact with someone infested with lice.
- Head lice are obligate human parasites and are not harbored in household pets.
- It should be stressed that all close contacts, including sexual contacts within the preceding month, should be informed about the lice infestation and advised to seek treatment.
- School nurses, caregivers, and the parents of a child's playmates should be notified about lice infestation in children.

- Patients should be reassured, especially parents of children infected with lice, that this disease affects individuals of all socioeconomic backgrounds.

SCABIES

Scabies is a cutaneous skin infestation caused by the mite *Sarcoptes scabiei,* which causes hypersensitivity with resultant cutaneous rash and pruritus.

Chief Complaint

Patients report excoriated papular eruptions accompanied by pruritus that tends to be more extreme at night.

Clinical Manifestations

- The primary skin findings of scabies include a linear or serpiginous, slightly elevated lesion, usually less than 1 cm in length, called a burrow. These burrows are caused by the female mite.
- Secondary lesions include scattered, excoriated, papular eruptions secondary to the intense pruritus and scratching.
- Symptoms first become evident 2 to 3 weeks after initial contact with the mite. However, a previously exposed individual may be already sensitized, thereby developing symptoms within 1 to 3 days.
- Typical distribution of lesions includes the lower abdomen, back, pubic and axillary areas and the classically observed lesions in the webs of the fingers, flexor portions of the wrists, and margins of the palm; beneath the breasts; and in the genital area, including the shaft of the penis.
- The lesions usually spare the face, scalp, palms, and soles of adult patients.
- Lesions occurring in infants may be found predominantly in areas that are spared in adults. Vesicular lesions, in particular, may be noted in the palms and soles of infants.
- The duration of these lesions may be weeks to months if left untreated.

Epidemiology

Scabies most commonly occurs among young, sexually active adults; however, any age may be affected.

Risk Factors

- Intimate skin-to-skin contact with an individual infested by the scabies mite is the major risk factor for this disorder.
- Individuals residing in institutional facilities such as nursing homes may be at increased risk for developing scabies.

PATHOLOGY

The life cycle of the scabies mite is approximately 30 days.

The female mite burrows into the stratum corneum within 1 hour of its arrival on the skin surface. Mites may burrow several millimeters to a few centimeters in length. During the burrowing cycle the female mite lays eggs that hatch in approximately 5 days. The newly hatched mites breed, burrow, and lay more eggs.

In the initial infestation hundreds of mites may be produced, although symptoms may not be noted. However, during the 2 to 3 weeks after infestation, the affected individual becomes highly contagious.

Both the rash and the pruritus are secondary to the allergic reaction caused by the presence of the scabies mite.

Diagnosis

- Diagnosis is based largely on patient history and physical examination. Patients describing a generalized rash and pruritus should be questioned about similar symptoms in family members or close personal contacts.
- The hypersensitivity reaction kills the majority of the mites; when symptoms become evident, there may be only 10 to 12 mites existing within the skin. To aid in identifying a mite burrow, the lesions may be marked with a black felt-tip marker and wiped with an alcohol swab. This procedure leaves a black dot or line where ink is absorbed by the burrow, making it identifiable.

Differential Diagnosis

See Table 19.3.

Diagnostic Tests

- Diagnosis can be confirmed by the isolation and microscopic observation of mites, eggs, egg capsules, or fecal matter in a scabies preparation.
- To perform a scabies preparation, a drop of mineral oil should be placed on the lesion. Ideal lesions are unscratched or unexcoriated burrows, usually found within the folds of the skin. The lesion is shaved, not scraped, with a No. 15 scalpel blade. Several lesions should be shaved because most lesions are secondary to allergic or hypersensitive reaction and do not contain mites. Shavings should be placed on a microscope slide with a drop of mineral or immersion oil and a coverslip. Examination is performed under 10× magnification.
- Mites appear as oval organisms that are approximately 0.5 mm in size, with eight legs grouped in four pairs. Eggs or egg capsules are egg-shaped structures, one-third to one-half the size of the mite. The fecal matter known as scybala are small, dark pellets approximately one-tenth the size of the eggs.
- Visualization of any one of these components confirms the diagnosis of a scabies infestation.
- Because of the allergic nature of this disorder, some patients demonstrate elevated immunoglobulin E (IgE) titers. This is an incidental finding and is not a specific diagnostic indicator.

Referral

Referral is indicated when the diagnosis is uncertain or the disorder is unresponsive to standard treatment modalities.

Management

Management is focused on the elimination of the mites and their eggs.

Medications

See Table 19.4.

For persistent pruritus, potent topical corticosteroids may be used (see Appendix A).

TABLE 19.3.   Scabies: Differential Diagnosis

Pyoderma	Areas of erythema, oozing, and crusting; no evidence of mites.
Pediculosis pubis	Nits and lice on hair; lack of burrows.
Winter's itch	Seasonal disorder; lack of burrows.
Dermatitis herpetiformis	Vesicular lesions with slightly different distribution; lack of burrows.
Eczema	Generalized pruritus and excoriated lesions.
	Lack of burrows; no evidence of mites.

T ABLE 19.4. **Medical Treatment of Scabies**

Permethrin 5% cream (Elimite)
Availability:	Prescription.
Dosage:	Apply to entire body, leave on for 8 to 14 hours, then shower off.
Duration:	Repeat in 7 days.
Comments:	May cause transient burning or stinging on initial application.
	Treatment of choice, safe enough to be used in children over 2 months of age.
	Pregnancy category B.

Lindane 1% lotion, cream, and shampoo (Kwell)
Availability:	Prescription.
Dosage:	Apply to the body from neck down, leave on for 8 to 12 hours, then shower off.
Duration:	Repeat in 7 days.
Comments:	Considered toxic.
	Alternate treatment for adults; not recommended for use in children or in pregnant or lactating women.
	May cause seizures in patients with history of seizures and children less than 2 years of age.

Crotamiton 10% cream (Eurax)
Availability:	Prescription.
Dosage:	Massage into skin from neck down; shower off 48 hours after *last* application.
Duration:	Repeat nightly for 3 to 5 nights.
Comments:	Combined scabicide and antipruritic.
	Alternate treatment in adults and children over 2 months of age.
	Cure rates reported at 50% to 100%.

Precipitated sulfur 6% in petrolatum
Availability:	Prescription.
Dosage:	Apply to entire body daily for 3 days, shower off 24 hours after last application.
Duration:	Repeat daily for 3 days.
Comments:	Messiness, stains, unpleasant odor.
	Treatment of choice in infants under 2 months of age and pregnant women.

Diphenhydramine (Benadryl)
Availability:	Over the counter.
Dosage:	*Adults:* 25 to 50 mg orally 4 times daily.
	Children: 5 mg/kg per day orally, divided every 6 hours orally.
Duration:	Use until pruritis resolves.
Comments:	Use to relieve pruritis.
	May cause sedation.

continued

T ABLE 19.4. *continued.* **Medical Treatment of Scabies**

Hydroxyzine HCl (Atarax)

Availability:	Prescription.
Dosage:	*Adults:* 25 to 50 mg orally, 4 times per day as needed.
	Children: 2 to 5 mg/kg per day orally, divided every 6 hours.
Duration:	Use until pruritis resolves.
Comments:	Use to relieve pruritus.
	May cause sedation.

Oral prednisone

Availability:	Prescription.
Dosage:	*Adults:* 40 to 60 mg orally daily for 2 to 3 days, then taper.
	Children: 1 to 2 mg/kg per day orally for 2 to 3 days.
Duration:	Taper over 7 to 10 days.
Comments:	Use to relieve severe pruritus. See PDR for side effects.

Cephalexin (Keflex)

Availability:	Prescription.
Dosage:	500 mg orally twice per day.
Duration:	10 days.
Comments:	For secondary bacterial infection.

PDR, *Physicians' Desk Reference.*

Other Treatment Modalities

Physical

Other antipruritic measures may include use of calamine lotion or colloidal oatmeal baths, such as Aveeno.

Environmental

- Scabies is not easily shed from skin; the mites can live away from humans for approximately 24 hours. Laundering with hot water, drying, and ironing are generally sufficient to kill the mites in clothes and bedding.
- Bed partners, sexual contacts (for 1 month before the onset of the rash), and all household members with whom the infested individual has had close personal contact should be treated at the same time as the initial patient.
- Nodular lesions, called nodular scabies, may occur in chronic infections and often respond to intralesional injections of corticosteroids (5 to 10 mg/mL triamcinolone in each lesion, repeated every 2 weeks if necessary).
- Scabies is often sexually transmitted; therefore these patients, especially those with scabies in the genital area, should be considered for testing to detect the presence of other sexually transmitted diseases.

Follow-up

Monitoring Disease Course

- Patients should be followed up in 10 to 14 days to detect the presence of reinfestation, new allergic lesions, or persistent pruritus.

- An additional visit 1 month after treatment is recommended to confirm complete remission.

Potential Problems and Complications

- Postscabies pruritus attributable to an allergic reaction is a common complication, often lasting 2 to 3 weeks after adequate treatment. Oral antihistamines, application of Eurax cream, or topical steroids may be indicated in these instances.
- Potential problems or complications as seen with scabies may include pyoderma and eczematous inflammation. Secondary infections may be treated with oral antibiotics, whereas persistent inflammation usually responds to treatment with topical steroids.

Patient Education

- Patients should be educated about the pathogenesis of scabies, including the route of transmission.
- Since this parasite cannot live away from the human host for more than 24 hours, only those clothes, towels, and bed linens used within the preceding 48 hours should be laundered.
- Compliance with the treatment modalities, including environmental and physical measures and treatment of contacts, helps to avoid recurrence and passing the scabies back and forth from one person to another.
- Treatment of any individuals who have close personal contact with the infected patient, even if those individuals are asymptomatic, should be emphasized.
- Patients should be educated that coats, walls, rugs, floors, furniture, and curtains need not be cleaned and treated in a special manner to eradicate any harboring mites within those materials, as the scabies mite is an obligate human parasite and does not live long (24 hours) when removed from its human host.
- Scabies is not transmitted by casual contact such as handshakes or medical examinations or by roommates (without intimate contact).
- Patients should be reassured that the persistent pruritus sometimes associated with scabies is not necessarily an indication that the treatment was unsuccessful. Pruritis may be controlled with the use of oral antihistamines and topical corticosteroids.

CERCARIAL DERMATITIS

Cercarial dermatitis, also known as "swimmer's itch" or "clam digger's itch," is an acute, pruritic, papular eruption at sites of cutaneous penetration by the cercariae of the *Schistosoma* parasite.

Chief Complaint

Patients report an acute episode of pruritus, followed hours later by the development of intensely pruritic papular or urticarial lesions.

Clinical Manifestations

- Cercarial dermatitis first appears as pruritus, followed by the development of pruritic papules, which may occasionally be surrounded by erythema at the points of contact (Figure 19.2, see color insert following page 170).
- Scattered, papular eruptions and urticaria are associated with erythema in a distribution consistent with areas directly exposed to the water and sparing those areas covered by the swimsuit.

- The pruritus and rash reach maximum intensity within the first 2 to 3 days of exposure, subsiding over the next 7 days.
- Because cutaneous manifestations are secondary to an allergic and hypersensitivity reaction, initial exposure may produce only minor symptoms, whereas reexposure of a previously sensitized individual brings about the typical reaction, which may be even more severe in hypersensitive patients.
- Excoriations caused by scratching with resultant secondary bacterial infection may also be observed.

Epidemiology
- Cercarial dermatitis is especially common among individuals residing in the states surrounding the Great Lakes.
- The disorder may be observed among individuals of any age, race or ethnic origin, or gender.

Risk Factors
Swimming in brackish, fresh, or salt water is a risk factor for cercarial dermatitis.

PATHOLOGY
Pathogenesis of the disorder is the cutaneous penetration by the cercariae of the *Schistosoma* parasite.

Microscopic larvae of the parasitic flatworm schistosome is released from a snail (its intermediate host) into the water, in which it seeks a warm-blooded host, usually some type of waterfowl. Human beings are not the typical hosts for these parasites. Larvae that come into contact with human skin begin to penetrate the skin as the water evaporates.

Initial symptoms, if noticed at all, are relatively minor, with the eruption occurring anywhere from 2 days to 2 weeks later. The hypersensitivity reaction caused by the cutaneous penetration kills the cercariae before inflicting damage aside from the typical dermatosis.

Diagnosis
Diagnosis is based on physical examination and patient history of swimming in a cercariae-infested body of water.

Differential Diagnosis
See Table 19.5.

Referral
Referral is indicated if the diagnosis is uncertain or the rash is unresponsive to standard treatment modalities.

Management
Cercarial dermatitis is a benign, self-limited disorder with symptoms that fade spontaneously over the course of a week.

Medications
See Table 19.6.

TABLE 19.5.   Cercarial Dermatitis: Differential Diagnosis

Sea bather's eruption	Rash occurs in areas covered by swimwear.
	Occurs only in salt water, primarily off the coast of Florida and the Gulf states.
Contact dermatitis	Diagnosis supported by discovery of substance in water to which patient is hypersensitive.

Other Treatment Modalities

Medication is targeted toward relief of pruritis. Colloidal oatmeal baths such as Aveeno, application of calamine lotion, or cool compresses may all be of use.

Follow-up

Close follow-up is usually unnecessary for the self-limited disorder. Patients may be advised to return in 10 to 14 days only if the rash does not regress completely.

Patient Education

- Patients may be reassured that cercarial dermatitis is a cutaneous, self-limited skin disorder with no complications to internal organs or long-term sequelae.
- Patients should be told that once they have been sensitized to the *Schistosoma* cercariae, they will continue to run the risk of repeat eruptions with each subsequent exposure, which may be of greater severity.
- There is no way to visibly determine whether one has been exposed to cercariae immediately after swimming. Attention should be paid to public health warnings posted at beaches or lakes. Swimming at a pool is another way to prevent this infection.
- Because the larvae generally penetrate the skin as the water is evaporating from the surface of the skin, towel drying immediately after swimming may aid in preventing penetration by the larvae and thus prevent the cutaneous manifestations and symptoms.

TABLE 19.6.   Medical Treatment of Cercarial Dermatitis

Diphenhydramine (Benadryl)

Availability:	Over the counter.
Dosage:	*Adults:* 25 to 50 mg orally 4 times per day as needed.
	Children: 5 mg/kg per day orally every 6 hours.
Duration:	Until pruritis resolves.
Comments:	May cause sedation.

Moderate-potency topical corticosteroids

Availability:	Prescription.
Dosage:	Apply twice per day.
Duration:	Until pruritis resolves.
Comments:	For intense inflammation.
	Use the lowest potency necessary to control pruritus.
	See Appendix A.

SEA BATHER'S ERUPTION

Sea bather's eruption is a pruritic skin eruption that appears on areas of the skin covered by swimming apparel.

Chief Complaint

Patients report a pruritic, papular, vesicular rash on areas of the body covered by swimwear.

Clinical Manifestations

- Sea bather's eruption appears as a monomorphic rash consisting of papules, vesicles, pustules, or urticaria accompanied by pruritus.
- Lesions are limited to areas of the body that were covered by a swimsuit.
- The course of the rash is relatively mild; however, there may be secondary skin findings of excoriations with erythema in cases of severe inflammatory reaction.
- Children with severe or extensive symptoms and lesions may also exhibit a low-grade fever.

Epidemiology

Sea bather's eruption commonly occurs among individuals who swim in salt water areas along the Gulf, Florida, and eastern coasts.

PATHOLOGY

Although a definitive specific cause of sea bather's eruption is unknown, the larvae of the thimble jellyfish *(Linuche unguiculata)* and exposure to planula larvae of the sea anemone *(Edwardsiella lineata)* have been proposed as likely causes.

Diagnosis

Diagnosis is based on patient history and physical examination.

Differential Diagnosis

See Table 19.7.

Referral

Referral is indicated if the diagnosis is uncertain or the rash is unresponsive to standard treatment modalities.

Management

Management is focused on relief of pruritis.

Medications

See Table 19.8.

Other Treatment Modalities

- Bathing in a colloidal oatmeal bath such as Aveeno may be useful to control pruritis.

T ABLE 19.7. Sea Bather's Eruption: Differential Diagnosis

| Swimmer's itch | Occurs after exposure to fresh water; lesions occur on areas not covered by swimwear. |
| Contact dermatitis | History of hypersensitivity to swimwear fabric or detergents used to launder clothing. |

- Sea bather's eruption may be prevented by avoiding swimming in infested areas, especially when public health warnings are posted on the beach indicating the potential for these etiologic agents to be in plentiful supply.
- If the etiologic agents of the disorder are in evidence, swimming in a pool will enable patients to avoid exposure.

Follow-up

Close follow-up is not typically necessary, because of the self-limited nature of this disease; however, patients should be advised to return for follow-up in 2 to 3 weeks if the rash has not completely resolved.

Patient Education

- Patients may be reassured that sea bather's eruption is a self-limited disorder brought about by a hypersensitivity reaction.
- On average, the lesions resolve spontaneously within 1 to 2 weeks.

T ABLE 19.8. Medical Treatment of Sea Bather's Eruption

Diphenhydramine (Benadryl)
Availability:	Over the counter.
Dosage:	*Adults:* 25 to 50 mg every 6 hours as needed.
	Children: 5 mg/kg per day orally divided into 4 doses.
Duration:	Until pruritis resolves.
Comments:	May cause sedation.

Prednisone
Availability:	Prescription.
Dosage:	*Adults:* 40 to 60 mg orally daily, initially for 2 to 3 days, then taper.
	Children: 1 to 2 mg/kg per day orally, initially for 2 to 3 days, then taper.
Duration:	Taper use over 7 to 10 days.
Comments:	See *Physician's Desk Reference* for side effects.

Moderate-potency topical corticosteroids
Availability:	Prescription.
Dosage:	Apply topically twice per day.
Duration:	Until pruritis resolves.
Comments:	For intense inflammation.
	Use the lowest potency necessary to control pruritus.
	See Appendix A.

- Patients may be informed that eruptions may become more severe and extensive with subsequent reexposure of previously sensitized individuals.
- The disorder is not contagious and can only be contracted by swimming in salt water infested with the suspected etiologic agents.

FLEA BITES

Fleas are small, jumping insects belonging to the order Siphonaptera. These parasites are about 2 to 6 mm long and are able to jump up to 30 cm. They feed on the blood of humans or domestic animals (dogs and cats) and can remain inactive in a cocoon in unfavorable conditions or if a host is unavailable, reactivating when the vibrations of a potential host are felt.

A severe pruritus develops from a delayed-type hypersensitivity reaction hours to days after the bite. The rash can be caused by either cat fleas *(Ctenocephalides felis)*, or dog fleas *(Ctenocephalides canis)*.

Chief Complaint

Patients report intensely pruritic papules on the lower extremities that have been present for a week.

Clinical Manifestations

- Flea bites initially appear as multiple hemorrhagic papules smaller than 1 cm. The initial lesions may become indurated or evolve to urticarial plaques or bullae after 12 to 24 hours (Figure 19.3, see color insert following page 170).
- Flea bites commonly occur in the lower extremities, such as the ankles, although bites may be seen on the trunk if the fleas are on the bed, as when infested dogs or cats sleep with humans.
- The anogenital area or axillae are usually spared.
- Excoriated lesions may be become secondarily infected with bacteria and may not resolve for weeks.
- Flea bites may heal with scars, hypopigmentation, or hyperpigmentation.

Epidemiology
Age
Flea bites may occur at any age, but are more common in children.

Seasonal
The lesions are seen during the summer in temperate climates.

Risk Factors
Allowing animals to sleep in one's bed is a risk factor for flea bites.

PATHOLOGY

Flea bites cause intercellular and intracellular epidermal edema. Dermis reveals a deep inflammatory infiltrate of eosinophils situated around blood vessels.

Diagnosis

Diagnosis is based on history and physical examination.

Differential Diagnosis

See Table 19.9.

Diagnostic Tests

• A *punch biopsy* can be confirmatory if the diagnosis is unclear.
• *Bacterial cultures* are indicated if the rash is secondarily infected.

Referral

Referral is usually unnecessary, but may be indicated if the diagnosis is uncertain or the rash is unresponsive to standard treatment modalities.

Management

• Management is focused on the relief of pruritis.
• The rash is the result of a delayed hypersensitivity reaction. Subsequent infestations cause the rash to appear more quickly with more severe signs and symptoms, including itching and blisters.
• Fleas may be vectors of many other diseases, such as bubonic plague, murine typhus (rat fleas), tularemia, Q fever, and tick-borne encephalitis.

Medications

See Table 19.10.

Other Treatment Modalities

Physical

• Lesions should be washed regularly with antibacterial soap to avoid secondary bacterial infection.
• Pruritis may be relieved by the use of calamine lotion.

Environmental

• The flea-infested animal should be treated with a flea bath.
• Dormant or active fleas may be eliminated from the household by spraying floors, carpets, furniture, bed and mattress, and basement with 1% malathion flea spray (nonprescription). The periphery of the floors and carpets should be sprayed more thoroughly than the central areas.
• The foundation of the house should be sprayed if an infested animal resides outdoors.

T ABLE 19.9.   **Flea Bites: Differential Diagnosis**

Allergic contact dermatitis	Lesions can occur anywhere on the body and are usually not bullous; patient has a history of exposure to the offending agent. Biopsy may be useful to differentiate the two.
Mite, bedbug, or mosquito bites	Pruritic papules appear on any part of body and usually disappear more quickly than the dermatosis from flea bites. Biopsy may be useful to differentiate the two.

T ABLE 19.10. Medical Treatment of Flea Bites

Potent topical corticosteroids

Availability:	Prescription.
Dosage:	Apply topically twice daily.
Duration of use:	Use until the rash is gone.
Comments:	Long-term use can cause skin atrophy or telangiectasia. See Appendix A for details.

Diphenhydramine (Benadryl)

Availability:	Over the counter.
Dosage:	*Adults:* 25 to 50 mg orally 4 times daily as necessary.
	Children under age 12 years: 5 mg/kg per day in 4 divided doses orally as necessary.
Duration:	Until pruritus is gone.
Comments:	Can cause drowsiness.

Hydroxyzine (Atarax)

Availability:	Prescription.
Dosage:	*Adults:* 25 to 50 mg orally 4 times daily as necessary.
	Children: 2 to 5 mg/kg per day orally in 4 divided doses as necessary.
Duration:	Until pruritus is gone.
Comments:	Can cause drowsiness.

Cetirizine (Zyrtec)

Availability:	Prescription.
Dosage:	*Adults:* 10 mg orally daily as necessary.
	Children 6 to 12 years of age: 5 to 10 mg (5 mg/5 mL) orally daily as necessary.
Duration:	Until pruritis is gone.
Comments:	Less sedating.

Loratadine (Claritin)

Availability:	Prescription.
Dosage:	*Adults:* 10 mg orally daily as necessary.
	Children 6 to 12 years of age: 5 to 10 mg (5 mg/5 mL) orally daily as necessary.
Duration:	Until pruritus is gone.
Comments:	Less sedating.

Calamine lotion

Availability:	Over the counter.
Dosage:	Apply daily.
Duration:	Until pruritus is gone.
Comments:	Minimal side effects, messy.

continued

T ABLE 19.10. *continued.* **Medical Treatment of Flea Bites**

Systemic corticosteroids **(in severe pruritus or extensive disease)**
Prednisone
Availability:	Prescription.
Dosage:	*Adults:* 40 to 60 orally initially, then taper over 7 to 10 days.
	Children: 1 to 2 mg/kg per day initially, then taper.
Duration:	Taper over 7 to 10 days.
Comments:	Long-term use can inhibit the pituitary-adrenal axis, which can cause severe systemic problems. Consult *Physician's Desk Reference* or internal medicine text for complete details.

Antibiotics **(for secondarily infected lesions)**
Topical agents
Mupirocin ointment (Bactroban) or polysporin ointment
Availability:	Bactroban, prescription; Polysporin, over the counter.
Dosage:	Apply topically to infected lesions daily.
Duration:	10 days.
Comments:	Minimal burning or stinging. Avoid in patients who are allergic to these agents.

Systemic agents
Availability:	Prescription.

Cephalexin (Keflex)
Dosage:	*Adults:* 500 mg orally twice daily.
	Children: 250 mg orally twice daily.

Erythromycin
Dosage:	*Adults:* 500 mg orally 4 times daily.
	Children: 250 mg orally 4 times daily.

Dicloxacillin
Dosage:	*Adults:* 250 mg orally 4 times daily.
	Children: 125 mg orally 4 times daily.
Duration:	10 days.
Comments:	See Chapter 16 for specific details.

Follow-up
Monitoring Disease Course
- Patients should be followed up in 5 to 7 days to check for secondary bacterial infection.
- If the rash does not disappear in several weeks, patients should be counseled to return to the physician for further treatment.

Potential Problems and Complications
The main complication is secondary bacterial infection with *Staphylococcus aureus* or streptococci.

Patient Education

- Patients should be advised that the key to the treatment of flea bites is controlling the flea population in any household pets.
- They should be cautioned that dormant fleas may be reactivated upon movement of potential hosts. When moving into a residence in which the previous owners had pets, treatment of the floors and carpets is advisable.
- Patients should be counseled to return for follow-up if bullae become purulent or more pain or erythema develops.

SPIDER BITES

Of more than 30,000 species of spiders, 50 have been shown to bite humans. Of these, only two species, the black widow spider and the brown recluse spider, cause significant damage.

Other species of biting spiders in the United States have smaller fangs or may only inject minute quantities of venom, thereby causing only minor symptoms, such as pruritus, erythema, and swelling.

Black widow spider (Latrodectus mactans).
- The black widow spider has a black, gray, or brown abdomen with a distinguishing ventral red hourglass abdominal marking.
- Females can be up to 4 cm long and cause a more symptomatic and dangerous bite than males.
- The spiders are found over the entire United States, but are more common in the South.

Brown recluse spider (Loxosceles reclusa).
- The brown recluse spider is commonly found in the central and south-central United States, predominantly in Tennessee, Arkansas, Missouri, and Kansas, but are present in all states.
- It is a light tan to dark brown spider with a small (1 to 2 cm) body and a characteristic violin-shaped marking on its abdomen.

Chief Complaint

Patients report painful bite marks on the extremities, often with little or no recollection of how the bite occurred (Figure 19.4, see color insert following page 170).

Clinical Manifestations
Black Widow Spider

- The initial bite of the black widow spider is painful, with redness or urticaria occasionally visible at the location of the bite.
- The bites cause pain in the back, abdomen, or legs secondary to the injected neurotoxin.
- Bites are usually located on lower extremities, hands, or forearms.

Brown Recluse Spider

- Brown recluse spider bites occur when patients encounter a spider in a dark place, such as under a rock or an article moved in an attic or a basement. The spiders may occasionally get into bed linens, or even into clothing or shoes, biting when an individual gets into bed or dresses.
- The bites are painless initially.
- Approximately 90% of bites cause no systemic problems.
- In severe bites, intense pain begins 2 to 8 hours later, with redness, edema, and tenderness at the bite site.

- The bites typically develop into a central, blue-black necrotic lesion surrounded by erythema. Observation shows the necrosis moving by gravity.
- Ulcers can develop at the necrosis site, healing in 6 to 8 weeks with resultant scarring on healing.
- Lymphangitis and a generalized maculopapular rash may also be present.
- Systemic symptoms are uncommon but may include fever, chills, nausea, vomiting, convulsions, hemolytic anemia, thrombocytopenia, and disseminated intravascular coagulation (DIC).

Epidemiology

Both the black widow spider and the brown recluse spider can be found anywhere in the United States and North America.

PATHOLOGY

The black widow spider delivers neurotoxic venom that produces acetylcholine depletion at motor nerve endings, which accounts for the muscle pain and abdominal cramping.

The brown recluse spider produces a necrolytic venom causing tissue destruction mediated by both its polymorphonuclear leukocyte–dependent and sphingomyelinase components, as well as a hemolytic toxin causing hemolysis, DIC, and fever.

Diagnosis

- Diagnosis is usually based on a recent spider bite and subsequent symptoms. However, in cases in which the patient does not recall receiving a spider bite, the presenting symptoms can be confused with acute respiratory distress, cardiac failure, shock, or acute appendicitis. These patients should be examined for two puncture sites on the lower extremities, buttocks, or hands.
- If the spider can be located, have the patient bring it to the physician to help in the diagnostic process.

Differential Diagnosis

See Table 19.11.

Referral

- Most black widow spider bites may be treated on an outpatient basis.
- Approximately 90% of brown recluse spider bites cause no major systemic medical problems, making referral largely unnecessary for these patients.
- Patients with severe systemic systems or pain following bites from either type of spider should be hospitalized.

Management

- Ice should be applied to the affected area to slow the activity and spread of the venom. *Avoid heat.*
- The wound should be cleansed with an antibacterial soap.

Medications

See Table 19.12.

Morphine should not be used for pain relief, since it can cause additive problems with hypotension and respiratory distress.

T ABLE 19.11. Spider Bites: Differential Diagnosis

Brown recluse spider	
DIC	May cause skin necrosis similar to the brown recluse bite; usually not painful. CBC, prothrombin time, PTT, fibrinogen level, and fibrin split product values are necessary to confirm the diagnosis.
Hemolytic anemia	May see hemolysis in both conditions. No history of spider bite or other dermatologic lesions.
Black widow spider	
Coronary artery disease	Chest tightness may occur in both conditions. CPK isoenzyme values and ECG changes may be useful to differentiate.
Acute appendicitis	Abdominal rigidity and pain similar to black widow spider bite. CBC is usually abnormal in acute appendicitis.

DIC, disseminated intravascular coagulation; CBC, complete blood cell count; PTT, partial thromboplastin time; CPK, creatine phosphokinase; ECG, electrocardiographic.

Other Treatment Modalities

- *Black widow spider.* Muscle relaxants may be used to relieve muscle spasms caused by the neurotoxin.
- *Black widow and brown recluse spiders.* Tetanus booster may be administered, if needed.
- *Environmental.* Patients living in endemic areas should use caution when putting on shoes and clothes. Before going to bed, the bed linens should be shaken to scare away any hiding spiders.

Follow-up

Monitoring Disease Course

Patients should be monitored daily for 2 to 3 days following initial presentation to detect the presence of systemic complications.

Potential Problems and Complications

- Both types of spider bites may cause severe systemic complications such as tissue necrosis, respiratory distress, renal failure, severe hypertension, hemolytic anemia, DIC, shock, coma, and convulsions.
- In rare instances, death may result from these bites, especially in very young or very old patients.

Patient Education

- Patients should be advised to stay quiet, apply ice to the bite site, keep the affected area elevated to keep the venom from spreading, and seek medical attention as soon as possible.
- They should also be cautioned that severe pain, fever, nausea, or vomiting following a spider bite signals severe systemic complications; these symptoms warrant immediate medical attention.
- Patients should attempt to locate and retrieve the spider, to facilitate diagnosis.

T ABLE 19.12. Medical Treatment of Spider Bites

Calcium gluconate 10% solution
Availability:	Prescription.
Dosage:	*Adults:* 10 to 20 mL intravenously.
	Children: 100 mg/kg per dose intravenously every 10 minutes.
Duration:	Repeat as needed.
Comments:	Useful for muscle spasms caused by neurotoxin.

Diazepam (Valium)
Availability:	Prescription.
Dosage:	*Adults:* 5 to 10 mg intramuscularly or intravenously.
	Children: 0.04 to 0.2 mg/kg per dose intramuscularly or intravenously every 2 to 4 hours, to a maximum of 0.6 mg/kg over 8 hours.
	Adults, oral dosage: 2 to 10 mg 3 to 4 times daily.
	Children, oral dosage: 0.12 to 0.8 mg/kg per day, divided in 3 or 4 doses.
Duration:	*Adults:* Repeat in 3 to 4 hours as needed.
	Children: Repeat every 2 to 4 hours as needed.
Comments:	Useful for muscle spasms.

Methocarbamol (Robaxin)
Availability:	Prescription.
Dosage:	*Adults:* 1 g intramuscularly or intravenously every 6 hours as needed; or 2 tablets (750 mg) orally, 4 times daily for 1 day, then 1 tablet 4 times daily.
	.Children: 15 mg/kg per day orally intramuscularly, or intravenously every 6 hours as needed.
Duration:	Intramuscular or intravenous administration should not exceed 3 days; however, tablets may be used until spasms resolve.
Comments:	Useful for muscle spasms.

Erythromycin or cephalexin
Availability:	Prescription.
Dosage:	*Adults:* 500 mg orally, 4 times daily.
	Children: Cephalexin 25–100 mg/kg/day orally divided in 4 doses. *Or* erythromycin 30–100 mg/kg/day orally divided in 4 doses.
Duration:	Use for 10 days.
Comments:	For secondary bacterial infection.

Dapsone
Availability:	Prescription.
Dosage:	50 mg orally, twice daily.
Duration:	10 days.
Comments:	Consider in brown recluse spider bites that are unresponsive to treatment. Contraindicated in G6PD-deficient patients.

continued

T ABLE 19.12.   *continued.*   **Medical Treatment of Spider Bites**

Antivenin antiserum (black widow)

Availability:	Prescription.
Dosage:	2.5 mL intramuscularly.
Duration:	One time only.
Comments:	To neutralize the neurotoxin.
	Consider in patients under 16 years of age or over 60 years of age; pregnant women; patients with stage 4 hypertension or respiratory distress; or patients with severe symptoms such as hemolysis or DIC.
	Side effects include serum sickness.

Meperidine (Demerol)

Availability:	Prescription.
Dosage:	*Adults:* 25 to 50 mg every 3 to 4 hours intramuscularly or intravenously.
	Children: 0.5 mg/kg per dose intramuscularly or intravenously every 3 to 4 hours.
Duration:	As needed for pain control.
Comments:	For pain relief in either spider bite type.

G6PD, glucose-6-phosphate dehydrogenase; DIC, disseminated intravascular coagulation.

BIBLIOGRAPHY

Brown S, Becher J, Brady W. Treatment of ectoparastitic infections: review of the English-language literature, 1982–1992. *Clin Infect Dis* 1995;20(suppl 1):S104–S109.

Elgart ML. A risk-benefit assessment of agents used in the treatment of scabies. *Drug Safety* 1996;6:386–393.

Haag ML, Brozena SJ, Fenske NA. Attack of the scabies: what to do when an outbreak occurs. *Geriatrics* 1993;48(10):45–53.

Orkin M, Maibach H. Scabies therapy: 1993. *Semin Dermatol* 1993;12(1):22–26.

Sterling GB, Janniger CK, Kihiczak G, Schwartz RA, Fox MD. Scabies. *Am Fam Physician* 1992;46(4):1237–1241.

APPENDIX A

Recommendations for Use of Topical Corticosteroids

BASICS

- Potent topical corticosteroids should be applied for a short term or intermittently to avoid local and systemic side effects such as skin atrophy, adrenal suppression, and steroid acne (Table Appendix A.1). Limit use of high-potency corticosteroids to twice daily for a maximum of 3 to 4 weeks.
- Sudden discontinuation of potent topical corticosteroids should be avoided to prevent a rebound phenomenon. When the rash is improving, switch to a less potent corticosteroid and taper off the low-potency topical agent.
- Low-potency topical corticosteroids should be used in children and in adults with a large area of skin to be treated or if the face, scrotum, or other areas susceptible to damage are to be treated.
- Choose the right vehicle for the type and site of lesion: lotions and creams for weeping lesions; lotions, creams, or gels for hairy areas or skin creases; and ointments for dry and chronic lesions.
- Choose one to two topical agents from each of the potency categories (guided by cost and cosmetic acceptability), and learn how to use them well.

TABLE APPENDIX A.1. Potential Adverse Effects of Topical Corticosteroids

Systemic effects

Pituitary–adrenal axis suppression
Cushing disease
Femoral head necrosis
Growth retardation—especially in children

Local effects

Formation of striae	Fungal infections
Skin atrophy	Candidiasis
Telangiectasia	Hypopigmentation
Erythema	Tachyphylaxis
Steroid acne	Hypertrichosis
Milia	Allergic contact dermatitis
Cataracts—rare	Purpura
Perioral dermatitis	

SKIN TYPES

- Thin or occluded skin such as that found on the face, eyelids, and genitalia may absorb more of the topical corticosteroids and is thus more susceptible to their adverse effects.
- Thicker skin such as that found on the palms and soles or in lichenified skin responds better to high-potency corticosteroids.
- The superhigh-potency agents are very well absorbed from the skin, and if used long term (e.g., more than 4 weeks) may cause both local and systemic side effects.
- Limit use of superhigh-potency corticosteroids to short periods (less than 2 weeks), to a limited area, and to thickened skin areas.

VEHICLE CHOICE

- Ointments are oil based and therefore greasy. They are inherently soothing and occlusive, which makes for better skin absorption.
- Creams have less oil and more alcohol, propylene glycol, and water in their vehicle, making them less greasy. This also makes them more cosmetically appealing. However, they may be slightly irritating to interrupted skin (causing stinging).
- Solutions contain more water and alcohol and less oil than creams. They are also more irritating to the skin. They are useful in hairy areas of the skin or when a large amount of skin must be covered.
- Gels contain more alcohol and less oil than other vehicles and are more drying. They are useful for the treatment of weeping or vesicular lesions (e.g., *Rhus* dermatitis).

RECOMMENDATIONS

- Ointments should be applied to lesions that are dry, in areas of thickened skin, or in rashes with plaque formation.
- Cream should be administered to wet or oozing lesions to dry them.
- Gels should be administered to oozing or vesicular lesions that need to be dried.
- Solutions should be applied to cover larger areas of skin or in hair-covered lesions.

STEROID RESPONSE

Some thicker-skinned areas, deep dermatoses, or areas of scar or lichenification can be unresponsive to the use of topical corticosteroids. Several treatment alternatives are useful.

Occlusion

Medium- to high-potency ointments applied under occlusive dressings can penetrate the skin better. However, caution should be taken to limit the use of occlusion to less than 2 weeks because of the increased potential for local and systemic side effects. Occlusion can be achieved with a simple adhesive strip (Band-Aid), a finger-cot, or the application of plastic wrap to an area. The recommendation is to use the occlusive dressing overnight to achieve at least 8 hours of improved skin absorption.

Intralesional Steroids

Localized areas of resistant skin disease can be treated by injecting a midpotency corticosteroid into the lesion. This treatment type is useful in inflamed lesions (cystic acne, trichilemmal cyst) or when attempting to thin connective tissue or scars. Local adverse skin effects can occur with this mode of treatment.

Systemic Corticosteroids

Systemic corticosteroids are useful for widespread disease or unusually resistant dermatoses. The authors suggest using a short course of systemic corticosteroids to minimize systemic effects. Oral prednisone is usually the drug of choice up to 60 mg/day in adults or 1 mg/kg per day in children, given over 7 to 10 days.

Topical Corticosteroids

See Table Appendix A.2.

TABLE APPENDIX A.2.   Topical Corticosteroids

Potency	Topical agent	Vehicle
Lowest		
0.25%–1%	Methylprednisolone acetate (Medrol)–generic	ointment
0.1%	Dexamethasone (Decadron Phosphate)	cream, aerosol
0.5%–1.0%ª	Hydrocortisone–generic	cream, ointment, lotion
2.5%	Hydrocortisone–generic	cream, ointment, lotion
1%	Hydrocortisone acetate–generic	cream, ointment
Low		
0.05%	Aclometasone dipropionate (Alcovate)	cream, ointment
0.01%	Betamethasone valerate (Valisone)	cream
0.05%	Desonide (Desowen, Tridesilon)	cream, ointment, lotion
0.01%	Fluocinolone acetonide (Synalar)–generic	cream, solution
Medium		
0.1%	Clocortolone pivalate (Cloderm)	cream
0.1%	Prednicarbate (Dermatop)	cream
0.1%	Hydrocortisone butyrate (Locoid)	cream, oinment, solution
0.1%	Hydocortisone buteprate (Pandel)	cream
0.025%	Betamethasone benzoate (Uticort)	lotion, gel, cream
0.1%	Betamethasone valerate–generic (Valisone)	cream, ointment, lotion
0.05%	Desoximetasone–generic (Topicort LP)	cream, gel
0.025%	Fluocinolone acetonide–generic (Synalar)	cream, ointment
0.2%	Hydrocortisone valerate (Westcort)	cream, ointment
0.1%	Mometasone furoate (Elocon)	cream, ointment, lotion
0.05% and 0.025%	Flurandrenolide–generic (Cordran, Cordran SP)	lotion, cream, ointment
0.1% and 0.025%	Triamcinolone acetonide–generic	cream, ointment, lotion
0.005%	(Aristocort A, Kenalog)	ointment
0.05%	Fluticasone propionate (Cutivate)	cream
0.025%	Halcinonide (Halog)	cream

continued on next page

T ABLE APPENDIX A.2. continued. Topical Corticosteroids

Potency	Topical agent	Vehicle
High		
0.1%	Amcinonide (Cyclocort)	cream, ointment, lotion
0.05%	Betamethasone diproprionate—generic (Diprosone, Maxivate)	cream, ointment, lotion
0.25%	Desoximetasone—generic (Topicort)	cream, ointment
0.05%	Diflorasone diacetate (Florone, Maxiflor)	cream, ointment
0.2%	Fluocinolone (Synalar HP)	cream
0.05%	Fluocinonide—generic (Lidex, Lidex-E)	cream, ointment, gel, solution
0.1%	Halcinonide (Halog, Halog-E)	cream, ointment, solution
0.5%	Triamcinolone acetonide—generic (Aristocort, Kenalog)	cream, ointment
Superhigh		
0.05%	Augmented Betamethasone dipropionate (Diprolene)	cream, ointment, gel, lotion
0.05%	Clobetasol propionate (Temovate)	cream, ointment, gel, solution
0.05%	Diflorasone diacetate (Psorcon)	ointment, cream
0.05%	Halobetasol propionate (Ultravate)	cream, ointment

ªNow available over the counter.

BIBLIOGRAPHY

Topical costicosteroids. *Med Lett* 1991;33(857)108-111.

Fisher DA. Adverse effects of topical corticosteroid use. *West J Med* 1995;162: 123-126.

Giannotti B, Pimpinelli N. Topical corticosteroids: which drug and when? *Drugs* 1992;44(1):65-71.

Hepburn DJ, Aeling JL, Weston WL. A reappraisal of topical steroid potency. *Pediatr Dermatol* 1996;13(3):239-245.

Ramsing DW, Agner T. Efficacy of topical corticosteroids on irritant skin reactions. *Contact Dermatitis* 1995;32(5):293-297.

Surber C, Itin PH, Bircher AJ, Maiback HI. Topical corticosteroids. *J Am Acad Dermatol* 1995;32(6):1025-1030.

APPENDIX B

....

Surgical Techniques

ANESTHESIA

- There are two groupings of local (intradermal) anesthetic agents: ester-linked and amide-linked agents (Table Appendix B.1). The ester-linked group causes more allergic problems and cross-reactivity, so they are not used as much in dermatologic surgery. The amide-linked agents are rarely associated with allergic problems and are widely used in dermatologic surgery.
- The anesthetic agent most widely used in dermatologic surgery is 1% lidocaine (Xylocaine) because the onset of anesthesia following injection is rapid (1 minute) with the duration of action about 30 to 60 minutes. This gives prompt anesthesia and allows the physician enough time to complete the office dermatologic procedure.
- The addition of epinephrine 1:100,000 to 1% lidocaine prolongs the duration of action of the anesthetic agent (2 to 6 hours), controls bleeding by vasoconstriction of local blood vessels, and reduces systemic toxicity. The addition of epinephrine to 1% lidocaine slows down the onset of action up to 5 minutes before anesthesia is achieved. The use of epinephrine with local anesthetic agents is contraindicated in the digits and penis because it may compromise blood flow in these confined spaces. Epinephrine may also be contraindicated in the earlobes and nose, and in patients with coronary artery or heart disease (inadvertent injection of epinephrine intravascularly could give rise to cardiac stimulation).
- Lidocaine toxicity can be seen if the dosage injected exceeds the maximum dosage. Toxicity can be manifested by confusion, dizziness, seizures, dysgeusia, coma, cardiac depression, and respiratory depression and arrest. The maximum dosage of lidocaine without epinephrine is 4 to 5 mg/kg (maximum total dose is 300 mg within a 1.5- to 2-hour period) or 7 mg/kg of lidocaine with epinephrine (maximum total dose is 500 mg within a 1.5- to 2-hour period). This translates to a dose of 30 mL of 1% lidocaine or 50 mL of 1% lidocaine with epinephrine that is safe to inject in an adult over a 1- to 2-hour period.
- Pain with injection is a common patient complaint. Techniques to reduce the pain include using 30-gauge needles (25-gauge is less preferable), injecting slowly and steadily, using buffered lidocaine [adding 1 mL of 8.4% sodium bicarbonate to 10 mL of lidocaine (1:10 ratio)], and using topical anesthetic agents such as ice, liquid nitrogen, or ethyl chloride spray. Pinching of the skin and psychological distraction may also be helpful.

TABLE APPENDIX B.1. List of Local Anesthetics

Ester-linked agents	Amide-linked agents
Procaine (Novacaine)	Lidocaine (Xylocaine)
Cocaine	Mepivacaine (Carbocaine)
Tetracaine (Pontocaine)	Bupivacaine (Marcaine)
	Prilocaine (Citanest)

- The injection of lidocaine should be conducted at an angle of 30 degrees to the skin into the subdermal space to raise a wheal and lift the lesion. A deeper injection will cause the lidocaine to diffuse into the subcutaneous fat, achieving little or no anesthesia.

COMPARISON OF DERMATOLOGIC SURGERY TECHNIQUES

The advantages and disadvantages of the various surgical techniques available are listed in the Table Appendix B.2.

Shave Biopsy
Purpose

To remove superficial lesions rapidly that reside in the epidermis and upper dermis or to obtain a specimen of the lesion to aid in the diagnosis.

Technique

- Prepare the skin with an alcohol-soaked cotton ball or gauze.
- Anesthetize the area with 1% lidocaine (use with or without epinephrine depending on location and patient history; see Anesthesia for details). A small wheal of anesthesia should be seen to lift the lesion, making it more amenable to shave biopsy.
- Use a No. 15 scalpel blade. Keeping it parallel to the surface of the skin, gently move the blade against the skin back and forth in a sawing motion. Avoid penetration of the dermis, which can result in more scar formation, by keeping the scalpel blade pointing upward.
- Place specimen in formalin to be sent for histopathologic examination.
- Hemostasis can be achieved with simple pressure, electrodesiccation, or topical solutions such as aluminum chloride hexahydrate (Drysol) or ferric subsulfate (Monsel solution). Ferric subsulfate solution should be used with caution, since the iron pigment could cause a tattoo (hyperpigmentation), which may be a cosmetic problem for the patient.
- After hemostasis is achieved, apply antibiotic ointment and dress the wound.
- Educate the patient on wound care (see Wound Care).

Complications

See Table Appendix B.2.

Punch Biopsy
Purpose

To remove a small lesion completely or to remove a small portion of a skin lesion to aid in the diagnosis.

Technique

- Anesthetize the area with 1% lidocaine (see Anesthesia for details).
- Use a skin punch of sufficient size to either completely remove the lesion or obtain sufficient amount of tissue to aid in the diagnosis. Punches are between 2 and 8 mm in diameter. Larger punches of up to 8 mm may make the skin closure more difficult by creating "dog-ears" at each end of the wound.
- Twirl the punch back and forth between the thumb and index finger while providing downward pressure. Also, apply tension to the skin with the other hand so that when the skin is cut and the tension is released, the wound will be elliptic rather than round, which will make it easier to close with sutures. Once the punch

T ABLE APPENDIX B.2.   Comparison of Dermatologic Surgery Techniques

Procedure	Advantages	Disadvantages	Lesions amenable to technique
Shave biopsy	Rapid removal of raised lesions.	Can bisect potentially dangerous lesions (i.e., melanoma), thus interfering with staging. Does not always get entire lesion (i.e., basal cell carcinoma). Scar formation. Slight chance for bleeding, infection, or nerve and artery damage.	Benign appearing melanocytic nevi, seborrheic keratosis, and keratoacanthoma.
Punch biopsy	Rapid removal of small lesions <4 mm in diameter. Useful when multiple biopsies are needed to make the diagnosis. Removes entire lesion.	Minimal scar formation. Minimal complications such as bleeding, infection, or nerve and artery damage.	Psoriasis, eczematous lesions, skin lesions of systemic disorders (lupus erythematosus), bullous skin disorders, skin cancers, and melanocytic nevi.
Excisional biopsy	Will be able to evaluate deep pathologic features of a visible lesion. Very sensitive diagnostic technique in removing a suspected melanoma; preserves the lesion for staging. Useful in totally removing larger lesions (>6 mm in diameter).	Skin defect at times can be large, creating a complicated closure (sometimes beyond the experience and training of some physicians). Creates a scar. Can cause bleeding, infection, or superficial skin, nerve, or arterial damage.	Skin cancer, melanoma, seborrheic keratosis, keratoacanthoma.

continued

TABLE APPENDIX B.2. *continued.* Comparison of Dermatologic Surgery Techniques

Procedure	Advantages	Disadvantages	Lesions amenable to technique
Cyst excision	Total removal for histopathologic evaluation of deeper lesions not visible at the surface.	Skin defect at time can be large, creating a complicated closure. Increased risk of bleeding, infection, or nerve and arterial damage.	Lipomas, cysts, fibrous lesions.
Snip excision	Sharp excision removing entire pedunculated lesion on skin surface.	Minimal bleeding, scar, or tissue damage.	Skin tags or pedunculated lesions.
Electrofulguration or electro-dessication	To totally remove or destroy benign lesions (if lesion is suspect for malignancy, use shave or excisional biopsy instead).	Does not preserve tissue for histopathologic evaluation. Relatively fast healing with low scar formation potential Hemostasis is achieved well.	Benign lesions such as warts, skin tags, pyogenic granuloma.
Cryosurgery	Rapid and safe procedure to treat and remove common skin diseases.	Can cause bleeding, infection, and nerve damage. Can cause nail dystrophy if periungual lesion is frozen too deeply.	Benign lesions such as warts, seborrheic keratosis, actinic keratosis, pyogenic granuloma.

gives, indicating that it is into the subcutaneous tissue, you may stop. Take an Adson forcep and lift the cylinder of tissue out from the wound. Cut the specimen with Iris scissors at its deepest connections. Take care not to damage or crush the punch material.
- Place the specimen in formalin and send it for histopathologic examination.
- Close the punch site with nonabsorbable, simple, interrupted sutures (see choice of suture size in Excisional Biopsy).
- Achieve hemostasis by direct, prolonged pressure to the wound, electrocauterization, or application of chemical cautery agent (see Shave Biopsy for details).
- Apply antibiotic ointment; then dress the wound.
- Counsel the patient on wound care (see Wound Care).

Complications
See Table Appendix B.2.

Excisional Biopsy
Purpose
To remove an entire lesion, which is visible at the surface, down to the subcutaneous level for complete pathologic evaluation.

Technique
- The path of the skin tension lines surrounding the lesion should be determined. Decide on the best route for the elliptical incision to run parallel to the skin tension lines.
- Prepare the skin with isopropyl alcohol 70% on a cotton ball or gauze, sterilize the skin with povidone-iodine (Betadine) solution or 5% chlorhexidene (Hibiclens), then drape the area in a sterile manner.
- Perform an elliptic excision with a No. 15 scalpel blade down to the subcutaneous level. Maintain the scalpel blade perpendicular to the skin surface at all times, which will help in skin closure and wound healing. The length of the ellipse should be about three times longer than the width. The ellipse should meet at either end at a 30-degree angle. Grasp one end of the ellipse with an Adson forcep and, using Iris scissors or a scalpel, separate the specimen from the subcutaneous layer. Keep the scissors or scalpel horizontal during this process.
- Place the specimen in formalin for histopathologic evaluation.
- For better closure and a thinner scar, undermine the margins of the wound with the Iris scissors, freeing the margin so they may be mobilized to close the wound with less tension on the skin.
- Close the wound in a layered fashion starting with the subcutaneous region. Use Dexon or Vicryl (absorbable), and bury the knots. Correct placement of these sutures causes less skin tension, which results in a thinner scar. The size of the suture depends on the location, as follows: face (5-0 or 6-0), trunk (3-0 to 5-0), and extremities (3-0 to 4-0).
- The skin can be closed with interrupted simple or vertical mattress sutures using Ethilon or Prolene. A subcuticular stitch could also be used. The suture should enter and exit the wound equidistant from the incision. Also, for ease of suture placement, place the first suture in the middle of the wound and the subsequent sutures half-way between the first suture and the end of the wound. Continue closure using this technique on both sides of the initial suture until the wound is closed. Suture size, again, depends on location.
- Clean and dress the wound; then apply an antibiotic ointment.
- Educate the patient about wound care (see Wound Care), signs of infections, and when to return for suture removal. Suture removal depends on location, as follows:

face (3 to 5 days), trunk (7 to 14 days), upper extremities (7 to 14 days), lower extremities (10 to 14 days), and scalp (7 to 10 days).

Complications

See Table Appendix B.2 for details.

Cyst Excision

Purpose

To completely remove lesions that are not visible in the epidermis for histopathologic evaluation.

Technique

- Alcohol should be administered with a cotton ball or gauze to cleanse the skin.
- Anesthetize the overlying skin in a manner similar to the procedure for excisional biopsy.
- Sterilize the skin with povidone-iodine, and drape the area.
- Place an elliptic incision around the majority of the lesion palpable below the skin surface. Place the ellipse parallel to the skin lines. Use a No. 15 scalpel to make the incision, making sure the blade is perpendicular to the skin throughout the incision.
- In the case of a cyst removal, do not cut into the cyst, since removing the cyst in toto is easier. The cyst wall must be removed entirely to prevent recurrence of the cyst.
- Place all specimens in formalin for pathologic evaluation.
- Before closure, achieve good hemostasis.
- Close the wound in a fashion similar to that described in the excisional biopsy section. If indicated, undermine the wound margins. Then clean the wound.
- Apply antibiotic ointment and dressing.
- The patient should be counseled about wound care (see Wound Care), signs of infection, and suture removal.

Complications

See Table Appendix B.2 for details.

Snip Excision

Purpose

To quickly and completely remove small to medium-sized pedunculated lesions.

Technique

- Alcohol should be administered with a cotton ball or gauze to cleanse the skin.
- Anesthesia is optional. The patient should be counseled about the advantages and disadvantages of using local anesthesia on these small lesions.
- Grasp the lesion with an Adson forcep, pulling to stretch the stalk for more visibility, and snip the lesion with scissors at the base.
- Not all skin tags need to be sent for pathologic evaluation. If the lesion has variegated coloration or is deeply pigmented, or if you are unsure of the diagnosis, place the specimen in formalin and send it for histopathologic evaluation.
- Aluminum chloride, silver nitrate, or electrocautery should be administered to achieve hemostasis. Local anesthesia is helpful to minimize the sting or burn from silver nitrate or electrocautery.
- Cleanse the wound; then apply antibiotic ointment and dressing.
- Counsel the patient about wound care (see Wound Care).

Complications

See Appendix Table B.2 for details.

Electrocautery or Electrodesiccation

Purpose

To remove or destroy (by electrical means) superficial skin lesions without preserving the capability of pathologic evaluation.

Technique

- Alcohol should be administered with a cotton ball or gauze to cleanse the skin. Make sure the alcohol is *completely vaporized* before using the electrocautery instrument, to lessen the chance of an alcohol fire on the skin.
- Anesthetize the skin in a fashion similar to that described for the excisional biopsy.
- In electrocautery, the metal tip is heated and becomes red-hot. This hot tip is applied to the tissue to be removed or destroyed. The remaining charred tissue can be removed with a curette (use 1- to 7-mm curette based on lesion size). The base of the lesion can be cauterized again if desired, to achieve further destruction or hemostasis, or both.
- In electrodesiccation (a unit called a hyfrecator is used), the tip of the instrument emits an electrical arc or spark destroying or removing the lesion as needed. A wet field (i.e., bleeding) does not allow the electrical current to flow well. Hemostasis must be achieved by placing pressure on the skin to reduce the blood flow. The resultant charred tissue can be curetted away. The remaining base can be fulgurated again if desired. It is best to use the least amount of electrical current to reduce perilesional tissue destruction. Also the tip of the unit should be disposable, in keeping with universal precautions to protect the patient from infection.
- No specimens are produced for pathologic evaluation in the process.
- Cleanse the wound, and apply antibiotic ointment; then dress the wound.
- Counsel the patient about wound care (see Wound Care for details).

Complications

See Table Appendix B.2 for details.

Cryosurgery
Purpose

To rapidly remove many common superficial skin lesions while still preserving the capability for pathologic evaluation.

Technique

- Use liquid nitrogen stored in a Dewar flask that can be conveniently doled out into a styrofoam cup; use a handheld spray unit for liquid nitrogen (Cry-Ac spray); or use a commercially available metal cryoprobe (several different sizes are available) for accomplishing the tissue freeze. The author's preferred method, because of the ease in application and storage, is liquid nitrogen stored in a bulk tank and applied using a cotton-tipped applicator, repeatedly dipping the applicator into a styrofoam cup for more liquid nitrogen.
- Localized anesthesia can be applied in the same manner as in the excisional biopsy.
- Frozen areas of the skin turn white immediately when the liquid nitrogen is applied to the skin by cotton-tipped applicator, probe, or spray. This area is called the freeze ball. The longer the area is frozen (duration of application of the liquid nitrogen), the deeper the freeze ball becomes. Remember, the freeze ball should

not extend beyond the dermal region, to decrease the potential of postfreeze pain and blistering. Destruction of the lesions is best with rapid freezing and slow thawing cycles.

- For thicker lesions (such as thick warts or seborrheic keratosis) freeze for as long as 40 seconds (measured by the amount of time the freeze ball is maintained before thawing occurs).
- Thin, flat lesions should be frozen for 5 to 10 seconds.
- For both thin and thick lesions, a 1- to 3-mm margin of frozen tissue (freeze ball) should be maintained around the lesion.
- Patience is needed to wait until the thaw cycle is completed (the freeze ball disappears entirely) before attempting a second freeze-thaw cycle.
- The second application of liquid nitrogen depends on the size and location of the lesion to destroy. Most lesions respond best to two freeze-thaw cycles.
- No special dressings are needed, although applying an adhesive strip over a wart aids in the disappearance of the wart.
- The patient should be counseled regarding potential complications.

Short term
- *Pain* is a variable problem. Lesions may be painful following cryosurgery as a result of the pressure caused by the edema from the tissue destruction and the expanding blister.
- *Edema* and *blistering.* The skin becomes swollen as the epidermis separates from the dermis. Blistering also becomes evident over the cryosurgery site.
- *Bleeding.* Often, the blisters fill with blood, creating a blood blister because the lesion was frozen deeper than the epidermis. This can occur when treating thicker lesions such as warts.
- *Infection* can occur, especially when the lesion is frozen deeper than the epidermis, causing a hemorrhagic blister. Patient should be informed about the signs of infection and proper wound care (see Wound Care).

Long term
- Nerve damage is a more serious complication in which the depth of the freezing has destroyed a superficial skin nerve. Caution is needed when freezing lesions where the skin nerves are superficial (along the sides of the fingers, the postauricular area, or along the distribution of the peroneal nerve). In these areas deep freezing should be avoided.
- Pigmentary changes can occur and should be explained to the patient before the cryosurgery. These can be especially disfiguring in African American patients.
- Hypertrophic scar formation. Thicker, more hypertrophic scars can be seen when freezing thick lesions or if lesions are frozen too deeply.
- Nail dystrophy. Dystrophic nails can occur because of disruption of the nail bed. This happens when periungual lesions are frozen too deeply. Caution should be taken to lightly freeze periungual lesions.

Wound Care
Purpose
To prevent wound infection and promote wound healing.

Technique
- In excisional biopsies, when the epidermal layer is being surgically penetrated, you should drape (sterile) the surgical area to maintain a sterile field.

- If a dressing is applied, leave the dressing on for at least 24 hours. If the dressing is loose or falling off, either reinforce the dressing or reapply a new dressing.
- Keep the wound clean and dry. For patients with occupations that involve grease and grime, use a protective glove or covering over the wound.
- Cleanse the wound once daily with hydrogen peroxide. Apply with cotton-ball gauze, or cotton-tipped applicator. Dry the wound with a clean, dry gauze.
- Apply a thin layer of antibiotic ointment such as Polysporin or bacitracin (Altracin) with a cotton-tipped applicator. Avoid Neosporin.
- Apply a bandage such as a Band-Aid or Telfa pad.
- If bleeding occurs, apply an ice pack on the wound for 20 minutes with pressure.
- If a blister ("water blister") develops (as in cryosurgery), leave the blister intact. Pop the blister only if the lesion is very painful. Always use a sterile lancet or needle.
- Watch for signs of infection such as erythematous, tender skin and increase in pain from the wound, or pus emanating from the wound. Instruct the patient to call or see the physician if these events occur, since they may indicate a wound infection.
- Pain control is best achieved with the use of acetaminophen because it does not interfere with hemostasis as does aspirin or nonsteroidal antiinflammatory drugs such as ibuprofen (Motrin) or naproxen sodium (Naprosyn). Sometimes the pain after cryosurgery can be helped by applying cold *tap water* (no ice or ice water) to the affected area and changing the water when it becomes warm.

BIBLIOGRAPHY

Achar S. Principles of skin biopsies for the family physician. *Am Fam Physician* 1996;54(8):2411–2418.

T ABLE APPENDIX C.   Treatment of Dermatoses Seen in Pregnancy

Rash	Clinical features	Treatment
1. Herpes gestationis (Plate Appendix C.1, see color insert following page 170)	Rash rare in pregnancy (1:10,000). May cause an increased risk of premature labor. Intensely pruritic. Not caused by a virus (herpes). Prodromal/systemic complaints include malaise, fever, nausea, and headaches. Rash comes and goes throughout pregnancy and postpartum period. Can recur in subsequent pregnancies. Rash begins as periumbilical initially, then spreads to trunk, extremities, palms, and soles. Spares mucous membranes. See circular red papules, plaques, and vesicles. Bullae can also occur.	Triamcinolone acetonide cream 0.1% tid topically. Prednisone 20 to 30 mg orally daily in moderate cases; 40 to 80 mg orally daily in severe cases (use after first trimester). Taper dose in last trimester and increase dose soon after delivery to prevent flare-up. Diphenhydramine 25 to 50 mg orally qid p.r.n. for pruritis.
2. Pruritic urticarial papules and plaques of pregnancy (PUPPP)	Unknown etiology. Seen in 0.5% to 1% of pregnancies. Occurs most commonly during third trimester of pregnancy (76% of patients are primigravida). Very pruritic. Warmth (i.e., hot baths) intensifies pruritus. Not likely to recur with subsequent pregnancies and regresses with delivery. Rash begins in striae distensae, then spreads to trunk and proximal extremities, usually over 1 to 2 weeks. See 1- to 3-mm red plaques and papules. May have pale halo surrounding isolated red lesions. Duration of rash is 6 weeks. Can be associated with polyhydraminos.	Use cool baths or showers. Triamcinolone acetonide cream 0.1% tid topically. Prednisone 40 mg orally daily, tapered over 7 to 14 days (use after first trimester). Diphenhydramine HCl orally 25 to 50 mg qid or Hydroxyzine HCl 25 to 50 mg orally qid as needed for pruritus (use after first trimester).
3. Melasma	See Chapter 11 for complete details.	See Chapter 11 for treatment details.

continued

TABLE APPENDIX C.   *continued.*   **Treatment of Dermatoses Seen in Pregnancy**

Rash	Clinical features	Treatment
4. Intrahepatic cholestasis of pregnancy	Can occur anytime during pregnancy. Resolves in approximately 2 days following delivery. No primary lesions. Severe pruritus begins on hands and feet and moves centrally, occurs most severely at night Excoriations can be seen secondary to pruritis. Abnormal serum bilirubin and liver function test results noted. In pruritus gravidarum, a normal bilirubin value is noted. Mild jaundice noted in 20% of patients. Some nausea or vomiting. Rash can recur in subsequent pregnancies in 50% of affected patients. Unknown fetal risk, though some reports indicate a risk of stillbirth or premature labor. Since liver function test values are elevated, recommend referral to gastroenterologist for evaluation.	No effective treatment. Can use cholestyramine. Use diphenhydramine HCl 25 to 50 mg orally qid or hydroxyzine HCl 25 to 50 mg qid orally p.r.n. for itching (use after first trimester). Aveeno (colloidal oatmeal baths) may be helpful bid–tid
5. Hyperpigmentation	Hyperpigmentation of areola, nipples, vulva, and linea alba (linea nigra) is common (90% of all pregnant women). Occurs after several months of pregnancy. Most prominent hyperpigmentation in patients with darkly pigmented skin. Hyperpigmentation gradually fades postpartum.	No treatment necessary.
6. Striae distensae (stretch marks)	Commonly occurs in pregnancy during the second or third trimester. Violaceous linear lesions found over the protuberant abdomen, breasts, buttocks, groin, or thighs. Stretch marks develop at right angles to the lines of tension in the skin. Color usually fades to flesh tones following delivery. Stretch marks remain, however, after delivery.	No effective treatment. Can use retinoic acid (Retin-A) topically 0.1% nightly until color and stretch marks diminish (improves appearance). Only use retinoic acid when *not* pregnant.

continued

TABLE APPENDIX C.   *continued.*   **Treatment of Dermatoses Seen in Pregnancy**

Rash	Clinical features	Treatment
7. Pruritus of pregnancy (pruritus gravidarum)	Occurs in 0.3% of all pregnancies. Occurs at 25 to 30 weeks of gestation. Persists about 3 months postpartum. Bilirubin level is normal. Very pruritic lesions. Red or skin-colored papules, 0.5 cm in diameter. Lesions become excoriated because of scratching. Lesions seen on extensor surfaces of extremities and trunk.	Clobetasone 0.05 % cream topically twice daily. Diphenhydramine HCl 25 to 50 mg orally qid as needed for pruritus.
8. Spider angiomas	Appear between 2nd and 5th month of gestation in up to 66% of white women and 10% of African American women. Small, red papules with radiating capillaries. Seen on the chest and upper arms. 75% of angiomas disappear within 2 to 3 weeks after delivery.	No specific treatment, since they are asymptomatic and angiomas usually regress spontaneously.
9. Palmar erythema	Seen during the first trimester. Probably caused by increased estrogen levels. Diffuse erythema of entire palmar surface or localized redness to thenar or hypothenar eminences. Disappears usually within 1 week following delivery.	No specific treatment, since it is asymptomatic and regresses spontaneously.
10. Gingivitis	Seen in the first trimester. Gingiva is enlarged, swollen, pink to red and can cause mild pain, bleeding, or ulceration. Usually regresses following delivery.	Proper dental hygiene (daily brushing and flossing). Avoid trauma to gingiva (vigorous brushing) and mouthwash. In severe disease with bleeding, dental referral may be necessary.
11. Pyogenic granuloma	Occurs on the gingiva in up to 2% of all pregnancies. Violaceous mass arising from the gingiva. Can cause bleeding or pain. If left untreated, will resolve after delivery.	Surgical intervention by a dentist is necessary to remove (especially if symptomatic).

From Errickson CV, Matus NR. Skin disorders of pregnancy. *Am Fam Physician* 1994;49(3):605–610; Fox GN. Pruritic urticarial papules and plaques of pregnancy. *Am Fam Physician* 1986;34(3):191–195; Fox GN. Pruritic folliculitis of pregnancy. *Am Fam Physician* 1989;39(3):189–193; and Sodhi VK, Sausker WF. Dermatoses of pregnancy. *Am Fam Physician* 1988;37(1):131–138, with permission.

A PPENDIX D

T ABLE APPENDIX D.   Treatment of Common Neonatal Rashes

Rash	Characteristics	Treatment
1. Mongolian spot	See Chapter 5 for complete details.	See Chapter 5 for complete details.
2. Erythema toxicum neonatorum	Affects 30% to 70% of term infants, less common in premature infants. Rash noted at 24 hours to 2 weeks after birth. Yellow/white macules, or vesicles, 1 to 2 mm in diameter seen on arms, legs, and trunk (not on palms and soles). Red, irregularly shaped macular rash surrounding the yellow papules/vesicles (flea-bitten appearance). Vesicles are negative for viruses, fungi, and bacteria. Regresses spontaneously in 1 to 2 weeks.	No specific treatment; resolves spontaneously. Reassure parents.
3. Transient neonatal pustular metanosis	Lesions present at birth. More common in African American infants. Superficial pustules noted on chin, neck, upper back (can be on palms and soles). Pustules rupture easily. White scale surrounding hyperpigmented macules. Pustular phase can occur in utero. Pustules are culture negative, although neutrophils can be identified on Gram stain. Regresses spontaneously within 3 months after birth.	No specific treatment; resolves spontaneously. Reassure parents.
4. Milia	See Chapter 7 for complete details.	See Chapter 7 for complete details.

continued

TABLE APPENDIX D.   *continued.*   **Treatment of Common Neonatal Rashes**

Rash	Characteristics	Treatment
5. Millaria	Two types: rubra and crystallina. Both occur in the intertrigenous areas, scalp, face, neck, or any occluded area such as the back of newborn. Millaria rubra: vesicular, pustular, or papular rash with associated erythema and distributed in a follicular pattern. Millaria crystallina: vesicular rash resembling water droplets that rupture easily and drain clear fluid. Both types resolve following the elimination of the environmental (excessive heat) and/or physical factors (occlusion).	Advise parents to avoid situations where child can become overheated or allowed to remain stationary on back for long periods.
6. Acne neonatorum	Appears around age 2 to 4 weeks. Occurs in response to maternal androgen stimulation. See papules, pustules, and closed comedones on face. Resolves spontaneously in 2 to 8 weeks.	Usually no treatment is necessary, since condition resolves spontaneously. If treatment is needed, use over-the-counter acne soap to cleanse face daily.
7. Seborrheic dermatitis (cradle cap)	See Chapter 2 for further details.	See Chapter 2 for further details.
8. Diaper dermatitis	See Chapter 17 for further details.	See Chapter 17 for further details.
9. Nevus simplex (salmon patch or stork bite)	Occurs in up to 70% of newborns at birth. See flat, pink vascular lesion at nape of the neck, glabellar area, and upper eyelids. Caused by dilated dermal capillaries. Erythema becomes more prominent when infants cries. Glabellar lesions regress spontaneously in 95% of cases, the neck lesions in 50% of cases, and the eyelid lesions 100% of the time.	No specific treatment; usually regresses spontaneously. Reassure parents.
10. Hemangiomas (strawberry hemangioma)	See Chapter 6 for further details.	See Chapter 6 for further details.

T ABLE APPENDIX D. *continued.* **Treatment of Common Neonatal Rashes**

Rash	Characteristics	Treatment
11. Nevus flammeus (port-wine stain)	Present at birth. Flat, red/blue rash most frequently on face. Lesion persists throughout life. Lesion can lighten as child ages. Rash can become nodular as patient becomes older. Associated with Sturge-Weber syndrome. Port-wine stain in this lesion involves the ophthalmologic branch of trigeminal nerve. Other anomalies include epilepsy, glaucoma, hemiplegia, and mental retardation. Glaucoma can occur with nevus flammeus even in the absence of Sturge-Weber syndrome when lesion surrounds the eye. In these cases, refer for ophthalmologic evaluation.	Refer early in childhood to a specialist trained with the pulsed-dye laser to remove the lesion and achieve good response. If lesion is bilateral or involves the ophthalmologic branch of the trigeminal nerve, consider Sturge-Weber syndrome. Workup includes EEG, MRI of the head, eye examination, and cerebral angiography.
12. Umbilical granuloma	Red, friable granuloma at umbilicus. Appears after umbilicus cord detaches (approximately 2 weeks of age). Can bleed easily.	Apply silver nitrate sticks to lesion daily for 3 to 5 days to resolve lesion.

EEG, electroencephalogram; MRI, magnetic resonance imaging.

From Treadwell PA. Dermatoses in newborns. *Am Fam Physician* 1997;56(2):443–450, with permission.

A PPENDIX E

T ABLE APPENDIX E. Treatment of Rashes Associated with Human Immunodeficiency Virus (HIV) Disease

Rash	Characteristics	Treatment
1. Exanthem of acute retroviral syndrome	Infectious mononucleosis-like syndrome with fever, lymphadenopathy, meningitis, GI tract symptoms, rash, and genital ulceration. 3- to 6-week incubation period before febrile illness. Rash begins 2 to 3 days after fever onset and lasts 5 to 8 days. Rash usually asymptomatic. Discrete morbiliform maculopapular rash up to 1 cm in diameter. Can see ulcers on penis or scrotum. Rash commonly located on upper chest, neck, face, arms, scalp, and palms. Can also cause rash on hard and soft palate which are round, shallow, 5- to 10-mm ulcers surrounded by a red halo. Lymphadenopathy can also be seen. Positive anti-HIV-1 antibodies within 3 weeks of illness.	Symptomatic and supportive treatment.
2. Eosinophilic folliculitis	Intensely pruritic red papular follicular eruptions 3 to 5 mm in size. Located on upper trunk, face, neck, and proximal extremities. Usually seen in advanced HIV disease. Pruitus can cause excoriation, which can lead to secondary bacterial infection. Will resolve into postinflammatory hyperpigmented lesions. Diagnosis made clinically but can confirm by punch biopsy (showing eosinophils). Bacterial cultures are usually negative. Chronic course with exacerbations and recurrences.	Use oral antihistamines for pruritis relief. Use potent topical corticosteroids for pruritis relief (see Appendix A). Isotretinoin 1 to 2 mg/kg per day orally used until rash is gone: effective in causing resolution of rash. Can also use oral prednisone to resolve lesions, 80 mg/day tapered by 5 mg/day over 14 days.

continued

379

TABLE APPENDIX E.   *continued.*   **Treatment of Rashes Associated with Human Immunodeficiency Virus (HIV) Disease**

Rash	Characteristics	Treatment
3. Kaposi sarcoma (Plates E.1 and E.2, see color insert following page 170)	Vascular neoplasm causing a violaceous mucocutaneous maculopapular rash on trunk, head, tip of nose, periorbital region, ears, scalp, penis, legs, palms, and soles. Usually asymptomatic. Sometimes lesions can ulcerate and bleed. Lesion on lower extremities cause edema. Can involve any organ system (GI tract, pulmonary, renal, etc.). Can also involve oral mucosa with lesions on gingiva, hard and soft palate, pharynx, and tongue. Can be confused with bacillary angiomatosis. A biopsy of the lesion and bacterial culture are helpful to differentiate.	Chemotherapy or radiotherapy
4. Bacillary angiomatosis (Plate E.3, see color insert following page 170)	Systemic infection with *Bartonella* species causing vascular tumors on the skin that can appear like Karposi sarcoma. Seen in advanced HIV disease almost exclusively. Predisposing factor: owning or being exposed to a cat. Lesions can be painful; in disseminated disease will see fever, malaise, and weight loss. Cherry-red papules/nodules that resemble angiomas surrounded by scales. Can be a solitary lesion or many (hundreds) lesions. Can occur on any site but sparring the palms, soles, and oral mucosa. Diagnosis can be made by lesion biopsy or bacterial culture. Can be fatal if untreated (become bacteremic).	Antibiotic treatment: Erythromycin 500 mg po qid *or* Ciprofloxacin 750 mg po bid *or* Doxycycline 100 mg po bid *or* Azithromcyin 600 mg po qd. Use for 8 to 12 weeks. Prevention: avoid contact with cats (harbor *Bartonella henselae*).
5. Oral hairy leukoplakia	See Chapter 4 for more details. Recommend HIV testing if this manifestation presents.	See Chapter 4 for treatment options.
6. Molluscum contagiosum	See Chapter 18 for more details.	See Chapter 18 for treatment options.

T ABLE APPENDIX E. *continued.* **Treatment of Rashes Associated with Human Immunodeficiency Virus (HIV) Disease**

Rash	Characteristics	Treatment
7. Herpes simplex infection	See Chapter 4 for more details on oral lesions. Can also cause chronic (>1 month in duration), large ulcerations in the anogenital region that are painful (one of the diagnostic criteria for AIDS). Diagnosed by Tzanck smear and/or viral culture.	See Chapter 4 for treatment options.
8. Recurrent aphthous stomatitis	See Chapter 4 for more details.	See Chapter 4 for treatment options.
9. Tinea unguium	Presents as a chalky-white proximal nail discoloration; rare in non–HIV-infected patients. Recommend HIV testing when this nail presentation is seen.	See Chapter 17 for treatment options.
10. Warts	See Chapter 18 for more details.	See Chapter 18 for treatment options.
11. Candidiasis: mucosal and vulvovaginal	See Chapter 17 for more details.	See Chapter 17 for treatment options.
12. Seborrheic dermatitis	See Chapter 2 for more details.	See Chapter 2 for treatment options.
13. Scabies	See Chapter 19 for more details. Usually infested by the Norwegian scabies mite with numerous mites causing crusting plaques on the genitalia. Diagnosed by a scabies preparation.	See Chapter 19 for more treatment options. May need to use oral ivermectin in recalcitrant infestation.

GI, gastrointestinal; HIV-1, human immunodeficiency virus type 1; AIDS, acquired immunodeficiency syndrome.
From Berger TA, Obuch ML, Goldschmidt RH. Dermatologic manifestations of HIV infection. *Am Fam Physician* 1990;41(6):1729–1741; and Khorenian SD, Lebwohl M. New cutaneous manifestations of systemic diseases. *Am Fam Physician* 1995;51(3):625–630, with permission.

BIBLIOGRAPHY

Arndt KA, Wintroub BU, Robinson JK, LeBoit PE. *Primary care dermatology.* Philadelphia: WB Saunders, 1997.

Ashton R, Leppard B. *Differential diagnosis in dermatology,* 2nd ed. Oxford: Radcliffe Medical Press, 1993.

Barone M, ed. *The Harriet Lane handbook,* 14th ed. Baltimore: Mosby, 1996.

Black MM, McKay M, Braude PR. *Color atlas and text of obstetric and gynecologic dermatology.* London: Mosby-Wolfe, 1995.

Briggs GG, Freeman RK, Yaffe SJ. *Drugs in pregnancy and lactation,* 4th ed. Baltimore: Williams & Wilkins, 1994.

Cohen BA. *Atlas of pediatric dermatology.* London: Mosby-Wolfe, 1993.

Cotran RS, Kumar V, Robbins SL. *Robbins pathologic basis of disease,* 4th ed. Philadelphia: WB Saunders, 1989.

Fitzpatrick TB, Eisen AZ, Wolff K, Freedberg IM, Austen KF, eds. *Dermatology in general medicine,* 4th ed. New York: McGraw-Hill, 1993.

Fitzpatrick TB, Johnson RA, Wolff K, Polano MK, Suurmond D. *Color atlas and synopsis of clinical dermatology: common and serious diseases,* 3rd ed. New York: McGraw-Hill, 1997.

Goldstein BG, Goldstein AO. *Practical dermatology,* 2nd ed. St. Louis: Mosby, 1997.

Goldsmith LA, Lazurus GS, Thorp MD. *Adult and pediatric dermatology.* Philadelphia: FA Davis, 1997.

Greenberger NJ, Coonrod S, Kauer C, Lawson M. *The medical book of lists: a primer of differential diagnosis in internal medicine,* 4th ed. St. Louis: Mosby, 1994.

Habif TP. *Clinical dermatology: a guide to diagnosis and therapy,* 3rd ed. St. Louis: Mosby-Year Book, 1996.

Hurwitz S. *Clinical pediatric dermatology: a textbook of skin disorders of childhood and adolescence,* 2nd ed. Philadelphia: WB Saunders, 1993.

Klippel JH, Weyand CM, Wortmann RL, eds. *Primer on the rheumatic diseases,* 11th ed. Atlanta: Arthritis Foundation, 1997.

Lawrence CM, Cox NH. *Physical signs in dermatology: color atlas and text.* London: Mosby-Wolfe, 1993.

Lynch PJ. *Dermatology,* 3rd ed. Baltimore: Williams & Wilkins, 1994.

Marks JG Jr, DeLeo VA. *Contact and occupational dermatology,* 2nd ed. St. Louis: Mosby-Year Book, 1997.

Pfenninger JL, Fowler GC, eds. *Procedures for primary care physicians.* St. Louis: Mosby, 1994.

Reeves JRT, Maibach H. *Clinical dermatology: illustrated and regional approach,* 2nd ed. Philadelphia: FA Davis, 1991.

Sams WM Jr, Lynch PJ, eds. *Principles and practice of dermatology,* 2nd ed. New York: Churchill Livingstone, 1996.

Sauer GC, Hall JC. *Manual of skin diseases,* 7th ed. Philadelphia: Lippincott-Raven, 1996.

White G. *Leven's color atlas of dermatology,* 2nd ed. London: Mosby-Wolfe, 1997.

SUBJECT INDEX

· ·

References followed by "f" indicate figures; those followed by "t" denote tables

385

color plate, *see* color insert following p. 170
definition, 58
diagnosis, 58 59
differential diagnosis, 59t, 247t
epidemiology, 58
follow-up, 59
management, 59, 59t 60t
pathology, 58
patient education, 60
referral, 59
risk factors, 58
Kerion, 284t
Ketoconazole
clinical uses
candidiasis, 307t
dermatophytic infections, 295t
infectious folliculitis, 250t 251t
onychomycosis, 294t, 299
pityriasis versicolor, 311t, 312t
seborrheic dermatitis, 45t
tinea barbae, 294t
tinea capitis, 294t
tinea corporis, 294t
tinea cruris, 294t
tinea manuum, 294t
tinea pedis, 294t
tinea unguium, 294t
side effects, 296t
Koebner phenomenon, 51, 143
Koilonychia, 197, 200t, 202t
Koplik spots, 317t

L
Lactic acid (Lac-hydrin), 57t, 59t
Lamisil. *See* Terbinafine
Laser
clinical uses
in Campbell-De Morgan spot, 94
in capillary hemangioma, 92
in pyogenic granuloma, 97
in resistant warts, 321
in spider angioma, 95
Lentigo maligna melanoma
clinical manifestations, 117
differential diagnosis, 77t, 82t
epidemiology, 118
risk factors, 118
Leprosy, 150t, 310t
Leukonychia, 196, 200t, 202t
Leukoplakia. *See* Oral hairy leukoplakia;
Oral leukoplakia
Lice. *See* Pediculosis
Lichenoid drug reaction, 145t
Lichen planus
chief complaint, 143
clinical manifestations, 143 144
color plate, *see* color insert following p. 170
definition, 143
diagnosis, 145
differential diagnosis, 109t, 139t, 142t,
145t, 304t 305t, 319t
epidemiology, 144
follow-up, 145, 147

management, 145, 146t
nail disorders secondary to
longitudinal ridging of nail matrix, 192
treatment, 201t
pathology, 144
patient education, 147
referral, 145
risk factors, 144
variations, 144
Lichen simplex chronicus
areas most commonly affected, 36t
chief complaint, 36
clinical manifestations, 36
color plate, *see* color insert following p. 170
definition, 35
diagnosis, 37
differential diagnosis, 37, 37t, 337t
epidemiology, 36 37
follow-up, 39
management, 37 39, 38t
pathology, 37
patient education, 39
referral, 37
risk factors, 37
Lidocaine, 363
for aphthous ulcer, 64t
for hand-foot-and-mouth disease, 325t
for herpangina, 72t
nongenital herpes simplex disease, 69
for Stevens-Johnson syndrome, 172
Lindane
for pediculosis, 338t
for scabies, 342t
Lipoma
chief complaint, 89
clinical manifestations, 89
color plate, *see* color insert following p. 170
definition, 89
diagnosis, 89 90
differential diagnosis, 90
epidemiology, 89
management, 90
pathology, 89
patient education, 90
referral, 90
risk factors, 89
Liquid nitrogen
for actinic keratosis, 107t
for granuloma annulare, 142t
Loratadine
for atopic dermatitis, 30t
for contact dermatitis, 35t
for dyshidrotic eczema, 48t
for exanthematous drug eruption, 228t
for flea bites, 351t
for lichen simplex chronicus, 38t
for nummular eczema, 41t
for urticaria, 163t
Lotrimin. *See* Clotrimazole
Lyme borreliosis
chief complaint, 271
clinical manifestations, 271 272
color plate, *see* color insert following p. 170